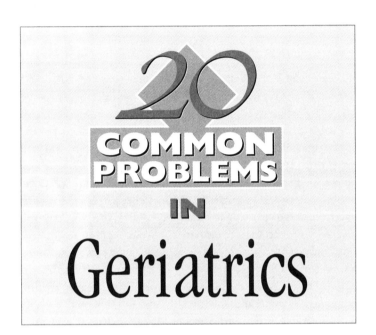

20 COMMON PROBLEMS IN Geriatrics

Notice

Medicine is an ever-changing science. As new research and clinical experience broaden our knowledge, changes in treatment and drug therapy are required. The editors and the publisher of this work have checked with sources believed to be reliable in their efforts to provide information that is complete and generally in accord with the standards accepted at the time of publication. However, in view of the possibility of human error or changes in medical sciences, neither the editors nor the publisher nor any other party who has been involved in the preparation or publication of this work warrants that the information contained herein is in every respect accurate or complete, and they are not responsible for any errors or omissions or for the results obtained from use of such information. Readers are encouraged to confirm the information contained herein with other sources. For example and in particular, readers are advised to check the product information sheet included in the package of each drug they plan to administer to be certain that the information contained in this book is accurate and that changes have not been made in the recommended dose or in the contraindications for administration. This recommendation is of particular importance in connection with new or infrequently used drugs.

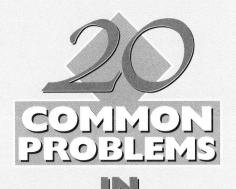

Geriatrics

EDITORS

ALAN M. ADELMAN, M.D.

Professor, Department of Family Practice and Community Medicine
Penn State University, College of Medicine, Hershey, Pennsylvania

MEL P. DALY, M.D.

Greater Baltimore Medical Center, Baltimore, Maryland

SERIES EDITOR

BARRY D. WEISS, M.D.

Professor of Clinical Family and Community Medicine
University of Arizona College of Medicine, Tucson, Arizona

McGraw-Hill
Medical Publishing Division

New York   St. Louis   San Francisco   Auckland   Bogotá   Caracas   Lisbon   London   Madrid
Mexico City   Milan   Montreal   New Delhi   San Juan   Singapore   Sydney   Tokyo   Toronto

McGraw-Hill

A Division of The **McGraw·Hill** *Companies*

20 COMMON PROBLEMS IN GERIATRICS

Copyright © 2001 by The **McGraw-Hill Companies**, Inc. All rights reserved. Printed in the United States of America. Except as permitted under the United States Copyright Act of 1976, no part of this publication may be reproduced or distributed in any form or by any means, or stored in a data base or retrieval system, without the prior written permission of the publisher.

1 2 3 4 5 6 7 8 9 0 DOCDOC 00

ISBN 0-07-000518-4

This book was set in Garamond by V&M Graphics, Inc.
The editors were Martin Wonsiewicz, Susan Noujaim, and Nicky Panton.
The production supervisor was Rohnda Barnes.
The cover designer was Marsha Cohen/Parallelogram.
The color insert was designed by Marsha Cohen/Parallelogram.
The index was prepared by Jerry Ralya.

R. R. Donnelley and Sons Company was printer and binder.

This book is printed on acid-free paper.

Library of Congress Cataloging-in-Publication Data

20 common problems in geriatrics / editors, Alan M. Adelman, Mel P. Daly.
    p. ; cm.
  Includes bibliographical references and index.
  ISBN 0-07-000518-4
  1. Aged—Diseases. 2. Geriatrics. I. Title: Twenty common problems in geriatrics. II. Adelman, Alan M. III. Daly, Mel P.
[DNLM: 1. Geriatrics. WT 100 Z999 2001]
RC952.A62 2001
618.97—dc21   00—020707

I dedicate this book to my parents,
Robert and Elaine, who started me on my journey;
and to my wife, Carol, who has been my companion, supporter, and friend.
—Alan M. Adelman—

This book is dedicated to the memory of my beloved father,
Denis Daly, who died last year.
—Mel P. Daly—

Contents

Part
3
Aches and Pains

137

Part
4
Neuropsychiatric Problems

185

Part
5
Other Common Problems   309

Color plates fall between pages 368 and 369.

Contributors

CARE AT THE END OF LIFE
(CHAPTER 2)
William Reichel, M.D.
Clinical Professor of Family Medicine
Georgetown University School of Medicine, Washington, DC
Adjunct Professor of Family Medicine
Brown University School of Medicine
Providence, Rhode Island

CAREGIVER ISSUES (CHAPTER 4)
Lisa Fredman, Ph.D.
Associate Professor
Department of Epidemiology and Biostatistics
Boston University School of Public Health
Boston, Massachusetts

**COMMON DERMATOLOGIC
PROBLEMS** (CHAPTER 18)
Alan M. Adelman, M.D., M.S.
Professor and Associate Chair
Department of Family and Community Medicine
Penn State University College of Medicine
Hershey, Pennsylvania

CONSTIPATION (CHAPTER 15)
Barbara Resnick, Ph.D., CRNP
Assistant Professor
School of Nursing
University of Maryland
Baltimore, Maryland

DEMENTIA (CHAPTER 12)
Mel P. Daly, M.D.
Greater Baltimore Medical Center
Baltimore, Maryland

**DEPRESSION AND OTHER MOOD
DISORDERS** (CHAPTER 11)
Joseph J. Gallo, M.D., M.P.H.
Department of Family Practice and Community Medicine
Department of Psychiatry
School of Medicine
University of Pennsylvania
Philadelphia, Pennsylvania

Junius Gonzales, M.D.
Clinical Economics Research Unit
Department of Medicine
Georgetown University Medical Center
Washington, D.C.
and
Chief, Services Research and Clinical
Epidemiology Branch
Division of Services and Intervention Research
National Institutes of Mental Health
Bethesda, Maryland

DIZZINESS (CHAPTER 20)
Alan M. Adelman, M.D., M.S.
Professor and Associate Chair
Department of Family and Community Medicine
Penn State University College of Medicine
Hershey, Pennsylvania

GAIT AND BALANCE DISORDERS
(CHAPTER 14)
Barbara Resnick, Ph.D., CRNP
Assistant Professor
School of Nursing
University of Maryland
Baltimore, Maryland

Michael Corcoran, M.D.
Assistant Professor
University of Maryland
School of Medicine
Baltimore, Maryland

Ann Marie Spellbring, Ph.D., RN
Associate Professor
School of Nursing
University of Maryland
Baltimore, Maryland

**HEALTH PROMOTION AND
DISEASE PREVENTION**
(CHAPTER 3)
Mel P. Daly, M.D.
Greater Baltimore Medical Center
Baltimore, Maryland

**HEARING AND VISUAL
IMPAIRMENT** (CHAPTER 13)
Alan M. Adelman, M.D., M.S.
Professor and Associate Chair
Department of Family and Community Medicine
Penn State University College of Medicine
Hershey, Pennsylvania

INFECTIONS (CHAPTER 17)
James P. Richardson, M.D., M.P.H.
Medical Director
Senior Care Services
Chief, Division of Geriatric Medicine
St. Agnes Health Care
Baltimore, Maryland

JOINT PAINS (CHAPTER 9)
Ursula McClymont, M.D.
Director of Family Medicine
Division of Geriatric Medicine
The Union Memorial Hospital
Baltimore, Maryland

Niharika N. Suchak, MBBS, MHS
Assistant Professor
Department of Geriatric Medicine
Oklahoma University College of Medicine
Medical Director, Extended Care Unit, UAMC
Oklahoma City, Oklahoma

MANAGING CHRONIC ILLNESS
(CHAPTER 1)
Alan M. Adelman, M.D., M.S.
Professor and Associate Chair
Department of Family and Community Medicine
Penn State University College of Medicine
Hershey, Pennsylvania

**NUTRITIONAL STATUS AND
INVOLUNTARY WEIGHT LOSS**
(CHAPTER 16)
Mel P. Daly, M.D.
Greater Baltimore Medical Center
Baltimore, Maryland

OSTEOPOROSIS (CHAPTER 8)
Luanne E. Thorndyke, M.D.
Associate Professor of Clinical Medicine
Department of General Internal Medicine
Penn State University College of Medicine
Hershey, Pennsylvania

**POLYPHARMACY AND
PRINCIPLES OF DRUG
THERAPY** (CHAPTER 5)
Robert J. Michocki, Pharm.D., BCPS
Professor, Department of Pharmacy Practice and Sciences
School of Pharmacy
Clinical Associate Professor
Department of Family Medicine
School of Medicine, University of Maryland
Baltimore, Maryland

PROSTATE DISORDERS
(CHAPTER 7)
Noel H. Ballentine, M.D.
Associate Professor
Department of General Internal Medicine
Penn State University College of Medicine
Hershey, Pennsylvania

SKIN ULCERS (CHAPTER 19)
Aubrey L. Knight, M.D.
Associate Professor of Clinical Family Medicine
University of Virginia School of Medicine
Director, Family Practice Education
Carilion Health System
Roanoke, Virginia

SLEEP DISORDERS
(CHAPTER 10)
Patrick P. Coll, M.D.
Associate Director, Center on Aging
Associate Professor, Family Medicine
University of Connecticut Health Center
Farmington, Connecticut

URINARY INCONTINENCE
(CHAPTER 6)
Barry D. Weiss, M.D.
Professor of Clinical Family and Community Medicine
University of Arizona College of Medicine
Tucson, Arizona

Preface

Perhaps the most important public health concern of the early 21st century is the exponential growth of the elderly population. Not only will the number of persons over 65 years double in the next 20 years (accounting for 1 in 4 Americans), persons who are now aged 65 years are, on average, likely to live for another 20 years.

Older persons represent approximately 1/8 th of the population (35 million), yet account for close to 40 percent of health care expenditures annually. Persons over the age of 65 account for 40 percent of all hospital admissions, and 40 percent of all prescription drug use. On average, persons over 65 years see primary care practitioners 9 times per year (compared to approximately 3 times per year for younger persons). Advice and interventions by primary care practitioners can have an important potential impact on the health of the rapidly growing older population.

There are many reasons why older persons visit primary care practitioners. Most often it is because of chronic illness, to refill prescriptions, or because of an acute episode of disease. Because older persons have multiple medical problems, frequently take many medications, and have many complicated social, neuropsychological, and financial difficulties, providing comprehensive care in a primary care setting can be challenging.

The implications for primary care practitioners are obvious. They will see increasing numbers of older patients in their practices. They will need to have the knowledge and skills that are unique to caring for an aging population. At a minimum, they will need to be familiar with the diagnosis and treatment of the most common problems.

About This Book

Given the number of problems that we deal with on a daily basis, we had a difficult time choosing *20 Common Problems*. Had we not narrowed our focus, we could easily have chosen *30* or *40 Common Problems*. We attempted to focus on problems and issues that are more unique to an elderly population. Although common, we did not devote chapters to several common chronic diseases such as cancer, hypertension, coronary artery disease, and chronic lung disease. This book is part of the *20 Common Problems* series, and as such, these topics are covered in other books in the series.

The 20 problems discussed in this text is in no way meant to comprehensively address the total spectrum of caring for older persons in primary care settings. Our hope is to present an overview of many of the most common issues in caring for older patients in primary care settings. We have divided the problems in to five sections. In section one (*General*), we deal with general issues including managing chronic illness, advance directives/end of life care, health promotion/disease prevention, caregiving issues, and polypharmacy. In section two (*Genitourinary Problems*), the common problems of urinary incontinence and prostate disorders are discussed. Section three (*Aches and Pains*), deals with a specific condition, osteoporosis, and a common symptom, joint pains. The fourth section (*Neuropsychiatric Problems*), deals with common neuropsychiatric problems including sleep disorders, depression, dementia, hearing/vision impairment, and gait disorders. The fifth and final section (*Other Common Problems*), deals with a variety of common problems including constipation, nutrition, infections, dermatologic conditions, wounds, and dizziness.

The purpose of this text is to provide the knowledge to care for problems common to an elderly population. We feel it will be of use to medical students, residents, nurse practitioners, physician assistants, and practicing physicians.

Thank You

We have asked well-respected experts and authors to contribute to this work and are grateful for their expertise. We would like to thank Barry Weiss, M.D., not only for his contribution as an author, but for his editorial advice and expertise as series editor. We would also like to thank all of our medical editors at McGraw-Hill: Joe Hefta who started us on this project; Susan Noujaim who has kept us going throughout almost the entire project; Andrea Seils and Nicky Panton who have helped us in the final stages. And finally, a special thanks to Diane Kocevar, Dr. Adelman's secretary at Penn State University College of Medicine for providing invaluable assistance in coordinating this work.

Part 1

General

Alan M. Adelman

Managing
Chronic Illness

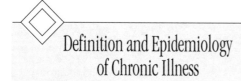

Definition and Epidemiology of Chronic Illness

The U.S. Centers for Disease Control and Prevention define chronic disease as "illnesses that are prolonged, do not resolve spontaneously, and are rarely cured completely." As the population ages, the prevalence of chronic illnesses climbs. The most common chronic conditions among noninstitutionalized persons are shown in Table 1-1. In the United States, more than 90 million persons have one or more chronic illnesses, and approximately 70 percent of the elderly population have multiple chronic conditions. Nearly 40 percent of elderly persons not living in nursing homes have a chronic condition that causes morbidity and limits function. Chronic illness is associated with considerable morbidity and mortality. Seventy percent of all deaths are attributed to chronic disease.

The cost of treating persons with chronic illnesses increases as the number of these illnesses increases. More than 60 percent of the total dollars spent on medical care in the United States is spent on the care of persons with chronic disease. It has been estimated that the average annual cost of caring for an enrollee in a health maintenance organization who does not have a chronic condition is approximately $925. The cost increases to approximately $2300 if the enrollee has one chronic condition and to more than $7000 if the enrollee has multiple chronic conditions.

The U.S. health care system has been geared toward acute, episodic care and not chronic care. In many health care systems, primary care providers spend 15 to 20 mins or less per patient because of scheduling constraints, making it difficult to deal with chronic conditions. Furthermore, Medicare does not generally reimburse comprehensive patient education for chronic conditions. It is only recently that patient education for diabetes mellitus has become a reimbursable service.

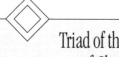

Triad of the Management of Chronic Illness

Figure 1-1 shows a model that may be useful in caring for patients with chronic illness. The figure depicts the triad of the clinician managing the illness, the patient also managing the illness, and the environment or structure of the care being provided. Traditional medicine has focused on the clinician managing the illness. However, to comprehensively address the needs of the elderly population with chronic illness, the health care system needs to expand its focus to deal with all components of the triad.

Managing the Illness

In 1983, Williams and Hadler proposed expanding the focus of the clinician in caring for geriatric

Table 1-1

Common Chronic Conditions of a Noninstitutionalized Elderly Population

CONDITION	PREVALENCE (%)
Arthritis	50
Hypertension	40
Heart disease	30
Vision impairment	10
Diabetes mellitus	5–10

Figure 1-1

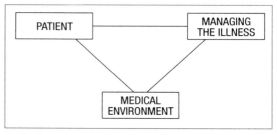

Model for managing patients with chronic disease.

Table 1-2

Principles of Medical Management of Chronic Illness

Start low, go slow
Focus on patient function
Identify reversible disease
Accept clinical uncertainty
Be aware of prognosis and natural history
Avoid polypharmacy
Be alert to the altered presentation of illness
Address psychosocial needs

patients. The traditional role of the clinician was primarily to search for a single cause of an illness and manage that single cause. This model worked well for many acute illnesses, such as uncomplicated infection. However, this approach is less likely to be useful in caring for patients with one or more chronic disorders. Chronic diseases usually are not curable and usually do not have a single cause. In many instances chronic diseases are the result of the interaction of multiple factors, including genetic, pathologic, iatrogenic, social, and environmental factors. Patients and families may struggle with and adapt to chronic illness for many years. The consequences are not only medical but also psychological.

To effectively deal with the challenges of managing chronic illnesses, clinicians need to develop a new model of medical care that involves dealing with many aspects of a patient's life (health, function, financial, social). Table 1-2 lists the areas in which clinicians may need to focus more attention to manage chronic conditions.

START LOW, GO SLOW

In general, the elderly are more sensitive to the effects of medications. The old adage, "start low, go slow," reminds clinicians to start at the lowest recommended dose and then cautiously titrate the dose upward as indicated by the patient's response. The goal is to use the lowest possible dose to achieve the desired outcome with little or no side effects. The effectiveness of the medica-

tion and the patient's tolerance of the medication must be assessed on a regular basis.

Many pharmacologic interventions are useful for older persons with chronic illnesses. Each intervention must be carefully evaluated and monitored for side effects and effectiveness. Clinicians must recognize that many older persons with chronic illnesses have already tried many different preparations and often are aware of the drugs that are available. These persons also often experiment with treatments that may be of controversial effectiveness.

FOCUS ON PATIENT FUNCTION

Clinicians often become focused on patients' illnesses rather than their functional abilities. An "illness approach" to elderly persons with chronic disease may be troublesome because the exact cause of the symptoms is not always found, and many symptoms experienced by elderly persons can be attributed to multiple factors. For example, a man's urinary incontinence may be caused by the combination of (1) a normally decreased bladder capacity; (2) the diuretic response to medication taken to control congestive heart failure (CHF); and (3) benign prostatic hypertrophy.

What frequently matters most to patients is their function, not necessarily the cause of the problem. Patients want to remain as active and as independent as possible. Their ability to perform day-to-day activities is of primary importance. Thus all energy must be focused on intervening to optimize function for patients with chronic illness.

IDENTIFY REVERSIBLE DISEASE

Although chronic illness is generally incurable, clinicians still must search for reversible disease or conditions. At the initial diagnosis of a condition, this search becomes especially important. A urinary tract infection, medication side effect, and drinking caffeinated coffee in the evening all are reversible causes of new-onset urinary incontinence (see Chap. 6). Identification of these factors may obviate further investigation. Optimizing a patient's therapy for arthritis, CHF, or benign prostatic hypertrophy may cure insomnia (see Chap. 10). Although most patients with dementia have a chronic, progressive course, some patients may have dementia that may be reversed with therapy for depression, vitamin deficiency, tertiary syphilis, or hypothyroidism (see Chap. 12).

A chronic condition can be exacerbated by an acute, reversible problem. For example, a patient with stable chronic obstructive pulmonary disease may become increasingly short of breath because of manageable conditions such as acute infectious bronchitis, pneumonia, or exacerbation of CHF. Acute urinary obstruction in a patient with previously stable benign prostatic hypertrophy may be caused by a manageable urinary tract infection (see Chap. 7). A sudden worsening of preexisting dementia may be caused by manageable acute infection or a reversible metabolic disturbance.

ACCEPT CLINICAL UNCERTAINTY

Clinical uncertainty is a common feature of primary care, especially in the treatment of patients with multiple chronic illnesses. Clinicians should be accepting of and comfortable with this uncertainty because a clear cause of the symptoms often is lacking. This was demonstrated by Kroenke and Mangelsdorff, who examined the records of patients at an internal medicine clinic. Among the 14 most common symptoms (chest pain, fatigue, dizziness, headache, edema, back pain, dyspnea, insomnia, abdominal pain, numbness, impotence, weight loss, cough, and constipation), the cause of symptoms could be determined with certainty for only 16 percent of the patients.

There may be a temptation to request laboratory or radiographic tests to exclude every possible cause of a problem. Although this approach may alleviate a clinician's anxiety and need to know, it may not help with formulating a diagnosis or developing a treatment program. For example, it may be of no value to a patient with end-stage chronic obstructive lung disease and hemoptysis to undergo a bronchoscopic procedure to rule out bronchogenic lung cancer. A patient without a focal neurologic deficit and a several-year history of slowly progressive confusion probably does not need a computed tomography of the head to exclude a diagnosis of a brain tumor or subdural hematoma. These decisions require clinical judgment in each case, but the clinician needs to question whether the proposed test will provide additional information that will alter treatment and be helpful to a patient's care.

BE AWARE OF PROGNOSIS AND COURSE OF DISEASE

Clinicians always need to take into consideration the course and prognosis of chronic illness when considering diagnostic and therapeutic interventions. For example, the course of most prostate cancers is slowly progressive disease. Prostate cancer often produces no symptoms at all (see Chap. 7). Treatment of an 80-year-old man for prostate cancer when the asymptomatic cancer is found during a routine digital rectal examination has to take into consideration the likelihood that the patient may die of something else before the prostate cancer becomes symptomatic. It also is questionable whether a disease prevention program should be recommended for a 72-year-old woman with moderate to severe dementia (see Chap. 3). It may not be reasonable or appropriate for her to undergo biannual mammography, yearly Hemoccult testing, or periodic flexible sigmoidoscopy.

AVOID POLYPHARMACY

Patients with single or multiple chronic illnesses probably are taking more than one medication. On average, older persons take four to eight medications on a regular basis and fill 10 to 14 prescriptions per year. Older persons frequently also take over-the-counter preparations such as antacids, aspirin, and acetaminophen. As the number of medications taken increases, the chance of adverse reactions and drug-drug interactions also increases (see Chap. 5). Polypharmacy will continue to be a difficult problem for clinicians to manage because the number of new medications available to manage chronic illnesses continues to grow. For example, 10 years ago, oral sulfonylureas and injectable insulins were the only medications available to treat a patient with type 2 diabetes mellitus. Today, in addition of oral sulfonylureas and injectable insulins, there are four new classes of oral hypoglycemic agents: meglitinides (repaglinide), α-glucosidase inhibitors (acarbose), thiazolidinediones (troglitazone), and biguanides (metformin). In the near future, an inhalable form of insulin is scheduled to be released.

Clinicians always should look for opportunities to safely reduce the dose of a medication, the number of medications prescribed, or both. Clinicians also should be mindful that many patients take not only prescription medications but also herbal preparations and over-the-counter medications. Polypharmacy is addressed in more detail in Chap. 5.

BE ALERT TO THE ALTERED PRESENTATION OF ILLNESS

Several factors influence the presentation of disease among the elderly (Table 1-3). First is a misperception of what constitutes normal aging and what constitutes disease among the elderly. Many elderly persons, and younger persons, believe that chronic illnesses are normal consequences of aging. Some misperceptions are that elderly persons normally experience memory loss, fatigue, urinary incontinence, constipation, and disability.

Table 1-3

Factors Influencing the Presentation of Disease Among Elderly Persons

Misperception of what is normal aging
Different physiologic response to disease
Effect of multiple chronic diseases
Polypharmacy

Elderly patients may not come to medical attention with the symptoms or signs of disease that occur among younger persons because of the different physiologic responses to disease among older persons. For example, older persons with pneumonia may not have a fever or leukocytosis (see Chap. 17). Symptoms of depression among older persons may include only apathy or memory loss without the classic symptoms of depression (see Chap. 11).

A third factor that may alter how illness occurs differently among the elderly is the concurrent effect of multiple chronic illnesses. One chronic illness may mask the symptoms of a coexisting chronic illness. For example, persons with diabetes mellitus are more likely to have a silent myocardial infarction, that is, infarction without chest pain. Patients with disabling arthritis or peripheral vascular disease may not have angina because they cannot engage in physical activities that sufficiently stress their hearts to produce chest pain.

ADDRESS PSYCHOSOCIAL NEEDS

Psychosocial health is a powerful predictor of overall health. Social support, ability to cope, self-confidence, mental health, and perceived health all are predictors of future health. Patients with chronic illnesses are subject to the daily stresses of living with a chronic illness. They and their caregivers also are subject to depression (see Chaps. 4 and 11). By not addressing these issues, clinicians miss an opportunity to improve the quality of life for patients and caregivers.

Patients as Managers of Their Own Illnesses: The Self-Care Model

Many providers have ignored patients as managers of their own health. There are many reasons for this attitude. First, clinicians traditionally have focused on searching for the cause of an illness and instituting the corresponding medical or surgical treatment with the patient being a passive recipient of care. Second, the medical community has only recently recognized alternative methods of treatment, so when patients self-administered alternative treatments, physicians did not consider it relevant to standard medical care. Third, medical care is largely fragmented in the current system of care, and most educational and preventive services are not reimbursable.

Clinicians and other health professionals see patients infrequently and for short periods of time. When patients leave a clinician's or other health professional's office, however, they must manage their day-to-day care. They must integrate all recommendations by clinicians into their daily routine. To optimally perform this task, patients need to be empowered and educated to assume the role of ultimate manager of their own health care.

Von Korff et al proposed several components of self-care and patient empowerment (Table 1-4). The model suggests that patients need to take the initiative to engage in activities that will promote their own health. Exercise, diet, and smoking cessation are a few examples of activities that can have an important effect on a patient's chronic illness. The patient–clinician relationship is important because if the clinician does not have the confidence of the patient, the patient is less likely to adhere to the agreed-upon treatment plan. Patients need to feel comfortable with their clinicians so that they can voice their concerns and raise issues that are important to them. They also need to feel that they will not be judged because of their concerns.

Patients are most familiar with their own emotional and physical health. This information can be valuable not only to the patient but also the clinician in managing the chronic illness and its sequelae. Patients need to recognize how their own emotional and physical health affects themselves and those around them. The incidence of mental health problems and physical disease among caregivers of patients with chronic illnesses is much greater than that among persons who are not caregivers. By recognizing that chronic illness affects patients and their caregivers, clinicians may be able to direct interventions that improve patient and caregiver outcomes (see Chap. 4). Putting all these skills together can help maximize the patient's functional ability.

Self-care should be viewed as complementary to the activities of the clinician. Von Korff et al proposed four essential elements of a collaborative management model (Table 1-5). Patients and clinicians first must agree on the problems to be addressed. Clinicians and patients frequently do not view illness in the same terms. Clinicians tend to focus on the diagnosis, interventions, and unhealthful behaviors. Patients are more likely to focus on symptoms and functional, mental, and general health. Clinicians and patients must communicate their perceptions about the chronic condition and issues to be addressed. One way to aid this process is for the clinician to share office notes with the patient.

Another important component of collaborative management is targeting, goal setting, and planning. Clinicians often are uncomfortable when asked to discuss issues such as prognosis or life

Table 1-4

Components of Self-Care

Performing activities that promote one's own health
Developing patient–clinician relationship
Following a mutually developed treatment plan
Monitoring one's own emotional and physical status
Recognizing how the illness can affect oneself and others
Maximizing one's own function

Table 1-5

Essential Elements of a Collaborative Management Model

Collaborative definition of problems
Targeting, goal setting, and planning
Creating a continuum of self-management training and support services
Active, sustained follow-up care

expectancy in chronic or terminal illness. Open discussion with a patient and the family often is useful in establishing realistic goals. Although clinicians may have their own targets that are determined by evidence-based goals and well-established algorithms, these plans often are not communicated or discussed with the patient. The management of diabetes mellitus is an example. Staged diabetes management, developed by Mazze et al, shows how these principles can be incorporated into practice. This management approach sets overall goals for care, specific targets for glycemic control, timetables to reach specific targets, and an overall master decision path. By reviewing the goals, timetables, and targets with the patient, the clinician can explore the patient's views about the disease and how they can work together in managing diabetes.

Another element of collaborative management is creating a continuum of self-management training and support services. Individuals differ in their learning styles and capacity to learn new skills. Training and support services should be individualized to best fit each patient's needs and abilities. The teaching modalities include written materials, audiovisual materials, and computer-assisted learning. The full potential of education and support services through the Internet should be explored. Individual and group teaching has been shown effective. The key is to recognize that a variety of methods are effective when tailored to meet an individual's needs.

A final element of collaborative management is active, sustained follow-up care. This follow-up care can be provided in the office and by telephone, electronic mail, or conventional mail. Rich et al showed that for patients with CHF, regular telephone follow-up sessions improved outcomes and decreased rehospitalization rates. Although not frequent today, house calls may be another way of providing ongoing medical care to homebound patients with chronic illnesses.

Patient education may be provided in a variety of ways, including handouts, brochures, videos, self-help groups, support groups, individual and group classes, computerized interactive learning, and the Internet. Each chapter in this book has a section on patient education, and many provide a listing of patient resources. There is extensive literature on the benefits of patient education programs directed at single diseases.

The arthritis self-management program developed by Lorig et al exemplifies the self-care model in a single chronic disease. Working with patients with arthritis, Lorig and associates developed a health education program that consisted of several elements (Table 1-6). The program was taught in six weekly, 2-h sessions led by trained lay leaders. Each participant received a copy of *The Arthritis Helpbook*, and the lay leaders received a training manual, *Arthritis Self-Management Leader's Manual*, revised. Patients who completed the program had a decline in pain and number of visits to a physician. They were also better able to cope with disability, fear, and depression. Their cost of care also declined.

Lorig et al developed a similar program for patients with chronic illnesses, but not targeted to a specific disease. Patients with heart disease, lung disease, stroke, or arthritis participated in this program with similar results as those enrolled in the single chronic disease (arthritis) program. The chronic disease self-management program improved time spent exercising, communication with physicians, self-reported health, and disability.

Table 1-6

Components of a Program for Self-Management of Chronic Illness

Knowledge of pathophysiologic mechanism of osteoarthritis and rheumatoid arthritis
Therapy for arthritis
Overview of arthritis medications
Individualized exercise program aimed at strengthening and increasing endurance
Relaxation program
Joint protection
Nutrition
Aspects of patient–physician communication
Problem solving
Relation between stress, pain, and depression

The Medical Environment

The environment may be divided into two separate components. The environment of medical practice includes the design of the office, information technology, and other support systems. The patient's environment includes family, caregivers, community, and social support networks. The patient's environment is discussed earlier and in Chap. 4. This section focuses on the medical environment.

MANAGING CHRONIC ILLNESS IN THE OFFICE SETTING

There are several ways of addressing the management of chronic illness in the office setting (Table 1-7). These methods can apply to any size group of physicians.

SET STANDARDS   Management guidelines exist for many chronic diseases, such as diabetes mellitus and CHF. These clinical guidelines are tools for the clinician and patient to keep up to date on the latest medical research applied to clinical practice. The best guidelines are evidence based and are updated on a regular basis. For example, the American Diabetes Association updates its guidelines on the management of diabetes mellitus on a yearly basis, and the guidelines are accessible on the Internet (www.diabetes.org).

Table 1-7

Steps to Improve the Management of Chronic Illness in the Office

Set standards
Involve patient
Involve staff
Develop office tools
Use the practice environment
Use every opportunity
Monitor compliance

Using a national guideline as a basis, an individual or group of clinicians can decide how the guidelines will apply to the practice of medicine in the office. This gains participation from the clinicians in the office. Practitioners may pick a few key recommendations as a beginning and then later adopt more recommendations as the first ones are implemented. The agreed-upon guidelines become the standard of care in the practice.

Evidence-based guidelines are available from a number of sources. Two excellent sources for clinical practice guidelines can be found at www.guidelines.gov and medicine.ucsf.edu/resources/guidelines. Many professional societies, such as the American College of Physicians, American Academy of Family Practice, and American Academy of Pediatrics, publish guidelines for their members. Government agencies, such as the U.S. Preventive Services Task Force and the National Heart, Lung and Blood Institute, have developed national guidelines for preventive services, lipid disorders, and asthma.

INVOLVE PATIENTS   Once the guidelines have been chosen, patients must be involved in implementing them. Discussion of guidelines may be a good way of getting patients involved in their care. This shows patients that the best available scientific evidence is being used in managing the illness. This may also be an opportunity to discuss the goals for the management of the illness.

INVOLVE STAFF   It is important to involve office staff in managing chronic illness. If appropriately educated and trained, staff members may be able to review a patient's chart before a visit to ensure that practice guidelines are being followed and appropriate laboratory tests and preventive measures are undertaken. Office staff can be helpful in the education process for patients. Every phase of the check-in and checkout process can be an opportunity to educate patients about practice guidelines. For example, nurses can request that patients with diabetes mellitus remove their shoes and socks before the clinician arrives.

DEVELOP OFFICE TOOLS In the absence of a computer reminder system or an electronic medical record, flow sheets can be developed that incorporate the office standards for a chronic illness. For example, a flow sheet to track a patient's prothrombin time and warfarin dose can facilitate the task of monitoring anticoagulation. Pocket cards may be an easy, quick reference for reviewing the recommendation of routine laboratory tests for a chronic disease. They can also summarize drug dosing, formulary recommendations, or diagnostic criteria.

USE THE PRACTICE ENVIRONMENT The practice environment presents many opportunities for patient education. Videotapes, computer-assisted learning materials, or brochures can be placed in the waiting room. Educational posters can be placed in key check-in and checkout areas, such as where the vital signs are taken or future appointments are scheduled. The examination room is another place where the patient may be exposed to posters or brochures. The formation of an education committee consisting of providers and office staff can develop and monitor patient education activities.

USE EVERY OPPORTUNITY Every office visit is an opportunity to promote chronic illness management. Many patients may visit for an acute problem such as an upper respiratory tract infection. At this time the chart can be reviewed to ensure the patient is up to date on immunizations, remind patients that influenza vaccination is recommended yearly in the fall, or schedule the next glycohemoglobin measurement for a patient with diabetes mellitus. A note may be placed in the chart to remind the provider what will be needed at the next visit, such as a routine foot examination or eye examination for a patient with diabetes mellitus.

MONITOR COMPLIANCE Once a practice guideline has been chosen, adherence to the guideline should be periodically monitored to assess performance. If a patient's medical record reveals that

the guideline has not been followed, every effort must be made to ensure compliance with the office standard of care.

Numerous organizations, such as the Health Care Financing Association (Medicare) are interested in performance of providers as measured against regional or national standards. These organizations publish standards of care. Clinicians can measure their own performance by auditing charts and comparing their performance against the national standards.

One example of such a program is the recently developed Diabetes Quality Improvement Project (DQIP). The DQIP is jointly sponsored by the American Diabetes Association, Foundation for Accountability, Health Care Financing Administration, and the National Center for Quality Assurance. The American College of Physicians, American Academy of Family Physicians, and Department of Veterans Affairs also have joined the effort. The hope is that the measures developed will be used to measure performance of clinicians in the provision of care to patients with diabetes (see Table 1-8).

Table 1-8

Clinical Measures in Diabetes Quality Improvement Program

Percentage of patients undergoing one or more glycohemoglobin tests per year

Percentage of patients with a glycohemoglobin level greater than 9.5 percent

Percentage of patients assessed for nephropathy

Percentage of patients undergoing a lipid profile once in 2 years

Percentage of patients with a low-density lipoprotein cholesterol level less than 130 mg/dL

Percentage of patients with blood pressure less than 140/90 mmHg

Percentage of patients undergoing a periodic dilated eye examination

Percentage of patients undergoing an annual documented foot examination

IMPROVING CARE IN LARGE GROUPS AND SYSTEMS

Disease management has become buzzwords in the health care system. Epstein and Sherwood defined disease management as "a systematic, population-based approach to identify persons at risk, intervene with specific programs of care, and measure clinical and other outcomes." Programs have been developed in many areas of the country and are reported to improve patient satisfaction and health outcomes. Diseases such as CHF and diabetes mellitus are frequent subjects of these programs.

A disease management program defines a population at risk and designs a program that best addresses the needs of the population. Interventions are not necessarily confined to traditional medical interventions. For example, many CHF programs include regular telephone follow-up sessions with patients enrolled in the program.

EXAMPLE OF A DISEASE MANAGEMENT PROGRAM: CONGESTIVE HEART FAILURE   Congestive heart failure is a common chronic illness. It affects 4 to 5 million Americans. More than 400,000 new cases are diagnosed every year, and it is the most frequent discharge diagnosis among Medicare patients hospitalized in the United States. The cost in terms of diagnosis, treatment, and frequent hospitalizations is massive for the health system. In the United States, more than 10 billion dollars per year is spent on this diagnosis. Rich et al reported that a multidisciplinary program could reduce the high readmission rate among persons with CHF and improve quality of life.

The example that follows is from the Penn State Geisinger Health Plan, a large health maintenance organization that provides care to approximately 300,000 persons in rural central and northern Pennsylvania. The health plan developed a disease management program for CHF. The components of the disease management program are shown in Table 1-9. A CHF team monitors the program. This team is multidisciplinary, including primary care clinicians, cardiologists who special-

Table 1-9

Components of Disease Management Programs

Identification of risk
Clinical guidelines
Patient and family education
Case management
Registries that produce reminders and feedback
Practitioner education

ize in the diagnosis and management of CHF, nurses, and dietitians. Participation in the program decreased the rate of rehospitalization, improved the quality of life of those enrolled, and saved the health plan millions of dollars.

Identification of Risk.   Patients with moderate to severe CHF are eligible for inclusion in the program. The health plan finds members for this program in a variety of ways, including referrals from inpatient case managers, clinicians, and the CHF clinic. Because patients hospitalized for CHF are at risk of frequent rehospitalizations, patients discharged from the hospital with a diagnosis of CHF are found through hospital discharge records. Health plan members also may self-refer for evaluation for the program.

Case Management.   Once it is identified that a member may be at risk, a case manager is assigned and begins an evaluation. The case manager collects information about symptoms of CHF, the diagnostic evaluation, measures of quality of life, and the patient's functional ability. This information is entered into a central registry maintained by the health plan. If the patient has moderate to severe CHF, the case manager enrolls the patient in the program. The case manager telephones the patient on a periodic basis to assess whether the patient is following the treatment plan.

Patient and Family Education.   The case manager initiates patient and family education. The educational program includes information on salt restriction, the importance of monitoring weight, and warning symptoms of worsening CHF failure. The case managers may do this themselves or they may request a health plan nurse or home health nurse to provide the necessary education.

Clinical Guidelines. A clinical guideline, based on a national CHF guideline developed by the Agency for Health Care Policy and Research, was developed. Members of the guideline development team included cardiologists who specialize in CHF, primary care clinicians, nurses, dietitians, and health educators. The guideline emphasizes the appropriate evaluation of CHF, and the treatment plan, including patient education, is outlined.

Practitioner Education. As part of the implementation process, clinicians are educated in the guideline and its use. The guideline is made available in printed form and on the health plan's Web site. Case managers are educated about the CHF guideline and often act as academic detailers for the guideline. Academic detailing is a process similar to pharmaceutical detailing whereby on a one-to-one basis an individual provides the clinician with information that supports the guideline. Detailing has been shown to be an effective method of influencing clinician prescribing and guideline use.

Registries That Provide Reminders and Feedback. The information collected by the case manager can be used in multiple ways. The registry contains a listing of telephone contacts and can be used to set a schedule of regular telephone follow-up sessions. Clinical information, including number of hospitalizations and rehospitalizations, use of angiotensin-converting enzyme (ACE) inhibitors, and use of cardiac ultrasonography, can be used to monitor the effectiveness of the program. For example, ACE inhibitors are underused in the management of CHF. The registry can find patients who are not taking an ACE inhibitor and send letters to the clinician to emphasize the beneficial effects of ACE inhibitor in the treatment of patients with CHF.

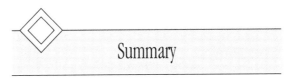

Summary

The difficulty in managing chronic illnesses will continue to grow as the population ages and the number of possible interventions for chronic illnesses grows. Although this chapter suggests ways of addressing the problem of caring for persons with chronic illnesses, many problems still exist. Physicians in individual practices do not have the resources to institute some of the programs described. A clinician may be capable of managing a few chronic disease guidelines or disease management programs at once, but managing 5 to 10 or more chronic illnesses at once may be quite difficult, if not impossible. One patient with multiple chronic illnesses may need several different algorithms of care and guidelines, and it is not clear how multiple disease management programs are effective when applied in concert. Furthermore, Medicare still does not reimburse case management or patient education programs, except for diabetes mellitus.

Implementing these systems of care will not be easy, and mixed success is reported in the literature. Coleman et al reported on the effectiveness of chronic care clinics. A half-day clinic was held every 3 to 4 months. The chronic care clinics incorporated many of the principles described in this chapter. The clinic included a visit with a physician, nurse, and pharmacist. There was also a patient self-management support group. Although patients reported high levels of satisfaction with the program, improved clinical outcomes could not be demonstrated.

Beck et al examined the effectiveness of group outpatient visits for patients with chronic disease. Patients attended a monthly group meeting with their physician and nurse. Health education and prevention were reviewed at the meetings. The meetings were conducted to allow socialization and mutual support. Patients could see the physician on a one-on-one basis if necessary. Patients who participated in this program had fewer emergency department visits, visits to subspecialists, and rehospitalizations. They demonstrated higher satisfaction with their care.

The results of these two studies show that the most appropriate and efficient system to deliver comprehensive care to patients with chronic illnesses has not yet been developed on a large scale. The principles presented are sound and if followed will improve care provided to persons with chronic illnesses. The question remains how best to incorporate these principles into systems of care.

Bibliography

Adelman AM, Harris RI: Improving performance in a primary care office. *Clin Diabetes* 16:54–159, 1998.

Beck A, Scott J, Williams P, et al: A randomized trial of group outpatient visits for chronically ill older HMO members: the cooperative health care clinic. *J Am Geriatr Soc* 45:543–549, 1997.

Bodenheimer T: Disease management: promises and pitfalls. *N Engl J Med* 340:1202, 1999.

Coleman EA, Grothaus LC, Sandhu N, Wagner EH: Chronic care clinics: a randomized controlled trial of a new model of primary care for frail older adults. *J Am Geriatr Soc* 47:775–783, 1999.

Davis RM, Wagner EH, Grover T: Managing chronic disease presents such challenges that the BMJ is devoting a special issue to it. *BMJ* 318:1090–1091, 1999.

Ellrodt G, Cook DJ, Lee J, et al: Evidence-based disease management. *JAMA* 278:1687–1692, 1997.

Epstein RS, Sherwood LM: From outcomes research to disease management: a guide for the perplexed. *Ann Intern Med* 124:832–837, 1996.

Fishman P: Chronic care costs in managed care. *Health Aff (Millwood)* 16:239–247, 1997.

Freudenheim D: *Chronic Care in America: A 21st Century Challenge.* Princeton, NJ: Institute for Health and Aging; 1996.

Hunter DJ, Fairfield G: Disease management. *BMJ* 215:50–53, 1997.

Konstam M, Dracup K, Baker D, et al: *Heart Failure: Evaluation and Care of Patients with Left-Ventricular Systolic Dysfunction,* Clinical Practice Guideline no. 11, AHCPR publication no. 94-0612. Rockville,

MD, US Department of Health and Human Services, Public Health Services, Agency for Health Care Policy and Research, 1994.

Kroenke K, Mangelsdorff AD: Common symptoms in ambulatory care: incidence, evaluation, therapy, and outcome. *Am J Med* 86:262–266, 1989.

Lorig K: *Arthritis Self-Management Leader's Manual,* revised. Atlanta: Arthritis Foundation; 1984.

Lorig K, Fries JF: *The Arthritis Helpbook.* Reading, MA: Addison-Wesley; 1990.

Lorig KR, Mazonson PD, Holman HR: Evidence suggesting that health education for self-management in patients with chronic arthritis has sustained health benefits while reducing health care costs. *Arthritis Rheum* 36:439–446, 1993.

Lorig KR, Sobel DS, Stewart AL, et al: Evidence suggesting that a chronic disease self-management program can improve health status while reducing hospitalization: a randomized trial. *Med Care* 37:5–14, 1999.

Mayfield J: Who cares about the quality of diabetes care? Almost everyone! *Clin Diabetes* 16:161–167, 1998.

Mazze RS, Etzwiler DD, Strock E, et al: Staged diabetes management: toward an integrated model of diabetes care. *Diabetes Care* 17(suppl 1):56–66, 1994.

Rich MW, Beckham V, Wittenberg C, et al: A multidisciplinary intervention to prevent the readmission of elderly patients with congestive heart failure. *N Engl J Med* 333:1190–1195, 1995.

Sobel DS: Rethinking medicine: improving health outcomes with cost-effective psychosocial interventions. *Psychosom Med* 57:234–244, 1995.

US Centers for Disease Control and Prevention, National Center for Chronic Disease Prevention and Health Promotion: About chronic disease: definition, overall burden, and cost effectiveness of prevention. Available at: http://www.cdc.gov/nccdphp/about.htm. Accessed April 23, 1999.

Von Korff M, Gruman J, Schaefer J, Curry SJ, Wagner EH: Collaborative management of chronic illness. *Ann Intern Med* 127:1097–1102, 1997.

Wagner EH: Managed care and chronic illness: health services research needs. *Health Serv Res* 32:702–714, 1997.

Wagner EH, Austin BT, Von Korff M: Improving outcomes in chronic illness. *Manag Care Q* 4:12–25, 1996.

Wagner EH, Austin BT, Von Korff M: Organizing care for patients with chronic illness. *Milbank Q* 4:511–544, 1996.

Williams ME: The approach to managing the elderly patient. In: Hazzard WR, et al (eds): *Principles of Geriatric Medicine and Gerontology,* 4th ed. New York: McGraw-Hill; 1999.

Williams ME, Hadler NM: Sounding board: the illness as the focus of geriatric medicine. *N Engl J Med* 308:1357–1360, 1983.

William Reichel

Chapter

Care at the End of Life

For everything there is a season,
And a time for every matter under heaven:
A time to be born, and a time to die

ECCLESIASTES 3:1-2

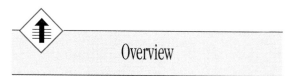

Overview

The last 5 years have seen many expressions that Americans are not happy with the American way of dying. Individuals and organizations and publications and other media reports all make it clear that patients' wishes do not receive attention, that clinicians shy away from discussing bad news, and that many patients suffer and die in pain. The good news is that progress has been made in the organization of hospice care and the advancement of palliative principles. Advance health care planning is progressing only slowly.

Corporate medicine, increasing use of new technologies, and the malpractice threat all create great societal angst. They have taken their toll on continuity of care and clinician-patient communication. Clinicians often simply do not have the time to come to know patients and stay connected with them. If a clinician spends only 12 mins with an elderly patient, can a clinician have time to learn about the patient's family situation, which may be characterized by estrangement from children, divorce, and children who live far away? Will the clinician discuss advance care planning at an early stage of the relationship or illness rather than during the last hospitalization? Does the clinician have any idea about the patient's religious or spiritual perspective or worldview? What issues does the patient want to process before he or she dies, such as reconciliation with a family member, or expression of love to an adult child or grandchild? Can the clinician properly evaluate suffering or pain or depression or fear? Is the clinician prepared to deal with these serious problems?

At worst, a primary care clinician may turn the patient's care over to an oncologist or cardiologist and no longer serve as the true primary care clinician. The primary care clinician may not know the patient's personal or family situation, life story, or religious or spiritual perspective. Advance health care planning may be overlooked, or if the patient's preferences have been documented, that information may not be retained in the clinical process, and the physicians involved may make decisions according to their own judgment and preferences. These are all negative aspects of the American way of dying. The positive advances and initiatives that follow should improve the care of the dying in America.

The work of Lynn and Byock and many others is leading us in a better direction. Lynn directs the Center to Improve Care of the Dying in Washington, DC, and she and her colleagues have made many contributions in this area. Byock directs the Missoula Demonstration Project, Missoula, Montana, and is author of the 1997 book *Dying Well*, which encourages reintegrating dying within living, allowing the prospect for growth at the end of life. Byock and others have written about dying well, physician-assisted living, and living while dying. Byock views the end of life as a time of love and reconciliation, a time of transcendence of suffering.

There have been a vast number of initiatives to improve the care of the dying, of which the Missoula Demonstration Project Quality of Life's End and the Center to Improve Care of the Dying at George Washington University are two. Last Acts is sponsored by the Robert Wood Johnson Foundation to improve care at the end of life and provides a resource center to the profession and the public (www.lastacts.org). The purpose of the Project on Death in America (www.soros.org) is to transform society and our experience of dying and bereavement through research, scholarship, and the humanities and art. The project, supported by the Open Society Institute, fosters new approaches in professional education, public policy, public education, and the provision of care. Americans for Better Care of the Dying (ABCD) (www.abcd-caring. com) is a coalition of the public and professionals dedicated to social and professional reform with the purpose of improving the care system for those who are dying and their families.

The National Hospice Organization (www.nho. org) in Arlington, Virginia, is the main organization representing hospice as described herein. Another hospice organization with similar themes is the Hospice Foundation of America (www.hospicefoundation.org).

The American Academy of Hospice and Palliative Medicine (www.aahpm.org) is the premier organization of physicians dedicated to the advancement of hospice and palliative medicine in the management of the terminally ill. Practitioners of many disciplines within medicine and nursing are studying the role of hospice and palliative care within their specialties. Geriatrics evolved the same way in the 1970s and 1980s. The American Academy of Hospice and Palliative Medicine offers a board certification examination in this area that is not part of the American Board of Medical Specialties. We can expect to see further developments within specialty areas as to the role that hospice and palliative medicine will play in each discipline.

The American Cancer Society (www.cancer. org) offers a plethora of resource material related to cancer and management of cancer pain to both the public and to professionals (1-800-ACS-2345).

The American Medical Association (AMA) (www.ama-assn.org) has established the Education for Physicians in End-of Life Care (EPEC) under its newly formed Institute of Ethics (at AMA Web site, go to Ethics, and go to EPEC). The EPEC project, supported by a grant from the Robert Wood Johnson Foundation, is designed to educate physicians across the United States on the essential clinical competencies that every physician should possess. An EPEC Curriculum is being disseminated through a series of national and regional conferences, the development of an EPEC Resource Guide, an EPEC Speakers List, and a self-directed learning manual, the *EPEC Monograph*, which will be distributed to physicians across the United States.

Other professional associations include the Hospice Nurses Association (www.hpna.org) and the Association of Oncology Social Workers (www.aosw.org).

A great paradigm shift is taking place in the United States that is affecting the professions and the public. With all of these efforts underway, our view of care at the end of life will be different, and our professional behaviors will change. The AMA has proposed the responsibilities of attending physicians in the care of patients at the end of life (Table 2-1).

It is no accident that so much societal action is taking place. Perhaps the increasing call for physician-assisted suicide is why many in the public and the professions are asking for a better way to care for the dying. It is perceived that death is not what it should be.

Physician-assisted suicide is a highly controversial subject. The practice of euthanasia in the Netherlands, according to studies conducted there, demonstrates a high percentage of involuntary euthanasia (failing to seek the patient's explicit request for termination of life) as opposed to voluntary euthanasia and of failing to follow certain criteria, such as seeking a second physician's

Table 2-1

Responsibilities of Attending Physicians in the Care of Patients at the End of Life

Signing the initial certification of terminal illness
Reviewing the hospice plan of care
Making ongoing visits with the patient
Prescribing medication for comfort care
Reviewing with hospice staff the condition and prognosis
Making telephone contact and house calls to the patient as necessary
Signing the death certificate

SOURCE: Adapted with permission from Department of Geriatric Health. *Medical Management of the Home Care Patient: Guidelines for Physicians*, 2nd ed. Chicago, American Medical Association, 1998; 18.

opinion. As U.S. medicine becomes more corporate and more focused on cost-containment, physician-assisted suicide may become an easy approach to reducing cost. It would be more convenient than denying days in the hospital or denying certain consultations or procedures. Woody Allen is often quoted in this debate. He said, "Think of death as cutting down on your expenses."

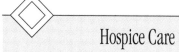

Hospice Care

Hospices are collaborations between a family and hospice professionals and volunteers to provide medical, psychological, social, and spiritual care for a person who is dying. Palliative medicine is meant to provide pain relief and relief of symptoms other than pain, such as nausea and vomiting, and depression.

Hospice care developed first in Great Britain and is exemplified by the seminal work of Cicely Saunders at St. Christopher's Hospice. Hospice moved to the United States in the early 1970s. The first U.S. hospice was the New Haven Hospice in New Haven, Connecticut, which later became the Connecticut Hospice. Hospice eventually spread throughout the country. Hospice care is a philosophy of management of pain and suffering associated with dying. The goal of hospice care is to support the quality of life of the patient and family while making possible a comfortable death at home. Palliative care manages the patient's pain with medication to guarantee that the patient is pain free. Physicians provide palliative care in treating patients throughout life, but palliative care at the end of life has grown in importance and urgency as a means of providing better end-of-life care.

Hospice is meant for patients whose life expectancy is 6 months or less. The physician must first recommend that hospice is an appropriate next step and that treatment has become ineffective and burdensome. Optimally the primary care clin-

ician who has monitored the entire progress of the illness has reached this decision in collaboration with an oncologist, cardiologist, or other specialists and will take the time to explain hospice in detail and why hospice is being recommended. It is helpful for the clinician to provide literature from the National Hospice Organization (bookstore 1-800-646-6460; www.nho.org) to explain hospice to patients and families. Hospice care can be provided in the home, in hospice beds in hospitals and nursing homes, or in a freestanding hospice.

In all of these environments, there is collaboration of an interdisciplinary team. The team works in concert with the patient and a designated primary caregiver (family member, friend, or neighbor). The principal focus is on pain management and symptom control. Clinical treatment and strategies that could prolong life are stopped. After the patient understands the recommendation for hospice, he or she signs a statement (the hospice elective form) choosing hospice care, which is covered by Medicare (see later), and waiving standard Medicare benefits for the terminal illness. Treatment of problems not related to the terminal illness, such as a broken arm, are covered by conventional Medicare benefits. The characteristics of hospice are listed in Table 2-2.

Physicians encounter patients who reject hospice. These patients demand maximal efforts for continuing life, even with very poor quality of life. There can be generational differences. An 80-year-old woman may reject home hospice for her 90-year-old husband because she believes she cannot handle the care at home. She needs help to understand the many supports that would make dying well at home a manageable option. The physician can suggest hospice options in other environments if the wife cannot accept home hospice.

There are many variations of hospice care in the United States. Some hospices are part of home health agencies or work in parallel with a home health agency or visiting nurse association. The hospice pays attention to the social, psychological, and spiritual aspects of care and provides case management and continuity if the patient moves between home and inpatient facilities.

Table 2-2

Characteristics of Hospice

Patient life expectancy is 6 months or less.

Coordination is by an interdisciplinary team, including nurse, social worker, physician, hospice, medical director, volunteers, aides, and a spiritual advisor such as a priest, rabbi, or minister.

Nurses are on call 24 h a day for home visits.

Pain management and symptom control are the primary focus.

Family counseling and bereavement services are available for 1 year after the patient dies.

The approach is palliative rather than curative.

Patients sign a statement choosing hospice care and waiving standard Medicare benefits for the terminal illness.

SOURCE: Adapted with permission from Department of Geriatric Health. *Medical Management of the Home Care Patient: Guidelines for Physicians*, 2nd ed. Chicago, American Medical Association, 1998; 19.

Hospice coverage is provided by Medicare throughout the United States, by Medicaid in 42 states, and by most private insurance plans. Hospice was funded as a capitated system under Medicare. In 1994, Medicare was the primary source of payment for two-thirds of hospice services, and other payers often use Medicare guidelines to set services (the financial arrangements are evolving under different managed care systems).

Medicare coverage of hospice provides supportive care and financial benefits not available in other programs. Home hospice services do not have to be categorized as skilled. Copayments usually are not required, and drugs related to the terminal illness are funded by Medicare.

Hospice is strongly interdisciplinary with required involvement by nursing staff, social workers, physicians, aides, clergy, and volunteers. Nearly one-fourth of the hospice team is home health aides and homemakers who provide services to lessen the family's heavy burden of care. In hospice, home hospice is the main locus of care. In fiscal year 1993, 87 percent of expenditures were for routine home hospice days.

The most common obstacle to early referral by physicians is difficulty determining life expectancy among persons with cancer or other chronic diseases. *Medical Guidelines for Determining Prognosis for Selected Non-Cancer Diseases*, second edition, published by the National Hospital Organization, 1-800-646-6460, is a useful tool for noncancerous disease. A similar set of guidelines is expected for cancer disorders. All hospice programs have cared for large numbers of patients not referred until the last week or two of life. Some patients live longer than the initial life expectancy of 6 months or less.

What are the responsibilities of the physician in hospice care? First, the physician must explain the recommendation of hospice to the patient and family and explain the decision to discontinue treatments that have become ineffective or burdensome. The physician must explain to patient and family that the decision to remain in hospice can be revoked, and the patient can return to traditional care under Medicare. For the patient to enter hospice, the physician must sign the initial certification of terminal illness. The physician must review the hospice plan of care for the specific patient. The physician is expected to visit the patient regularly and prescribe medications for comfort care. The physician must review the patient's condition and prognosis with hospice staff. The physician's staying in telephone contact and making house calls as necessary maintains the connection that patient and family need. A random phone call asking the patient or the caregiver how things are going is of great benefit and is appreciated. And the physician must sign the death certificate.

The hospice movement has grown with much vigor in the United States as it has in Great Britain, Australia, New Zealand, and Canada. It is taking on new forms under managed health care plans. Overall, hospice provides hope for dying well. Primary care physicians can join this process and participate in improving health care to dying patients in the United States.

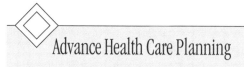

Advance Health Care Planning

The Study to Understand Prognoses and Preferences for Outcomes and Risk of Treatments (SUPPORT) showed first in a 1995 study that interventions failed to improve care or patient outcomes. The interventions included physicians' receiving information about prognosis and functional disability and the service of a specially trained nurse who was in contact with patient, family, physician, and hospital staff to elicit preferences, improve understanding of outcomes, encourage attention to pain control, and attempt to facilitate advance health care planning and patient-clinician communication. Many articles quantify the limited use of advance directives, but the 1995 study concluded that to "improve the experience of seriously ill and dying patients, greater individual and societal commitment and more proactive and forceful measures may be needed."

Lynn and associates demonstrated that advance directives did not substantially improve clinician-patient communication about resuscitation. Advance directives when placed in the medical records of seriously ill patients did not provide meaningful guidance. Even when specific instructions were present, care often was inconsistent. Teno et al stated that one principal conclusion was that "Future work to improve decision-making should focus upon improving the current pattern of practice through better communication and more comprehensive advance care planning."

The Legal History of Advance Directives

The legal history of advance directives begins with the events involving Nancy Cruzan, a young woman in a persistent vegetative state. The Cruzan family asked the U.S. Supreme Court to hear their case after the Missouri Supreme Court ruled against the family's request to withdraw a gastros-tomy tube that had been providing nutrition and hydration to Nancy Cruzan for 6 years. Although Nancy Cruzan had discussed wishes regarding medical care with her family and friends, the Missouri Supreme Court decided reports of these discussions were insufficient to justify removal of the tube. The U.S. Supreme Court upheld the decision of the state supreme court that there was a lack of clear and convincing evidence. Although the Cruzans lost their case, the U.S. Supreme Court ruling increased awareness of the rights of individuals to refuse life-prolonging medical treatment, including nutrition and hydration. It was highlighted that individuals do not take advantage of opportunities to express their wishes or preferences through a living will or durable power of attorney.

The Cruzan case was a stimulus for new legislation, the Patient Self-Determination Act (PSDA), which was passed by Congress in 1990 and became federal law on December 1, 1991. The law requires all hospitals, nursing homes, home health agencies, hospices, and health maintenance organizations that receive Medicare or Medicaid funding to ask patients whether they have signed an advance directive. There are to be no negative consequences if patients have not signed one. The law also requires that patients receive a written statement of their rights under state law to accept or refuse medical treatment, to provide information about advance directives, and to encourage patients to write one.

Although it was hoped that the PSDA would encourage patients to consider writing advance directives, that has not been the case. Many Americans, young and old, have postponed this step. Many Americans receive a living will or advance directive while preparing their financial will with their lawyer. Clinicians may have simple forms in their offices but have not entered into discussions of advance care planning with their patients. Many hospitals conform with the PSDA simply by asking patients at admission whether they have a living will. Unfortunately, if the answer, is "yes," many admitting offices do not request a copy of the living will or advance directive.

A living will is a statement allowing a person to indicate that life-prolonging medical treatment be withdrawn or withheld in the future. The durable power of attorney gives a designated person the legal authority to make decisions on the patient's behalf, for example, in financial management, even if the designated person becomes incapacitated. A separate durable power of attorney for health care is an instrument giving a designated person the legal authority to make decisions specifically about health care. A proxy or health care surrogate is the person designated to serve as an agent under a durable power of attorney for health care.

Any advance directive remains in effect but can be revoked at any time. Only the person who signed the advance directive can revoke it. It can be revoked partially or totally. The person can create and sign a new advance directive that replaces any previous one.

The Values History

The advance directive in Table 2-3 is a Values History, originally developed by Doukas and McCullough. This document is intended to complement a living will or durable power of attorney for health care by focusing on a person's beliefs, preferences, and values, particularly those important in the event of a terminal illness, coma, or persistent vegetative state. Particular details regarding specific medical treatments are stated in this advance directive. Ideally the patient should take the Values History home, reflect on it, and return to the clinician's office alone or with a family member to discuss the issues involved. The clinician's role in counseling the patient is to explain components of the Values History and to answer questions about events or procedures that are abstract or not comprehended by the patient, particularly if the patient is well. This type of dialogue should take place before the patient's finalizing and signing the Values History. The Values History and any advance directive can be revoked at any time.

If the physician receives an advance directive from a patient, the minimal response may be to place it in the patient's chart for safekeeping and to place a label on the chart "Patient's Advance Directive Is Filed in This Chart" with the date the directive was received.

Problems in the Use of Advance Directives

There are several problems in using advance directives and a Values History. First, discussing the need for an advance directive is not yet a high priority in the daily work of clinicians. Many clinicians are simply not trained or accustomed to discussing advance directives. Some clinicians may become focused on the current disorder or chief complaint and may not be thinking of a broader biopsychosocial-spiritual model, or of future scenarios in which an advance directive would benefit the patient. Time pressures and the uncertainty of payment for this type of counseling are part of the current health care environment. Physicians working in managed care or corporate medicine may be precluded from providing such counseling by demands of productivity. At the same time, managed health care organizations may be sending letters to all the patients in their system recommending that they complete an advance directive.

Patients may not realize the importance of this type of planning. Patients who use an attorney may receive a durable power of attorney, a living will, and a durable power of attorney for health care as additional instruments when they start work on a will or living trust. Some of the public may be sophisticated enough to value the importance of advance directive instruments, and others may not. Many people learn about advance directives as part of their estate planning and not on recommendation from their physicians.

Many patients do not fully understand the role of living wills or advance directives. They may fear signing a living will in case aggressive, life-saving treatment be withheld in the course of a nonterminal illness, such as a first heart attack. Some patients may fear being placed on a machine or

Table 2-3
Values History

Patient's name:

This Values History serves as a set of my specific value-based directives for various medical interventions. It is to be used in health care circumstances when I may be unable to voice my preferences. These directives shall be made a part of the medical record and shall be used as supplementary to my living will and/or durable power of attorney for health care if I am terminally ill or in a persistently vegetative state.

I. Values Section

There are several values important in decisions about end-of-life treatment and care. This section of the Values History invites you to identify your most important values.

A. Basic Life Values

Perhaps the most basic values in this context concern length of life versus quality of life. Which of the following two statements most accurately reflects your feelings and wishes? Write <u>your initials</u> and the <u>date</u> next to the number you choose.

_____ 1. I want to live as long as possible, regardless of the quality of life that I experience.

_____ 2. I want to preserve a good quality of life, even if this means that I may not live as long.

B. Quality-of-Life Values

There are many values that help us to define for ourselves the quality of life that we want to live. The following values appear to be those most frequently used to define quality of life. Review this list and <u>circle</u> the values that are most important to your definition of quality of life. Feel free to elaborate on any of the items in the list, and to add to the list any other values that are important to you.

1. I want to maintain my capacity to think clearly.
2. I want to feel safe and secure.
3. I want to avoid unnecessary pain and suffering.
4. I want to be treated with respect.
5. I want to be treated with dignity when I can no longer speak for myself.
6. I do not want to be an unnecessary burden on my family.
7. I want to be able to make my own decisions.
8. I want to experience a comfortable dying process.
9. I want to be with my loved ones before I die.
10. I want to leave good memories of me for my loved ones.
11. I want to be treated in accord with my religious beliefs and traditions.
12. I want respect shown for my body after I die.
13. I want to help others by making a contribution to medical education and research.
14. Other values or clarification of values above:

II. Directives Section

Some directives involve a simple yes or no decision. Others provide for the choice of a trial of intervention. Write your <u>initials</u> and the <u>date</u> next to the number for each directive you complete.

_____ 1. I want to undergo cardiopulmonary resuscitation.

___ Yes

___ No

Why?

Table 2-3
Values History *(continued)*

_____ 2. I want to be placed on a ventilator
   ___ Yes
   ___ Trial for the time period of _____.
   ___ Trial to determine effectiveness using reasonable medical judgment.
   ___ No
   Why?

_____ 3. I want to have an endotracheal tube in order to perform items 1 and 2.
   ___ Yes
   ___ Trial for the time period of _____.
   ___ Trial to determine effectiveness using reasonable medical judgment.
   ___ No
   Why?

_____ 4. I want to have total parenteral nutrition administered for my nutrition.
   ___ Yes
   ___ Trial for the time period of _____.
   ___ Trial to determine effectiveness using reasonable medical judgment.
   ___ No
   Why?

_____ 5. I want to have intravenous medication and hydration administered. Regardless of my decision, I understand that intravenous hydration to alleviate discomfort or pain medication will not be withheld from me if I so request them.
   ___ Yes
   ___ Trial for the time period of _____.
   ___ Trial to determine effectiveness using reasonable medical judgment.
   ___ No
   Why?

_____ 6. I want to have all medications used for the treatment of my illness continued. Regardless of my decision, I understand pain medication will continue to be administered including narcotic medications.
   ___ Yes
   ___ Trial for the time period of _____.
   ___ Trial to determine effectiveness using reasonable medical judgment.
   ___ No
   Why?

_____ 7. I want to have nasogastric, gastrostomy, or other enteral feeding tubes introduced and administered for my nutrition.
   ___ Yes
   ___ Trial for the time period of _____.
   ___ Trial to determine effectiveness using reasonable medical judgment.
   ___ No
   Why?

Table 2-3

Values History *(continued)*

_____ 8. I want to be placed on a dialysis machine.
      ___ Yes
      ___ Trial for the time period of _____.
      ___ Trial to determine effectiveness using reasonable medical judgment.
      ___ No
      Why?
_____ 9. I want to have an autopsy done to determine the cause(s) of my death.
      ___ Yes
      ___ No
      Why?
_____ 10. I want to be admitted to the intensive care unit.
      ___ Yes
      ___ No
      Why?
_____ 11. If I am in a long-term care facility or receiving care at home and experience a life-threatening change in health status, I want 911 called in case of a medical emergency.
      ___ Yes
      ___ No
      Why?
_____ 12. Other directives.

I consent to these directives after receiving honest disclosure of their implications, risks, and benefits from my physician, being free of constraints, and being of sound mind.
Signature:_____ Date: _____
Witness: _____
Witness: _____
13. Proxy Negation: I request that the following persons not be allowed to make decisions on my behalf in the event of my disability or incapacity:

_____

_____

Signature:_____ Date: _____
Witness: _____
Witness: _____
14. Organ Donation:
[Insert here your state's version of the organ donor card.]
15. Durable Power of Attorney for Health Care:
[Insert here your state's version of the durable power of attorney for health care.]

Source: Adapted from Doukas D, McCullough L: The Values History: The evaluation of the patient's values and advance directives. *J Fam Prac* 1991; 32:145–153. Doukas DJ, Reichel W: *Planning for Uncertainty: A Guide to Living Wills and Other Advance Directives for Health Care.* Baltimore: Johns Hopkins University Press: 1993. Reprinted with permission of Appleton and Lange, Inc. and Johns Hopkins Press.

use of other technology, when that mechanical support might be life saving in an acute, nonterminal illness. Most important, patients must understand that living wills and advance directives apply only to terminally ill patients.

Another problem is that the advance directive may not specifically address the situation that may eventually be the actual dilemma. In addition, if decision-making is the responsibility of a designated proxy, that person may not be in a position to truly represent the preferences, beliefs, values, or wishes of the patient. The designated proxy or his or her alternate may not be capable of making a sound decision. There may not have been any discussion of these issues in advance, and there may be no written directives stating preferences, beliefs, or wishes. Although the clinician can encourage a patient to instruct the proxy on specific issues, the patient may want simply to turn the decision-making over to a loved and trusted proxy. I have seen a number of situations in which the patient has said, "Doctor, I don't want to discuss any of these issues. Please let my wife [or husband] decide everything." This type of response has been noted among patients with ordinary chronic illnesses and those with terminal illnesses.

The following scenario poses the problem of where the physician should draw the line in his or her desire to benefit a patient. On the chart of an elderly hospitalized patient with congestive heart failure was a do not resuscitate order. She went into cardiac arrest, and her cardiologist who happened to be present believed she could be helped. The physician performed cardiac resuscitation with a defibrillator, and the patient survived. Although this scenario makes an appealing argument for a paternalistic response by the clinician, do not resuscitate orders and advance directives should be respected.

A patient's written directive may appear foolish or unreasonable to an attending physician. The directive might request that everything possible be done when the patient has reached a point of futile, burdensome, and ineffective care. What should the physician do?

In general, if a patient has written reasonable instructions and directives to his or her proxy or agent, these instructions and directives should be followed. If the physician reviews these instructions and finds an element or elements that are not reasonable, the time to discuss and negotiate the matter is when the patient is as well and competent as possible. The physician can provide a valuable service in reviewing the written directives and instructions and discussing them with the patient.

The patient's family members may be unaware of the exact instructions in the living will or advance directive. They may have different opinions and request that the physician take another course. The physician is bound ethically and legally to follow the instructions of the advance directive. It is optimal for the physician to review the details of the advance directive when the patient has written the instructions. The physician may advise the patient to review the instructions with at least the proxy or agent, if not with the entire family.

I witnessed a situation in which the patient asked that life-prolonging measures be discontinued in the case of futile and burdensome care. The entire family and the hospital ethics committee agreed with the interpretation of the patient's living will. A cousin from out of town, who had not been seen for more than 5 years, arrived and demanded that everything possible be done to save his cousin. Was his response related to guilt or grief? He said that the clinician and hospital were at fault because they wanted to reduce costs or expenses, and he threatened legal action. In the face of a properly completed advance directive that has been discussed and reviewed with the physician, and in some cases with others such as the patient's lawyer or pastor, the physician is doing the right thing in following the instructions of the advance directive.

When a properly completed advance directive is available, it is the physician's responsibility to write the orders that reflect the patient's instructions and wishes. The physician can explain these orders and the patient's advance directive to other physicians, nurses, and other professional staff.

The orders should be carried out in a caring and compassionate manner with palliation and comfort care provided to the patient. The patient's family should be assured that the treatment underway is specifically what the patient, their loved one, had requested.

The clinician should be attentive to the possibility that the proxy's decisions may be based on self-interest or deceit. The clinician should be comfortable that the surrogate agent's decisions are in harmony with what the patient truly requested. Could the proxy decision maker benefit from a prolonged life, as in a persistent vegetative state, or from a premature death? The physician's role includes considering these possibly selfish motives. A safeguard in the Values History is the proxy negation that allows the patient to direct that certain persons *not* be allowed to make decisions on the patient's behalf in the event of the patient's disability or incapacity. This anticipatory measure would seem prudent as part of an advance directive.

Clinicians are ideally situated to discuss and review the living will and other advance directives with patients when the patients are well and competent. The physician knows and understands conditions such as dementia, coma, persistent vegetative state, stroke, and malignant disease. The physician understands the use of life-prolonging modalities such as ventilation, cardiopulmonary resuscitation, dialysis, antibiotics, and feeding tubes or gastrostomies. Ideally the advance directive should be discussed in the physician's office or the patient's home over a period of time before life-limiting illness occurs. Ideally the patient alone or with family should have time to reflect on the issues involved in the advance directive, even before meeting with the physician.

Communication Enhancement

Doukas and Brody call for communication enhancement. They state that primary care physicians need to be experts at communication to facilitate discussions about health care planning among family members. Advance directives ideally should be discussed as part of general preventive health maintenance for all competent adults. Tulsky et al believe that time must be allotted for this type of counseling in a practitioner's busy schedule. Physicians must be forthright in truth telling about a life-threatening or terminal illness. This is often difficult in the presence of certain chronic diseases, such as congestive heart failure. The prognosis may appear fair, but the patient may die suddenly of arrhythmia. The primary care physician and physicians in general live with a certain degree of uncertainty.

Physicians should explore the patient's values, beliefs, life view, and religious or spiritual beliefs or worldview. Matthews et al stated that physicians do not routinely ask patients in a nonintrusive way, "What role does religion play in your life? Do you belong to a particular faith community? Are there any religious or spiritual questions that you want to discuss? Should your family members or pastor be brought into the discussion?"

After values and concerns are discussed with the patient, the following issues should be discussed if appropriate with family members and religious advisor: independence and dependence, such as whether the patient can continue living alone; pain and suffering; economic issues; and religious or spiritual questions. Is there a need to discuss estate planning with family members or an attorney? The clinician should be careful to hold any of these discussions with family members only with the competent patient's consent. If the patient is mentally incompetent, it would be appropriate to deal with the proxy or surrogate agent. In the case of partial mental impairment, complex ethical issues arise concerning confidentiality and decision-making.

The clinician may ask about the funeral home or memorial service. What types of prayers or hymns or rituals does the patient want? The clinician might ask the patient and family to think it over to discuss again. It can occur that when such discussions do not take place, the patient's funeral is not conducted according to the religious perspective the patient would choose. There should be honest communication about the issues while the patient is best able to participate in such deliberations.

The clinician should help identify and mediate any conflicts between the patient's wishes, preferences, and values and wishes of the family. The physician should be available to facilitate discussion of conflicted issues and concerns between patient and family. This type of discussion might best take place during a home visit. Finally, in communication enhancement, physicians should be aware of their own values and beliefs regarding end-of-life care and should be open to sharing any differences with the patient and family in a nonintrusive or noncoercive way.

As suggested by the work of Lynn and associates and Doukas and Brody, the goal is better communication and more comprehensive advance care planning. We can anticipate societal, legislative, and regulatory measures to achieve these goals.

Palliative Care: Pain Management

The most common symptoms at the end of life include pain, fatigue and cachexia, depression, nausea and vomiting, confusion, dyspnea, restlessness, and constipation.

Pain management is essential for good care at the end of life. One common definition is: "Pain is what the patient says hurts." There are many barriers to good pain management, and these should be surmounted. In general, pain medication is grossly underused in the care of dying patients. We are capable of eliminating pain at the end of life.

Societal Barriers in Pain Management

A societal pressure on physicians is the fear of causing drug addiction. Physician barriers include a widespread lack of experience in pain management and symptom control that is an outgrowth of traditional medical education and fear of violating drug enforcement regulations. Many physicians withhold opioids until death is imminent. Patient barriers include reluctance to report pain to family, clinicians, or nurses; not wanting to bother the physician; and the fear that the need for pain medication indicates the presence of more advanced disease. There is also fear of the sedation that may be caused by pain medication.

Physicians can be informed to respond to these concerns. Fears of addiction or tolerance can be allayed, and predictable side effects with good pain management can be discussed. For example, sedation from opioids is short-lived because the patient develops tolerance to the sedative effects. Many patients in hospice care can function at a much higher level when pain is relieved.

Pain Assessment

The first step is reassuring patients and families that most pain can be relieved safely and effectively. Clinicians should assess and reassess patients for pain.

One type of pain that the patient may not discuss openly is chronic pain. The pain is always there and interfering with the patient's functioning, but the patient is so accustomed to the pain, that he or she does not discuss it. This pain can be relieved, and the patient can return to normal activities and function.

A valuable resource, *Management of Cancer Pain*, Clinical Practice Guideline No. 9 (Agency for Health Care Policy and Research, 1994),* offers an easy assessment mnemonic, ABCDE. *A*sk about pain regularly and *A*ssess pain systematically. *B*elieve the patient and family in their reports of pain and what relieves it. *C*hoose pain control options appropriate for the patient, family, and setting. *D*eliver interventions in a timely, logical, and coordinated way. *E*mpower patients and their families and enable them to control their course to the greatest extent possible.

*Available from the American Cancer Society (1-800-ACS-2345).

An Approach to Pain Management

A simple, effective, and well-validated approach to the management of pain was reported by the World Health Organization. The WHO ladder describes a stepped approach to the management of pain (Fig. 2-1). The drugs that correspond to the steps are shown in Table 2-4. The five incremental principles in the WHO ladder of drug therapy for cancer pain are by the mouth, by the clock, by the ladder, for the individual, and with attention to detail. This stepwise adjustment of medications must be individualized to the patient undergoing treatment. The simplest dosage schedules and least potent pain management modalities should be used initially.

Pain is a manageable condition. Every effort should be made to ensure that the patient is comfortable and free of pain. Some hospices and hospitals are reassuring patients that they will receive a prompt response for severe pain: 15 min in the hospital and 1 h at home. This can be very reassuring to the patient.

STEP 1: MILD TO MODERATE PAIN

The first step starts with the use of acetaminophen, aspirin, or nonsteroidal anti-inflammatory drugs (NSAIDs) for mild to moderate pain. Although it does not cause gastrointestinal irritation, acetaminophen can cause hepatotoxicity and lacks anti-inflammatory activity. The clinician should watch for adverse effects of NSAIDs, including gastrointestinal irritation and bleeding, gastric ulceration, renal failure, and hepatic dysfunction.

Figure 2-1

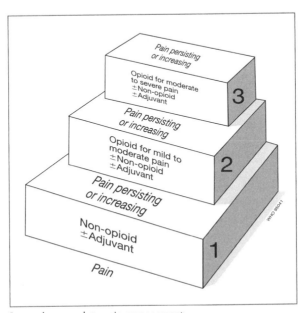

Stepped approach to pain management.

SOURCE: Reproduced with permission from *Cancer Pain Relief and Palliative Care: Report of a WHO Expert Committee*. World Health Organization Technical Report Series 804. Geneva, World Health Organization, 1990;9.

Table 2-4

Drugs Used in the Stepwise Approach to Pain Management

		USUAL STARTING DOSE	
DRUG	BRAND NAME	ORAL	PARENTERAL
NONOPIOID ANALGESIC			
Aspirin	—	325–650 mg every 4 h	—
Ibuprofen	Advil, Motrin	400 mg qid	—
Acetaminophen	Tylenol	325–1000 mg every 4 h	—
Naproxen	Naprosyn	275 mg 3–4 times daily	—
Choline magnesium trisalicylate	Trilisate	1000 mg 3 times daily	—
STEP 2 OPIOID ANALGESIC			
Codeine*	—	60 mg every 3–4 h	60 mg every 2 h IM or SC
Hydrocodone*	Lorcet, Lortab, Vicodin	10 mg every 3–4 h	
Oxycodone*	Percocet, Percodan	10 mg every 3–4 h	—
STEP 3 OPIOID ANALGESIC			
Morphine	MSIR	30 mg every 3–4 h	10 mg every 3–4 h
Morphine, sustained release	Oxycontin, MS Contin, Oramorph	90–120 mg every 12 h	—
Oxymorphone	Numorphan		1 mg every 3–4 h
Hydromorphone	Dilaudid	6 mg every 3–4 h	1.5 mg SC or IM every 4–6 h 3-mg suppository every 6–8 h
Fentanyl	Duragesic	—	25 µg every 72 h
ADJUVANT AGENTS			
Amitriptyline	Elavil	10 mg daily	—
Nortriptyline	Pamelor	10 mg daily	—
Desipramine	Norpramin	10 mg daily	—
Carbamazepine	Tegretol	200 mg twice daily	—
Gabapentin	Neurontin	300 mg per day[†]	—
Clonazepam	—	0.5 mg 3 times per day	—

*Combined with aspirin or acetaminophen.

[†]Increased to 300 mg twice daily on day 2 and then 300 mg 3 times daily on day 3.

SOURCE: Dosing recommendations for analgesics are from *Management of Cancer Pain*. Clinical Practice Guideline no. 9, AFKPR publication no. 94-0529. Rockville, MD, US Department of Health and Human Services, Public Health Service, Agency for Health Care Policy and Research, 1994. Dosing recommendations for adjuvant agents are from *Management of Cancer Pain* and manufacturer's recommendations.

STEP 2: MODERATE PAIN

When pain persists or increases, a step 2 opioid should be added, such as codeine, hydrocodone, or oxycodone. Hydrocodone and oxycodone are commonly available as a combination opioid-acetaminophen preparation. Administration generally is started at 10 mg of opioid every 3 to 4 h. Doses of pain medication may have to be adjusted in the care of patients with hepatic or renal insufficiency or other conditions affecting drug metabolism. Doses also may have to be decreased for patients who weigh less than 50 kg.

The combined use of opioids and acetaminophen or another NSAID often results in greater analgesia than use of either of the drug classes alone. The addition of an NSAID or acetaminophen to opioid analgesia may achieve a drug-sparing effect thus lower doses of opioids may produce pain relief with fewer side effects.

Opioid tolerance and physical dependence are to be expected with long-term use of the opioid drugs and should not be confused with addiction (psychological dependence) and drug abuse behavior. The adverse effects of opioids include constipation, nausea and vomiting, sedation, and rarely, respiratory depression. Constipation is almost universally a result of opioid use, so all patients should take a prophylactic stimulant laxative unless specifically contraindicated. For a further discussion of constipation and its management, see Chap. 15.

Sedation is a frequent initial response to opioid use, but tolerance to the sedative effects usually develops. Respiratory depression is of special concern among persons with pulmonary disease, especially with carbon dioxide retention. Most patients, however, do become tolerant of the respiratory depression caused by long-term use of opioids.

STEP 3: SEVERE PAIN

Persistent or moderate to severe pain should be managed by means of increasing the dose or changing to a step 3 agent. Medications for persistent pain should be administered around the clock with additional as needed or breakthrough doses. Regular dosing maintains a constant drug level and helps to prevent a recurrence of pain. In addition to the breakthrough dose, when the pain worsens, a third type of dose is an incident dose. An incident dose is given when the patient needs additional medication for pain caused by regular incidents such as the daily bath or shower.

The step 3 opioid of choice is immediate-release morphine. With a starting dose of 30 mg every 3 to 4 h, a steady state is reached within 20 to 24 h. When pain control is satisfactory, a sustained-release morphine preparation can be used. Immediate-release morphine is much less expensive than longer-acting morphine products. The dose of morphine used is continually titrated. In a ladder manner, the dose is increased 25 to 50 percent and, if necessary, by 50 to 100 percent. For example, it may be necessary to increase morphine from 60 mg to 90 mg to 120 mg to prevent pain.

USE OF TRANSDERMAL FENTANYL Opioids do not have an analgesic ceiling effect, and therefore the dose can be titrated to achieve maximal benefit. The oral route of administration of opioids is preferred for its convenience and lower cost, except for persons who cannot take or tolerate oral medication. When patients are unable to take medications orally, an easy route is transdermal. Fentanyl is an opioid available as a transdermal patch in doses of 25, 50, 75, and 100 (μg). A patch dose is roughly equivalent to one-half the total daily dose of a sustained-release morphine preparation. Fentanyl has a long duration of action of 72 h. Fentanyl also can accumulate, so the patient can be overnarcotized. Meperidine is not indicated in the management of chronic pain because of its short duration of action (2.5 to 3.5 h) and its toxic metabolites that can cause adverse central nervous system effects.

SUSTAINED-RELEASE OPIOIDS Sustained-release products can be used as indicated. Brand names include MS Contin, Oxycontin, and Oramorph SR. To change to therapy with a prolonged-release product, one-half the total daily dose of immediate release morphine is administered as a prolonged-release product every 12 h. If breakthrough pain occurs, about 15 percent of the total daily dose is given every 2 to 4 h. If there are more than three instances of breakthrough pain per day, the basal dose is increased in a ladder manner. With the use of various opioid drugs, clinical response must be monitored and titrated to the level of pain control. Cross-tolerance varies among the drugs available for use.

PARENTERAL MORPHINE Parenteral treatment is effective in many situations when pain is not controlled with oral medication. If it is necessary to convert from oral to parenteral morphine therapy, the total daily dose should be calculated, including breakthough doses. The hourly infusion rate is determined by dividing the total daily dose of parenteral morphine by 24.

Continuous intravenous infusion provides the most steady level of analgesia and is easy to provide for patients who have a permanent intravenous line for other purposes, such as hydration. If intravenous access is not available or desirable, continuous subcutaneous infusion offers an alternative for use in the hospital or at home. The usual starting dose of parenteral morphine is 10 mg every 3 to 4 h.

ADJUVANT THERAPY

Adjuvant therapy may be added for pain management at any of the three stages. The purpose of adjuvant therapy, through its independent effects on pain, is to enhance the pain relief provided by other analgesic medications. The medications listed in Table 2-4 are used primarily for neuropathic pain. Tricyclic antidepressants may have the additional benefits of controlling depression and insomnia.

PATIENT-CONTROLLED ANALGESIA

Patient-controlled analgesia (PCA) allows patients to control the amount of analgesia they receive. Most of the opioid dose used in PCA is delivered by the subcutaneous or intravenous route. The patient may administer PCA boluses if needed to manage breakthrough pain and to allow more accurate titration of the continuous infusion rate. Subcutaneous or intravenous PCA is well accepted by patients but requires special infusion pumps and education by professional staff. PCA would not be appropriate for patients with delirium or dementia.

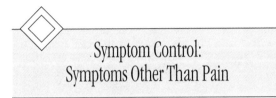

Symptom Control: Symptoms Other Than Pain

In addition to pain management, palliative care requires control of symptoms other than pain.

Nausea and Vomiting

Nausea and vomiting are common among patients with advanced cancer. Nausea may exist without vomiting. There are many causes of nausea and vomiting, but there is no single universal treatment. Nausea and vomiting related to opioids, NSAIDs, chemotherapy, and radiation therapy may be controlled with antiemetics, such as prochlorperazine or chlorpromazine. Metoclopramide, ondansetron, or granisetron also can provide relief. Ondansetron or granisetron is particularly effective in preventing nausea and vomiting induced by chemotherapy or radiation therapy. They are serotonin antagonists that bind to 5-hydroxytryptamine (5-HT$_3$) receptors. Combination topical agents (lorazepam, haloperidol, diphenhydramine, metoclopramide) also may be effective. In the use of chemotherapy and radiation therapy, the serotonin antagonists are the most effective antiemetics, but they are expensive. If emesis is associated with bowel obstruction, octreotide, a long-acting analog of somatostatin, may be helpful. If the patient has uremia, chlorpromazine may be effective for the nausea. The medication doses of the commonly prescribed antiemetics are listed in Table 2-5.

Constipation and Impaction

Constipation and impaction are managed by means of increasing fiber consumption and administration of milk of magnesia, bisacodyl, standardized senna concentrate, or hyperosmolar agents such as lactulose or sorbitol. Enemas (soap suds or mineral oil) and manual disimpaction sometimes are necessary. For a full discussion of the evaluation and management of constipation, see Chap. 15.

Restlessness and Confusion

Restlessness and confusion have many causes, but medication should be considered first. A change in opioid used may be helpful, for example, transdermal fentanyl may cause less confusion than morphine. Hypoxia, hypercalcemia, other metabolic causes, anxiety, and psychosis also are possible causes of confusion. Subcutaneous haloperidol frequently provides some relief. Anxiety is a common cause and often responds well to oral, sublingual, or subcutaneous benzodiazepines such as lorazepam (0.5 mg to 2 mg 6 to 8 h). It may be necessary to accept confusion, and sometimes the presence of a companion can be beneficial.

Bowel Obstruction

If lower bowel obstruction occurs, a low-residue diet may provide comfort. If obstruction occurs higher in the intestinal tract, discontinuation of oral intake and placing ice chips in the patient's mouth may be beneficial. Although it often is inappropriate therapeutic intervention, nasogastric aspiration or suctioning may help alleviate symptoms such as drooling or vomiting. However, a suction machine often makes matters worse. Many bowel obstructions open spontaneously.

Intestinal obstruction has multiple causes, including hypokalemia from vomiting, peritoneal seeding of tumor that affects gastrointestinal motility or causes loops of bowel to adhere and kink, and paraneoplastic effects of tumor that cause autonomic neuropathy. Intestinal obstruction also may be caused by mechanical blockage.

Table 2-5
Antiemetic Drugs

DRUG		DOSE	
GENERIC	BRAND	ORAL	PARENTERAL
Chlorpromazine	Thorazine	10–25 mg every 4–6 h	50–100 mg rectally every 6–8 h or 25–50 mg IM every 3–4 h
Metoclopramide	Reglan	10 mg 4 times daily	
Prochlorperazine	Compazine	5–10 mg 3–4 times daily	2.5–5 mg IV or 5–10 mg IM every 3–4 h or 25 mg rectally twice daily
Promethazine	Phenergan	25 mg every 4–6 h	25–50 mg IM or rectally every 4–6 h
Trimethobenzamide	Tigan	—	200 mg IM or rectally 3–4 times daily

Surgery is of limited usefulness to relieve intestinal obstruction in patients with advanced cancer. The goal is to relieve cramps, pain, and nausea and vomiting. This can be accomplished in most cases with analgesics and anticholinergic and antiemetic drugs and without nasogastric tubes, surgery, or intravenous administration fluid. The following management of intestinal obstruction is recommended:

- Pain: Strong opioids
- Nausea: Haloperidol, phenothiazines (anticholinergic effect), antihistamines. Avoid metoclopramide that stimulates gastric emptying.

Dry Mouth

Dry mouth is a common problem related to dehydration, debility, mouth breathing, and oral thrush or candidiasis. Dry mouth also is related to treatment, such as radiation therapy to the facial area, antidepressants, narcotics, phenothiazines, and antispasmodics. Mouth washes and frequent stimulating drinks are essential. Candidal infections should be treated initially with a toothbrush and dilute hydrogen peroxide, but may necessitate other treatments such as oral nystatin suspension held in the mouth for a while and then swallowed. Other treatments are available if these are not satisfactory or if the esophagus is involved.

Cachexia, Wasting, and Weight Loss

No effective remedy has been found for cachexia. Small portions of easily swallowed, nourishing, favorite foods might be offered. If nasogastric feeding is considered, it should be on a trial basis. In general, a dying patient does better staying dry at the end of life. Using large amounts of hydration is usually poorly tolerated by patients who are dying. A continuous subcutaneous saline infusion (1 L or less over 24 h) may provide comfort. For patients with weight loss and poor appetite, the clinician should consider the presence of depres-

sion. Corticosteroids may be tried in the care of patients whose fatigue is related to the use of opioids. Amphetamines, such as methylphenidate (Ritalin) starting at 5 mg once a day, may be helpful for relief of weakness and fatigue.

Incontinence

Always a source of embarrassment and discomfort, incontinence calls for careful assistance with frequent toileting, use of absorbent pads, condom drainage, or use of catheters. For a full discussion of the evaluation and management of urinary incontinence, see Chap. 6.

Pressure Ulcers

A risk among wasted, dependent, and incontinent patients, pressure ulcers should be reduced with the use of sheepskins, soft foam "egg crate" pads, and special mattresses to reduce pressure on prominent body parts. Regular turning and attention to skin surfaces with protection of early changes can play an important role. For further discussion of the evaluation and management of pressure ulcers, see Chap. 19.

Dyspnea

Dyspnea often is overlooked. Some patients benefit from opioids and even from benzodiazepines. Bredin et al described patients with breathlessness helped by a nursing clinic intervention that combines breathing control, activity pacing, relaxation techniques, and psychosocial support. Nonpharmacologic interventions that may be helpful in the treatment of patients with dyspnea are as follows:

- Instruction to family and staff on positions to make breathing easier
- Elevation of the head of the bed
- Provision of a fan to circulate the air in the patient's room

- Swabbing the patient's face with a cool, wet cloth
- Use of oxygen
- Emotional support
- Elimination of smoke and allergens

Pharmacologic interventions are as follows:

- Opioids such as codeine, morphine sulfate (e.g., 5 to 10 mg up to every 4 h), nebulized morphine, prolonged-release opiates (10 to 20 mg every 12 h), all to be titrated appropriately
- Bronchodilators
- Diuretics
- Antianxiety medication with a benzodiazepine such as lorazepam (0.25 to 2 mg every 6 h) for mild anxiety or midazolam (starting 1 to 2 mg/h and increasing to 2 to 5 mg/h subcutaneously or intravenously) for more severe anxiety, all to be titrated appropriately

Anxiety and Depression

Care providers should listen to the feelings expressed by the patient, whether fear, anger, anxiety, depression, pain, or other suffering. Anxiolytic medications are useful in the management of anxiety. Depression at the end of life should not be overlooked, and many patients benefit from antidepressant therapy. Although medications are useful, it is most important to allow patients to express their fears or other manifestations of suffering. Spiritual counseling is an integral part of terminal care and helps alleviate suffering.

Other Problems

HYPERCALCEMIA

Hypercalcemia associated with terminal cancer can be managed with hydration, saline diuresis, or pamidronate. Most patients with hypercalcemia initially are volume depleted and need adequate hydration. Once the patient has been rehydrated, calcium excretion can be promoted by means of saline infusion. Pamidronate, a biphosphonate, inhibits bone resorption and often is used to manage hypercalcemia. It usually takes 2 to 3 days before an effect is seen. Prednisone can be used to control hypercalcemia caused by hematologic malignant disease or multiple myeloma. Although it is not as effective as pamidronate, plicamycin can be used to control hypercalcemia due to cancer.

MALIGNANT PLEURAL EFFUSIONS

Thoracentesis usually is performed to relieve shortness of breath due to pleural effusions. The patient may be also undergoing chemotherapy or mediastinal radiation. If effusion recurs, chemical pleurodesis may be considered to control malignant pleural effusions. Talc, doxycycline, and bleomycin are sclerosing agents that are introduced into the pleural space. The resulting pleural inflammation causes the pleural surfaces to stick together to reduce the potential for reaccumulation of the pleural effusion. If pleural effusions continue to recur despite these measures, the comfort measures for dyspnea are indicated (see earlier section on treatment of dyspnea).

METASTATIC BONE PAIN

Basic principles of pain management apply to alleviating the pain of bone metastasis. In addition to analgesia, radiation therapy helps patients with localized bone metastasis from cancer of the breast, prostate, or lung. Bone metastases from multiple myeloma also may respond to radiation therapy. For diffuse bone pain, hemibody irradiation, which is used to manage multiple metastases, may be appropriate. Several radiopharmaceuticals have been been used to alleviate pain from bone metastasis. Iodine-131 has been used in the management of multiple bone metastases from thyroid cancer. In about 80 percent of patients with pain from bone metastasis from tumors of the breast and prostate, phosphorus-32-orthophosphate has provided partial or complete relief.

Summary: Death and Bereavement

Care at the end of life is improving in the United States. We are learning more about pain and management. Advance health care planning and clinician-patient communication at the end of life can improve as a result of societal, educational, and legislative initiatives. Clinicians can provide more support to the patient and family and help the patient and family find meaning, love, and reconciliation at this stage.

Clinicians should communicate as good listeners. Some patients and families are more comfortable if the patient is sedated; others value the patient's being awake even if agitated or delusional. Clinicians can use the telephone to stay in frequent touch with the patient and family or caregiver to discuss this and similar issues. Clinicians also can ask about the funeral or memorial service. They need to ask about pain, children, and the role of religion. Who is the appropriate surrogate agent or proxy at the end of life? If the patient were to die soon, what would be left unattended? Is there a family matter, financial issue, religious concern, or opportunity for reconciliation or expression of love that has not been addressed or fulfilled? In the bereavement period, there should be follow-up contact, at least one call to ask about how the family is doing. This communication is highly rewarding. Most of all, clinicians should know their patients. This knowledge is the standard of care throughout life and is certainly the standard at the end.

Bibliography

Bredin M, Corner J, Krishnasamy M, et al: Multicentre randomized control of nursing intervention for breathlessness in patients with lung cancer. *BMJ* 318:901, 1999.

Byock I: The nature of suffering and the nature of opportunity at the end of life. *Clin Geriatr Med* 12: 237, 1996.

Byock I: *Dying Well: The Prospect for Growth at the End of Life.* New York, Riverhead Books, 1997.

Crigger BJ (ed): Series, Giving life to patient self-determination. *Hastings Center Report* 23:12, 1993.

Cruzan v Director, Missouri Department of Health, in *Supreme Court Reports* 110:2841–2892, 1990.

Department of Geriatric Health: *Medical Management of the Home Care Patient: Guidelines for Physicians,* 2nd ed. Chicago: American Medical Association; 1998; 18–19.

Doukas DJ, Brody H: Care at the twilight: ethics and end-of-life care. *Am Fam Physician* 52:1294, 1995.

Doukas DJ, Reichel W: *Planning for Uncertainty: A Guide to Living Wills and Other Advance Directives for Health Care.* Baltimore: Johns Hopkins University Press; 1993.

Doyle D, Hanks GWC, MacDonald N (eds): *Oxford Textbook of Palliative Medicine,* 2nd ed. Oxford, UK: Oxford University Press; 1998.

Horgan J: Seeking a better way to die. *Sci Am* 276:100, 1997.

Lattanzi-Licht M, Mahoney JJ, Miller GW: *The National Hospice Organization Guide to Hospice Care. The Hospice Choice.* New York: Simon & Schuster; 1998.

Levy MH: Pharmacologic treatment of cancer pain. *N Engl J Med* 335:1124, 1996.

Lynn J: Caring at the end of our lives. *N Engl J Med* 335:201,1996.

Lynn J: Measuring quality at the end of life: a statement of principles. *J Am Geriatr Soc* 45:526, 1997.

Management of Cancer Pain. Clinical Practice Guideline no. 9, AHCPR publication no. 94-0529. Rockville, MD, US Department of Health and Human Services, Public Health Service, Agency for Health Care Policy and Research, 1994.

Matthews DA, McCullough ME, Larson DB, et al: Religious commitment and health status. *Arch Fam Med* 7:118, 1998.

McCann RM, Hall WJ, Groth-Jancker A: Comfort care for terminally ill patients: the appropriate use of nutrition and hydration. *JAMA* 272:1263, 1994.

McCullough LB, Doukas DJ, Holleman WL, et al: Advance directives. In: Gallo JJ, Busby-Whitehead J, Rabins PV, Silliman RA, Murphy J (eds): Reichel's *Care of the Elderly: Clinical Aspects of Aging.* 5th ed. Philadelphia: Lippincott William & Wilkins; 1999; 813.

Moulin DE, Johnson NG, Murray-Parsons N, et al: Subcutaneous narcotic infusions for cancer pain: treatment outcome and guidelines for use. *Can Med Assoc J* 146:891, 1992.

National Hospice Organization: *Medical Guidelines for Selected Non-Cancer Diseases*, 2nd ed. Arlington, VA: National Hospice Organization; 1996.

SUPPORT Principal Investigators. A controlled trial to improve care for seriously ill hospitalized patients. *JAMA* 274:1591,1995.

Teno JM, Licks S, Lynn J, et al: Do advance directives provide instructions that direct care? *J Am Geriatr Soc* 45:508, 1997.

Teno J, Lynn J, Connors AF, et al: The illusion of end-of-life resource savings with advance directives. *J Am Geriatr Soc* 45:513, 1997.

Teno J, Lynn J, Wenger N, et al: Advance directives for seriously ill hospitalized patients: effectiveness with the Patient Self-Determination Act and the SUPPORT intervention. *J Am Geriatr Soc* 45:500, 1997.

Tulsky JA, Fischer GS, Rose MR, et al: Opening the black box: how do physicians communicate about advance directives? *Ann Intern Med* 129:441, 1998.

World Health Organization: *Cancer Pain Relief and Palliative Care: Report of a WHO Expert Committee.* World Health Organization Technical Report Series, 804. Geneva, Switzerland; World Health Organization; 1990.

Mel P. Daly

Chapter

3

Health Promotion and Disease Prevention

Overview

Persons who reach the age of 65 years can expect to live for many more years because of advances in the medical care of coronary artery disease, infection, and other conditions that previously caused premature death. Women 65 years of age will live an average of 20 additional years, men an average of 17 years. The human life span of approximately 100 years is not likely to be prolonged by means of advances in the management of chronic disease. Life expectancy decreases markedly after the age of 80 years because of the increased likelihood of age- and disease-associated illnesses. Strategies for health promotion and disease prevention must consider age, pathologic process, and life expectancy.

The approach to developing health promotion and disease prevention interventions for older persons must be individualized. Many older persons are motivated to enhance their health and well-being. Many older persons, especially young-old (65 to 75 years) persons, are enthusiastic about planning for a healthy life over their remaining decades and are well informed about the suggestions of many expert agencies or organizations and about public opinion. These persons are exposed to peer groups, newspapers, television, and other sources of information about potential benefits of all kinds of interventions that may improve their quality of life and life expectancy. This information may be influential in how a person develops strategies for approaching their older years from a health perspective. In contrast, some older persons are less than enthusiastic about taking the steps necessary to promote or improve their health.

There is no consensus about a health promotion and disease prevention strategy that is widely applicable to older persons. Little rigorous research data are available about the effectiveness of such interventions, and when making recommendations, clinicians have to extrapolate on data from studies involving middle-aged persons. There also are conflicting recommendations from specialty organizations about whether a screening intervention is beneficial, and if it is, how often it should be done. Examples are prostate-specific antigen (PSA) testing, stool testing for occult blood, and Papanicolaou testing.

Clinicians historically have not received reimbursement for time spent counseling patients about risk factors for disease and strategies for prevention and health promotion. Clinicians who care for older patients thus have been more likely to spend time performing reimbursable services such as physical examinations and writing prescriptions, rather than counseling about diet, exercise, or cigarette use.

A pervasive ageism exists among older persons and clinicians. This creates a perception that preventive intervention may be an exercise in futility because the person is already old. Older persons and clinicians often perceive that although they recognize that smoking, obesity, or a sedentary lifestyle may be deleterious to health, there is little purpose in changing their behavior because they are already old and it is too late to make a difference.

Clinicians are often unwilling to suggest that older persons undergo tests that may be potentially harmful or have side effects, unless the benefit of testing is proved. For example, colonoscopy can be used as a screening test for early detection of colorectal cancer. The preparation for this test involves drinking a gallon of the laxative polyethylene glycol (Golytely) and sitting on a toilet to clear the colon for endoscopic examination. This often is difficult and uncomfortable for older persons. The examination itself may be embarrassing and is not without complications (bleeding and in rare instances perforation of the colon). Therefore, without firm evidence that colonoscopic screening is beneficial, many physicians are reluctant to recommend it.

Excellent evidence supports the benefits of health promotion and disease prevention interventions in reducing the incidence, morbidity, and mortality of many diseases. The age-adjusted mortality for cerebrovascular disease has decreased 50 percent since the 1950s, because hypertension was recognized as a major risk factor and treatment was instituted. The mortality from invasive cervical cancer also has decreased because of the widespread use of Papanicolaou (Pap) smears. Polio, tetanus, and rubella have been all but eliminated because of population-wide use of vaccines against these infections.

Although there is less evidence supporting the effectiveness of such interventions in the care of older adults, in many instances enough evidence exists to recommend that certain interventions be instituted for older persons. Clinicians must be aware that some interventions are considered the standard of care, such as screening mammography every 1 to 2 years. Clinicians may be liable in lawsuits brought by patients should these standards not be met.

Targeting groups at high risk is most likely to be beneficial in reducing morbidity and mortality. Interventions should focus on the major causes of death and the major illnesses among older persons (Tables 3-1 and 3-2). The goal of prevention among older persons should be to enhance the quality of life.

Table 3-1

Common Causes of Death Among Older Persons

Disease of the heart
Cancer
Stroke
Lung disease
Accidents
Pneumonia and influenza
Diabetes mellitus
Suicide
Kidney disease
Chronic liver disease and cirrhosis

Table 3-2

Most Common Illnesses Among Older Adults

Hypertension
Arthritis
Hearing impairment
Vision impairment
Coronary artery disease
Chronic lung disease
Diabetes mellitus
Peripheral vascular disease
Cancer
Cognitive impairment
Parkinson's disease
Cerebrovascular disease
Multiple coexisting conditions

Primary Prevention

Primary prevention refers to preventing illness before it develops in persons who have no symptoms and who have no evidence of the disease. Primary prevention usually includes identifying risk factors of a disease and instituting interventions to reduce the likelihood that the disease will develop. Common primary prevention interventions include vaccination, behavior change, injury prevention, and chemoprophylaxis.

Vaccination

The fourth leading cause of death among elderly persons is respiratory illness due to chronic lung disease (emphysema) complicated by bacterial pneumonia and influenza. There is good evidence that the incidence of and rate of hospitalization for influenza and pneumonia among persons vaccinated against pneumonia and influenza are significantly lower than among persons who have not been vaccinated. This is especially true if programs are developed to target for influenza and pneumonia vaccination older persons, especially those at risk, such as older persons who have been discharged from the hospital after a respiratory illness and persons with chronic diseases.

INFLUENZA

Epidemic or endemic infectious outbreaks of influenza occur annually in the United States. Virus strains change annually because of antigenic shifts and drifts. The Centers for Disease Control and Prevention conducts surveillance of virus strains that are likely to cause infection in the United States and develops a vaccine to combat the strains of influenza likely to cause an outbreak during a given year.

More than 20,000 deaths occur during influenza epidemics, and most of these deaths occur among elderly persons. Older persons with chronic illnesses, such as chronic obstructive pulmonary disease, diabetes mellitus, chronic renal failure, and older persons living in long-term facilities are at greatest risk of influenza. The illness causes respiratory and systemic symptoms that can be debilitating. The most common complication of influenza is pneumonia, which can be fatal.

The vaccine usually is administered in October or November to allow recipients to develop antibody protection in anticipation of influenza occurring in December, January, and February. It takes about 2 to 3 weeks for protective antibody levels to develop, and titers decline over 2 to 3 months. The only contraindication to influenza vaccination is an allergy to egg protein (the vaccine is developed in an egg protein base). Side effects are minimal, usually only minor muscle aches or redness at the site of injection, and the vaccine is well tolerated.

Some older persons believe that the vaccine can cause influenza; however, this is impossible because the vaccine contains no live virus. Influenza-like symptoms that occur around the time a person receives the vaccine are most likely caused by a non-influenza virus that causes respiratory symptoms or influenza that was contracted

before the patient developed antibodies as the result of vaccination.

PNEUMOCOCCAL VACCINE

Pneumonia is four times more common among older persons than younger persons and is more likely to cause death. This may be because older persons are less likely to have classic signs and symptoms of pneumonia (fever, sputum production, and cough), and the diagnosis is missed or made late. A 23-valent vaccine has been available since the 1980s that provides protection against most strains of pneumococci that cause disease in the United States. This vaccine provides protection for up to 8 years, so most persons need only receive the vaccine once or twice. Many older persons received an earlier version of the vaccine that was available in 1970s. The effectiveness of this vaccine has waned, and these persons should be revaccinated. There is no increased danger of an allergic or other reaction if these persons are vaccinated with the newer vaccine.

TETANUS

Tetanus is uncommon in the United States because most Americans have been vaccinated. However, immunity wanes 10 years after vaccination or booster injection. Therefore, the incidence and mortality of tetanus are higher among elderly persons, who often are not up to date on tetanus vaccination.

All older persons should receive booster tetanus toxoid injections if they have not done so in the last 10 years. A primary series of tetanus immunization should be administered if an older person has not undergone this series of injections.

Behaviors

CIGARETTE SMOKING

Cigarette smoking is a major risk factor for morbidity and mortality among older persons. Cigarette smoking is implicated as a direct cause of one in three deaths in the United States, and one in six deaths from cancer. Cigarette smoking is a risk factor for cardiovascular disease; cerebrovascular disease; cancer of the lung, oropharynx, esophagus, stomach, pancreas, and bladder; chronic obstructive pulmonary disease; peripheral vascular disease; and renal disease. Risk of disease and mortality from cigarette smoking are directly related to the amount of tobacco smoked and the type of tobacco inhaled. Older men are more likely to be at risk of cigarette-related illness because they are more likely to start smoking at an earlier age and to have smoked and inhaled tobacco-related carcinogens from stronger cigarettes manufactured in past decades.

There is good evidence that stopping smoking is beneficial even among older persons. The increased risk of a serious cardiac event is reduced to that of a nonsmoker after 5 years, even among older heavy (1 pack per day) smokers. Discontinuing cigarette smoking improves pulmonary function immediately and enhances the sense of well-being. Bronchoconstriction, coughing, and circulating carboxyhemoglobin levels are reduced. The risk of lung cancer from cigarette smoking decreases 30 to 50 percent 10 years after cessation of smoking.

Older persons often are unwilling to stop smoking and may do so only when they sustain a sentinel event, such as myocardial infarction or a cerebrovascular accident, that they relate to smoking. Recidivism is common, and many older persons who try to stop smoking succeed only after many attempts.

All older persons should be told to stop smoking by their physicians (Table 3-3). Strategies should be agreed upon to facilitate cessation. Physician and patient should determine a cessation date, and frequent contacts should be made thereafter to ensure conformance. Family and friends may have to become involved for support, and support groups may be helpful. Nicotine patches and gum may be useful but should be used with caution by elderly persons because of potential cardiac side effects, such as tachycardia, arrhythymias, and elevated blood pressure.

Table 3-3

Strategies to Help Patients Stop Smoking

Inquire about cigarette smoking

Explain risks of continuing smoking

Outline the benefits of stopping

Insist that patients stop

Be an advocate

Agree on a cessation date

Enroll family members and other loved ones as supports

Provide self-help materials

Provide information and contact persons for support groups

Make contact to assess conformance at 1- and 2-week intervals

Arrange follow-up visits

Conduct a follow-up visit 1 month after the cessation date

Consider prescribing nicotine patches or recommending nicotine gum

ALCOHOL USE

The prevalence of alcohol use among older persons is unknown. Alcoholism may be common among older persons because of loneliness, boredom, and loss. Alcohol excess among older persons is associated with an increased incidence of falls; car crashes; changes in mental status, including dementia and behavioral outbursts; peptic ulcer disease; and malnutrition.

All older persons should be asked about how they use alcohol and whether they have had any problems related to alcohol use. Standardized screening tests such as the Michigan Alcohol Screening Test or CAGE test can be administered if suspicions of alcohol abuse arise.

PHYSICAL ACTIVITY

Most older persons are sedentary or engage in minimal physical activity. A sedentary lifestyle is associated with a greater risk of all-cause mortality, cardiovascular disease, obesity, insulin resistance, diabetes mellitus, osteoporosis, and a greater likelihood of hip fracture and functional decline.

Many benefits have been demonstrated among older persons who engage in regular physical activity programs (Table 3-4). Even the very elderly experience these benefits. Older persons, however, are less likely than younger persons to agree to participate in these programs despite encouragement by physicians and others.

Older persons should be instructed to exercise at least three times per week and should do so for at least 30 to 40 min at a time (Table 3-5). They should start by warming up and stretching (5 to 10 min), followed by aerobic or resistance exercise (20 to 30 min), and concluding with a cooldown period (walking, stretching). For motivated elderly persons, the goal may be to achieve 70 percent of age-specific maximum heart rate (220 minus age in years) for 45 min three to four times per week.

There are few contraindications to participation in an exercise program. Cardiovascular disease that causes symptoms during normal activity should be investigated further before the patient

starts an exercise program. For most older persons who do not have cardiac risk factors, exercise is safe. Some older patients who start an exercise program may develop orthopedic problems, such as strains, sprains and muscle aches, especially when exercise is overly aggressive.

DIET

Many older Americans are overweight, but after the age of 80 years the prevalence of protein-

Table 3-5
Exercise Prescription

Endurance
Walking
Stair climbing, steps exercise
Swimming
Cycling
Goal: 30–45 min at least 3 times per week at a moderate level of exertion. For motivated older persons, 70% maximum heat rate (220 minus age) is ideal.
Strength
Free weights
Isometric and isotonic weight lifting
Goal: 2–3 times per week (3 sets per muscle group, limited by fatigue). For motivated older persons, weight and repetitions can be increased as tolerated each week.
Balance
Tai Chi
Posture (yoga, balance, dance)
Goal: 2–3 times per week to improve posture and sense of verticality
General
Warm-up for 10 min (stretching, range of motion)
Exercise for 20–30 min within tolerance
Cool-down for 10 min

Table 3-4
Benefits of Exercise Programs for Older Persons

Improved aerobic capacity
Reduced mean arterial blood pressure
Reduced resting heart rate
Increased maximum oxygen consumption
Increased muscle mass and strength
Increased bone density
Increased flexibility
Improved gait velocity
Improved lipoprotein profile, especially increases in high-density lipoprotein cholesterol levels
Reduced platelet adhesiveness
Improved sense of well-being

calorie undernutrition increases. Obesity is a major risk factor for cardiovascular disease, cerebrovascular disease, and diabetes mellitus. Undernutrition is a risk factor of death, infection, and osteoporosis.

The elderly are less likely to follow strict dietary guidelines such as those recommended by the American Heart Association (AHA). There is no good evidence that counseling older persons about dietary indiscretions results in changes in dietary habits and behaviors. It makes plausible and intuitive sense, however, to recommend that all older persons eat sensibly and healthfully.

Most older persons should be encouraged to maintain their body weight within 10 percent of their age-adjusted normal weight. They should be encouraged to reduce fat intake and to eat lean and white meat or fish. Total calories from fat should be restricted to less than 30 percent of all calories and saturated fats to less than 10 percent of calories. Although hypercholesterolemia is a risk factor for coronary artery disease, there is inconclusive evidence that efforts to reduce serum cholesterol levels are of benefit in reducing the risk of or mortality from coronary artery disease among persons older than 75 years. All should be encouraged to eat fresh fruits and vegetables. Intake of dietary fiber, calcium, and vitamin D should be optimized. These types of general recommendations are more likely to be followed by older persons than are suggestions to count calories and calculate fat, protein, and supplement intakes.

Physicians who prescribe restricted diets must be mindful of the risks of undernutrition. Hypocholesterolemia among very elderly persons is associated with increased mortality. Many older persons are not ingesting adequate calories and nutrients, and placing further dietary restrictions may exacerbate the risk of undernutrition.

Injury Prevention

Unintentional injury (falls; automobile crashes; fires; burns and scalds; and shootings) is the fifth leading cause of death among the elderly.

FALLS

It is estimated that one in three community-dwelling elderly persons falls in any given year. Falls, especially noninjurious falls, are underreported by the elderly because falls are regarded as an admission of frailty. Most older persons who fall do so repeatedly. About 5 percent of falls result in a fracture or other soft-tissue injury (strain, sprain, hematoma) that forces inactivity or bed rest. The inactivity is likely to compound functional decline and the risk of falling.

One of the more serious consequences of falling is hip fracture. As many as 25 percent of persons who fracture their hip die as a result. Of those who survive, 20 to 30 percent have to live in a more restricted living arrangement, such as a nursing home, because of inability to function as well as they did before the fracture.

Most falls occur in the home and usually are the result of a combination of age-associated changes (decreased visual acuity, decreased proprioception), disease factors (weakness, Parkinson's disease, hypotension), medications (long-acting benzodiazepines, tranquilizers, antihypertensive agents), and an environment that is unsafe (cluttered, dark, wet). For a detailed review of falls, see Chap. 14. The incidence of falling may be reduced with interventions that modify any risk factors that can be identified. This may involve discontinuing or changing medications, performing a home safety evaluation, or recommending physical therapy.

AUTOMOBILE CRASHES

The elderly are involved in more automobile crashes than any other age group except new teenage drivers, even though on average older persons drive fewer miles. Most crashes occur during twilight hours when light is fading or when the older person is performing a potentially dangerous maneuver, such as making a left turn across a four-lane highway. The many factors that contribute to the higher number of motor vehicle accidents include age- and disease-related reductions in visual acuity, slower reaction times when quick action is required, impaired visuospatial perception, use of alcohol, not wearing safety belts, and the presence of comorbid disease that may interfere with function (weakness, sensory loss, Alzheimer's disease).

Older persons are not likely to volunteer that they are having difficulties with driving. Family members are more likely to bring it to the physician's attention. Older persons are unwilling to relinquish their driver's licenses even after a crash and often vehemently deny that they have any difficulties.

Physicians always should ask whether an older person is driving and whether they are experiencing any difficulties driving. All older drivers should be counseled to wear safety belts at all times. Physicians may be compelled by the department of transportation to request that a person's license be revoked. Independent driver testing can be arranged through the American Association of Retired Persons (AARP) or through the occupational therapy departments of most hospitals. Driver education classes are widely available for older persons who may need to relearn skills. Many groups, including the AARP, are investigating ways to enhance older persons' abilities to drive safely.

FIRES, SCALDS, AND BURNS

Many older persons live in homes that were built before 1950. These homes often do not have smoke detectors or have improperly functioning detectors. In some instances even when there is a functioning smoke detector, an older person may not hear it sound during a fire because of age and disease-related hearing loss. It is important to advise older persons and their families about the risk of fire and insist that they check that they have an operational smoke detector. For persons with hearing loss, the local fire department should be contacted for advice about other types of fire alarms, such as sprinkler systems or flashing lights.

The upper temperature setting of many water heating systems often is higher than is safe for older persons, especially those whose manual dexterity or vision is impaired. Adjusting the upper temperature setting to less than 130°F (54.4°C) can prevent many scalds and burns among the elderly.

FIREARM INCIDENTS

Many older persons keep firearms for protection. Unintentional shootings occur when these firearms get into the hands of toddlers or infants and are discharged. Intentional shootings also are a problem among the elderly. The incidence of suicide is greatest among older men, and the method of choice is self-inflicted shooting. More deaths from suicide by self-inflicted gunshots occur than homicides by firearms in the United States.

If an older person possesses a firearm, it should have a working safety mechanism and should be regularly maintained. Older men who are depressed or recently bereaved and at risk of major depression should be asked whether they have a firearm. If they are at risk of suicide or have suicidal ideation or a plan for suicide, family members or friends should be apprised of the risk and the firearm removed from the home.

Chemoprophylaxis

Data supporting the use of aspirin as a prophylaxis of cardiovascular and cerebrovascular disease among elderly persons are not available. Data suggesting a beneficial effect among middle-aged men are at best inconclusive.

Most experts suggest using aspirin is beneficial in reducing risk among persons at high risk of these conditions. This includes men; those with a family history of cardiovascular disease; cigarette smokers; persons with hypertension, diabetes mellitus, previous myocardial infarction, or angina pectoris; and persons with hypercholesterolemia. No data exist to support a beneficial effect among women.

Aspirin in a dosage of 81 to 325 mg every day usually is well tolerated. An additional beneficial effect of aspirin may be a reduced incidence of colorectal polyps and colorectal carcinoma, which has been shown among persons taking aspirin in this dosage.

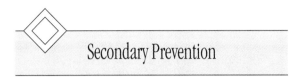

Secondary Prevention

Secondary prevention interventions are those used to detect diseases in early and asymptomatic stages and prevent them from becoming symptomatic. Testing to detect cancer in early stages is a good example of screening. Screening may be useful if the condition being screened for has a high morbidity or mortality, occurs commonly, can be detected with acceptable and cost-effective testing (acceptable sensitivity and specificity of tests), and can be effectively treated if the condition is detected at an early stage. Conditions that occur infrequently (brain tumors) and diseases for which there is no cure (lung cancer) are not appropriate for screening interventions that are likely to be cost-effective among older persons.

There is some evidence that screening interventions may result in improved outcomes for older persons if appropriately delivered. Evidence for effectiveness is lacking for persons older than 70 years. Older persons have been underrepresented in studies of outcomes of screening interventions for cancer and other conditions. Many of the currently suggested recommendations are based on extrapolations from studies of younger adults and expert opinions based on available evidence of benefit. Common secondary prevention interventions focus on hypertension, cancer, and several other chronic diseases.

Hypertension

Hypertension is the one of the most common chronic conditions among older adults. An estimated 60 million persons have hypertension. The incidence of hypertension, especially systolic hypertension, increases with age. Systolic and diastolic hypertension together and independently are major risk factors for coronary artery disease, stroke, peripheral vascular disease, and renal failure. There is excellent evidence from randomized, controlled, prospective studies of older populations that treating patients for hypertension significantly reduces the likelihood of cerebrovascular events and coronary artery disease.

All persons older than 65 years should have their blood pressure measured at every office visit and at least annually. The Joint National Committee recommends that patients with blood pressure readings consistently (three readings) greater than 140/90 mmHg be treated. The U.S. Preventive Services Task Force (USPSTF) recommends that patients with blood pressure readings consistently higher than 160/90 mmHg be treated.

Cancer

CERVICAL CANCER

The incidence of cervical cancer increases with advancing years, and the mortality from invasive cancer of the cervix also increases with age. This is largely because as many as 50 percent of older women have never had a Pap smear and as many as 75 percent have not undergone regular screening for cervical cancer. Two of the many risk factors of cervical cancer are relations with multiple sexual partners and infection with the human papilloma virus (HPV). Most older persons who are sexually active are monogamous and are no longer at risk of new HPV infection. Increased risk exists only because older persons are unlikely to have undergone adequate screening to detect cervical dysplasia or carcinoma in situ before it develops into invasive cervical cancer.

Older persons who have not undergone a Pap test in recent years should do so. This test should be repeated annually at least twice. If the result is negative at each testing, further screening probably can be discontinued because the risk of new cancer of the cervix or HPV infection is very low.

BREAST CANCER

The incidence of breast cancer increases with each decade after the age of 50 years. The risk of breast cancer increases among women who have a family history of breast cancer, had an early menarche or a late menopause, are nulliparous, or have had breast disease (benign adenoma, previous carcinoma).

There is good evidence that screening for breast cancer among women without symptoms results in a markedly reduced mortality rate. In the past, older women, especially minorities, were less likely to have undergone screening with mammography or clinical breast examination by a clinician. Recent data suggest that more older women are undergoing screening. Medicare provides coverage for biennial mammograms for persons older than 65 years. All women older than 65 years should undergo annual clinical breast examinations and annual or biennial mammography.

Controversy exists regarding when to discontinue screening for breast cancer. In older women breast cancer is often a less aggressive disease and if detected usually is successfully managed by means of lumpectomy or tamoxifen therapy. Many physicians suggest that annual and biennial mammography be discontinued at 75 years of age unless life expectancy is estimated to be more than another 7 years.

COLORECTAL CANCER

The incidence of colorectal cancer increases with each decade after the age of 50 years. Risk increases if there is a family history of colorectal cancer, a history of adenomatous polyps, familial polyposis coli, or ulcerative colitis. Early detection of colorectal cancer is likely to improve the survival rate, although lead-time and length of time biases may confound conclusions about survival benefits of early detection.

There is evidence from three large randomized trials that screening for colorectal cancer by means of fecal occult blood testing (FOBT) reduces mortality. Other data suggest that periodic screening by means of flexible sigmoidoscopy reduces mortality from colorectal cancer. FOBT is a sensitive test for detection of bleeding, but it has a high false-positive rate for detection of cancer. The positive predictive value of FOBT is in the range of 5 to 10 percent. More than 90 percent of persons who have positive results of screening tests of stool for occult blood do not have colorectal cancer. Thus many persons may be subjected to further testing (colonoscopy, air-contrast barium enema) to rule out colorectal cancer as the cause of a positive stool test result for occult blood.

Current evidence suggests that it is reasonable to recommend that all persons older than 65 years should undergo annual FOBTs and flexible sigmoidoscopy every 3–5 years. If the result is positive, colonoscopy should be performed. Medicare pays for a screening whole-bowel evaluation every 10 years on the basis of evidence that adenomatous polyps (if detected) may undergo malignant transformation over this time. Studies are evaluating the effectiveness of screening interventions for detecting and possibly reducing mortality from colorectal cancer.

PROSTATE CANCER

Prostate cancer is second only to lung cancer as a cause of mortality from cancer among older persons. About 15 percent of all men eventually have cancer of the prostate; however, most men with cancer of the prostate die of other causes. African American men have twice the age-adjusted incidence of prostate cancer of white men. The disease is more likely to be diagnosed at a more aggressive or advanced stage among African American men and thus is associated with a higher mortality. For most men prostate cancer is most often an indolent condition; however, for a small percentage the disease can be aggressive.

Screening for prostate cancer by means of digital rectal examination and prostate-specific antigen (PSA) testing for all men older than 50 years is recommended by the American Cancer Society and the American Urological Association. Other groups recommend that screening not be conducted because there is a high incidence of false-negative and false-positive results from currently available screening modalities, including ultrasonography, and there is uncertainty about the effectiveness of therapy for even early-stage disease. Studies are evaluating the effectiveness of screening tests such as PSA testing, PSA density, PSA velocity, age-specific PSA testing, and ultrasonography. Randomized controlled trials are in progress to evaluate the benefits and risks of screening.

For now there is little evidence to support routine screening for prostate cancer among older persons who are otherwise at low risk of prostate cancer. For further discussion of screening for prostate cancer, see Chap. 7.

SKIN CANCER

Basal and squamous cell cancers are prevalent among older adults. One million new cases are diagnosed each year. Risk factors for these cancers include advanced age, substantial cumulative sun exposure, and light skin. Both basal and squamous cell cancers are slow growing, rarely metastasize, and are treatable.

Malignant melanoma is the most serious skin condition that a clinician sees in the office. Risk factors include white race, family or personal history of skin cancer, and melanocytic precursor or marker lesions, such as atypical moles. Malignant melanoma is most frequently missed by primary care clinicians who fail to examine the back or other clothed areas. Early-stage melanoma usually has a good prognosis whereas late-stage disease usually is fatal.

The recommendations for screening for skin cancer vary depending on the professional organization. The USPSTF states that there is insufficient evidence for or against routine screening. The American Cancer Society and the American Academy of Dermatology recommend periodic screening. The American Academy of Family Practice recommends screening for persons at high risk.

OVARIAN CANCER

Ovarian cancer is the fourth leading cause of cancer death among older women and is most common among women older than 60 years. Most women come to medical attention with advanced disease that is associated with a poor prognosis. Currently available methods for detection of ovarian cancer include bimanual pelvic examination, transvaginal ultrasonography, and transabdominal ultrasonography. None of these techniques is useful in detecting early-stage disease. Assessment of tumor markers such as CA-125 is not useful as a screening measure because is has a low positive predictive value (3 percent). Screening for ovarian cancer is not recommended at this time.

OTHER CANCERS

Screening for cancer of the pancreas, lung, liver, esophagus, stomach, kidney, and spleen is not likely to be beneficial.

Other Conditions

DEMENTIA

Although dementia is common among older adults and causes great morbidity and formidable health care expenditures, there are currently no good screening tests that are sensitive and specific enough to detect dementia. The most commonly used tests are the Folstein Mini-Mental State Examination and the Short Portable Mental Status Questionnaire. Although these tests may be specific, they lack sensitivity to detect dementia, especially in the early stages. These tests are less useful for testing minorities and persons of lower educational levels. Even if dementia is detected, treatment options are limited. Pharmacological agents such as donepezil may be of potential benefit in treating patients with Alzheimer's disease (see Chap. 12).

DEPRESSION

The prevalence of depression among ambuatory older persons is in the range of 5 to 10 percent. Clinicians therefore should have a high index of suspicion for depression among older persons who have a history of depression or a family history of depression, who have had a loss such as bereavement, loss of a job, financial problems, or illness. There are no data to support screening for depression except among groups at high risk. Screening instruments have been developed and may be useful in helping make the diagnosis in these situations (see Chap. 11).

Older persons with depression are at increased risk of committing suicide, and older persons who have successfully committed suicide had seen their primary care physician in the prior month. Suicidal ideation and intent should be assessed in all encounters with an older person with depression.

DIABETES MELLITUS

As many as 20 percent of persons older than 65 years (8 million persons) have diabetes mellitus, and many cases have not been diagnosed. Diabetes mellitus is associated with a greater likelihood of patients' development of coronary artery disease and other complications such as retinopathy, neuropathy, and nephropathy. Risk factors of diabetes mellitus among the elderly include obesity (insulin resistance), family history of diabetes, African American race, and hypertension.

There is excellent evidence that "tight" glycemic control among younger insulin-dependent patients with diabetes mellitus results in great reduction in the incidence of complications from diabetes. Such evidence does not exist for older persons who have non-insulin-dependent diabetes mellitus.

The American Diabetes Association recommends that screening for diabetes be done every 3 years and that interventions instituted if fasting blood glucose levels are greater than 125 mg/dL. The USPSTF suggests that there is insufficient evidence to recommend screening for diabetes mellitus. Clinicians may choose to screen for diabetes among groups at high risk.

HEARING LOSS

Hearing loss is the most common sensory deficit that occurs among older persons. As many as 60 percent of persons older than 80 years have substantial impairment. High-tone frequency loss is the most common deficit. This type of loss decreases the ability of the older person to appreciate spoken words, especially in crowded rooms, where there is considerable background noise. Hearing loss affects physical, social, emotional, and psychological functioning. There is evidence that if hearing loss is detected and an older person is willing to use an aid, function improves markedly (see Chap. 13).

Clinicians should check the hearing of their older patients with either a screening questionnaire or an office audiometer. If the results are abnormal, formal audiometric testing is indicated.

VISION LOSS

Vision loss is second to hearing loss as a sensory deficit among older persons. The most common pathologic conditions are cataracts, macular degeneration, and glaucoma. Age-associated presbyopia occurs among all persons after the age of 50 years. It is characterized by an inability to focus on near objects. Many older persons are unaware that they have impaired vision (see Chap. 13).

Corrective lenses can improve the visual acuity of persons with presbyopia. Iridectomy and placement of an intraocular lens helps to improve vision for patients with cataracts, unless there is coexisting retinal disease, glaucoma, or macular degeneration. Evidence is less than convincing that early detection and management of glaucoma improves vision appreciably. In many cases patients with macular degeneration cannot be treated if the condition is identified. Studies are investigating the effectiveness of screening for and treating patients with these conditions.

Older persons should undergo an annual visual acuity test. Clinicians can perform this test with a Snellen chart and refer the patient for further testing if abnormalities are detected. Screening for glaucoma and macular degeneration is controversial. There is no evidence that primary care clinicians should screen for these conditions.

ASYMPTOMATIC CAROTID ARTERY STENOSIS

Whether routine screening to detect asymptomatic carotid stenosis is effective is unknown. Some patients with high-grade stenosis may benefit from surgery. There are two screening tests: carotid artery auscultation and carotid Doppler studies. Although auscultation is easy to perform, the presence of a carotid bruit has relatively low sensitivity (63 to 76 percent) and specificity (61 to 76 percent). In addition, 40 to 75 percent of persons with an asymptomatic carotid bruit do not have clinically significant carotid artery stenosis. Although carotid Doppler studies are more accurate than auscultation, the cost of carotid Doppler studies is substantial.

ABDOMINAL AORTIC ANEURYSM

Almost 9000 deaths each year are caused by abdominal aortic aneurysm (AAA). Most of these deaths occur among the elderly. Risk factors of AAA are male sex, hypertension, cigarette use, and atherosclerotic coronary or carotid vascular disease. Rate of rupture is related to the size of the aneurysm and the rate of increase in size of the aneurysm. The accuracy of the clinical examination for detecting AAA is unknown. Ultrasonography is sensitive and specific for detecting AAA, but it is expensive.

There are no data to show that screening for and intervening for AAA are worthwhile. However, elective surgical therapy for AAA is effective if an aneurysm is detected. The mortality of emergency surgical management of ruptured AAA is approximately 50 percent.

Summary

There are two important goals for implementing health promotion and disease prevention strategies among the elderly population. The first goal is to prolong life. This is accomplished by removing the risk of disease through primary prevention and by identifying diseases in an early stage, when the prognosis is good, through secondary prevention. The second goal of prevention is to avoid or delay the onset of dependency. How well people live is as important to many persons as how long they live. The disability caused by many diseases can be avoided by implementing health promotion and prevention strategies. Primary care clinicians need to invest the time and effort to promote these strategies.

Bibliography

AAFP recommendations for periodic health examination. Reprint no. 510. Kansas City, MO: American Academy of Family Physicians; 1998.

Ades PA, Ballor DL, Ashiga T, et al: Weight training improves walking endurance in healthy elderly persons. *Ann Intern Med* 124:568, 1996.

Balducci L, Schapira DW, Cox CE, et al: Breast cancer of the older woman: an annotated review. *J Am Geriatr Soc* 39:1113, 1991.

Campos-Outcalt D: 20 *Common Problems in Prevention.* New York: McGraw Hill; 2000.

Carter TL: Age-related vision changes: a primary care guide. *Geriatrics* 49:37, 1994.

Cho CY, Alessi CA, Cho M, et al: The association between chronic illness and functional change among participants in a comprehensive geriatric program. *J Am Geriatr Soc* 46:677, 1998.

Cobbs EL, Ralapatti RA: Health of older women. *Med Clin North Am* 82:127, 1998.

Coley CM, Barry MJ, Mulley AG: Screening for prostate cancer. *Ann Intern Med* 126:480, 1997.

Eekoof JA, deBock GH, deLaat JA, et al: The whispered voice: the best test for screening for hearing impairment in general practice? *Br J Gen Pract* 46:473, 1996.

Feussner JR, Oddone EZ, Wong JG: Screening for cancer. In: Cassel CK, Cohen HJ, Larson EB, et al (eds): *Geriatric Medicine*, 3rd ed. New York: Springer; 1997;231.

Fiatarone MA, Marks EC, Ryan ND, et al: High-intensity strength training in nonagenarians: effects on skeletal muscle. *JAMA* 263:3029, 1990.

Fleming MF, Barry KL, Manwell LB, et al: Brief physician advice for problem alcohol drinkers: a randomized controlled trial on community-based primary care practices. *JAMA* 227:1039, 1997.

Garber AM, Littenberg B, Sox HC, et al: Costs and health consequences of cholesterol screening for asymptomatic older Americans. *Arch Intern Med* 151:1089, 1991.

German PS, Burton LC, Shapiro S, et al: Extended coverage for preventive health services for the elderly: response and results in a demonstration population. *Am J Public Health* 85:379, 1995.

Guralnik JM, Ferrucci L, Simonsick EM, et al: Lower-extremity function in persons over the age of 70 years as a predictor of subsequent disability. *N Engl J Med* 332:556, 1995.

Guralnik JM, Fried LP, Salive ME: Disability as a public health outcome in the aging population. *Annu Rev Public Health* 17:25, 1996.

Hazzard WR: Weight control and exercise: cardinal features of successful preventive gerontology. *JAMA* 274:1964, 1995.

Kronborg O, Fenger C, Olsen J, et al: Randomized study of screening for colorectal with faecal-occult-blood test. *Lancet* 348:1467, 1996.

Marine WM, Kerwin EM, Moore EE, et al: Mandatory seat belts: epidemiologic, financial, and medical rationale from the Colorado matched pairs study. *J Trauma* 36:96, 1994.

Mouton CP, Espino DV: Health screening in older women. *Am Fam Physician* 59:1835, 1999.

Muldrow CD, Lichtenstein MJ: Screening for hearing impairment in the elderly: rationale and strategy. *J Gen Intern Med* 6:249, 1991.

Physical activity and cardiovascular health. NIH Consensus Development Panel on Physical Activity and Cardiovascular Health. *JAMA* 276:241, 1996.

Popelka MM, Cruickshanks KJ, Wiley TL, et al: Low prevalence of hearing aid use among older adults with hearing loss: the Epidemiology of Hearing Loss Study. *J Am Geriatr Soc* 46:1075, 1998.

Potter J, Scott DJ, Roberts MA, et al: Influenza vaccination of health-care workers in long-term hospitals reduces the mortality of elderly patients. *J Infect Dis* 175:1, 1997.

Ransahoff DF, Lang CA: Suggested technique for fecal occult blood testing and interpretation in colorectal cancer screening. *Ann Intern Med* 126:808, 1997.

Recognition and Initial Assessment of Alzheimer's Disease and Related Dementias. AHCPR publication no. 97-0702. Rockville, MD., US Department of Health and Human Services, Public Health Service, Agency for Health Care Policy and Research, 1996.

Rooks DS, Kiel DP, Parsons C, et al: Self-paced resistance training and walking exercise in community-dwelling older adults: effects on neuromotor performance. *J Gerontol* 52:M161, 1997.

Rowe JW, Kahn DL: *Successful Aging*. New York: Pantheon; 1998.

Sixth report of the Joint National Committee on prevention, detection, evaluation, and treatment of high blood pressure. *Arch Intern Med* 157:2413, 1997.

Smoking Cessation Clinical Practice Guideline Panel: The Agency for Health Care Policy and Research smoking cessation clinical practice guideline. *JAMA* 275:1270, 1996.

Stuck AE, Aronow HU, Steiner A, et al: A trial of in-home comprehensive geriatric assessment for older people living in the community. *N Engl J Med* 338:1184, 1995.

Tinetti ME, Baker DI, McAvay G, et al: A multifactorial intervention to reduce risk of falling among elderly people residing in the community. *N Engl J Med* 331:821, 1994.

Tinetti ME, Innouye SK, Gill TM, et al: Shared risk factors for falls, incontinence, and functional dependence: unifying the approach to geriatric syndromes. *JAMA* 273:1348, 1995.

US Preventive Services Task Force: *Guide of Clinical Preventive Services*, 2nd ed. Baltimore: Williams & Wilkins; 1996.

Weissman MM, Olfson M: Depression in women: implication of health care research. *Science* 269:799, 1995.

Woolf SH: Screening for prostate cancer with prostate-specific antigen: an examination of the evidence. *N Engl J Med* 333:1401, 1995.

Lisa Fredman

Caregiver Issues

Overview

Informal caregivers are persons who provide unpaid assistance or supervision with personal (ADLs) and instrumental (IADLs) activities of daily living, such as bathing, dressing, and shopping, to someone who cannot function independently because of physical, cognitive, or psychiatric impairment. Formal caregivers are persons who are paid for providing this help, such as home health aides and nursing home aides. The estimated number of informal caregivers of frail elderly persons in the United States increased from 2.2 million in 1982 to more than 7.3 million in 1989. These figures probably underestimate the number of caregivers because they do not include caregivers of persons with cognitive impairment who need only general supervision or to persons with psychiatric disorders or other chronic illnesses.

Caregivers present a paradox to health care providers for several reasons. Recipients of care benefit from having caregivers because they live longer, are less likely to be placed in nursing homes, and have better physical and psychological well-being. Caregivers also benefit health care providers by being a link for the elderly patient who may forget, misinterpret, or be physically unable to implement medication regimens; by alerting the health care provider to problems that the care recipient may not have mentioned; and by ensuring compliance with medical interventions. However, caregivers themselves report more stress and psychological problems than do persons who are not caregivers and often have physical health problems that may compromise the quality of care they provide.

Identification by clinicians of caregivers and caregiver-related problems is hampered by two factors. First, many clinicians view caregivers solely in terms of the help they provide to the elderly patient. Second, caregivers often are reluctant to reveal caregiving-related problems. Thus caregivers often are referred to as *hidden patients.*

Caregiver-related problems are important in primary care practice, although they differ from some of the distinct clinical entities discussed in this book. Primary care clinicians often are in the best situation to identify problems among caregivers because the caregiver generally brings the care recipient to office visits. According to demographic projections of the elderly population in the United States, these physicians will be encountering more caregivers because of the growth of the oldest-old population and the increasing number of elderly persons who will be caregivers of elderly spouses and parents. Primary care clinicians' knowledge of long-term care services puts them in an ideal position to help caregivers make decisions about care options.

Statistics on Elderly Caregivers of Elderly Adults

More than one-third of all caregivers are 65 years and older. They actively perform ADL and IADL tasks for a dependent elder. Sixteen percent of elderly persons are potential caregivers of a spouse or other relative with functional limitations. Although 46 percent of caregivers are spouses of the care recipients, 29 percent are an adult daughter and 25 percent are another relative or friend. Seventy-five percent of caregivers live with the care recipient, and 25 percent perform caregiving activities 5 or more hours per day.

Trends suggest that more elderly persons will become caregivers for a variety of reasons. These include the growth of the aged population, especially persons older than 85 years (the oldest old), a higher prevalence of cognitive and functional impairment among older age groups, technologies that prolong living with disabilities, and health care policies that result in more community- and home-based care for persons with these disabilities. By 2050, the white population 85 years and older will be five times larger than it was in 1990, and the same-aged black population will be eight times larger. As the population ages, a larger number of elderly persons will need caregiving because of their health needs, and more will become caregivers.

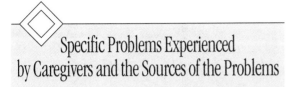

Specific Problems Experienced by Caregivers and the Sources of the Problems

Caregiver-related problems include those stemming directly from caregiving, from methods caregivers use to cope with the stresses of caregiving, and from factors that impede the caregiver's ability to provide optimum care. Problems stemming directly from caregiving include emotional problems and stress, lack of sleep, and physical problems such as strain from lifting the care recipient. Problems stemming from coping methods include the caregiver's use of psychotropic medications, alcohol, cigarettes, and mood-altering drugs. All of these problems may jeopardize the caregiver's ability to provide optimum care, as do factors such as the caregiver's physical health impairments, other family and work obligations, difficulty gaining access to community resources to assist with caregiving, and financial and time constraints.

Psychological Morbidity

A review of studies of caregivers of persons with dementia found consistently higher levels of depressive symptoms and psychological distress among caregivers than among persons who were not caregivers. Caregivers of persons with other conditions, such as stroke, also report high levels of depression and stress. Higher levels of stress and depression are more likely among caregivers who care for someone with more limitations in ADL and cognitive impairment. Caregivers who spend more hours per day performing caregiving activities, who assist the care recipient with more ADLs and IADLs, and who need respite from caregiving activities also have more psychological

morbidity than do those who spend less time in caregiving activities. The curve of length of time involved in caregiving appears to have a U-shaped association with stress and depression. Caregivers are more stressed if they have been caregiving for a short time (1 year or less) or a long time (4 or more years).

Whether a caregiver becomes stressed or depressed may vary with the relationship between caregiver and care recipient. One study found more emotional and social distress among daughter caregivers compared with wife caregivers. In two other studies, a patient's need for more help was associated with both higher stress and higher satisfaction among adult-child caregivers but was not related to stress among spouse caregivers and was associated with stress among husbands but not among wives or daughters. These results may be due to greater willingness of middle-aged adults to admit to depressive symptoms and stress than are elderly adults and to greater familiarity and acceptance of helping others with ADLs among women than among men. Standardized instruments such as the Patient-Caregiver Functional Unit Scale (PCFUS) may help primary care clinicians to identify caregiving activities that are a source of emotional stress to the caregiver (see Table 4-3).

The relationship between the care recipient's symptoms and the amount of caregiver stress may vary over time according to the course of the patient's condition, caregiver adaptation to caregiving, or the influence of other factors. For example, among caregivers of persons with stroke, the care recipients' degree of disability was significantly associated with caregiver depression during the first year of follow-up but not during the second year. However, another study of caregivers of persons with stroke found that one-third of caregivers were stressed because of patients' behaviors, such as confusion, depression, or irritability at baseline and after 1 year of follow-up.

The results of these studies suggest that caregiver stress and psychological problems may be predicted better by patients' functional and cognitive status than by the patient's diagnosis. Primary care clinicians' assessment of these factors would be important in detecting and preventing psychological problems among caregivers. It would also be important for preparing persons in the early stages of caregiving for problems that can develop as the patient's condition worsens, such as incontinence, being wakeful at night, or disruptive behaviors, and that are associated with stress and depression.

Physical Morbidity

There is less evidence that caregiving is associated with physical morbidity than there is for psychological morbidity. However, caregivers have been shown to have poorer physical health than persons who are not caregivers, according to measures such as self-ratings of health status, immunologic and cardiovascular indicators, and functional status. Caregivers consistently rate their health poorer than do persons who are not caregivers and poorer than does the general population. Caregivers' self-rated health is poorer when they are burdened, depressed, and psychologically strained and when they care for persons with more cognitive symptoms.

Caregiving may affect physical health status through the effects of stress on immune status or cardiovascular reactivity. This hypothesis is based on results of laboratory studies in which experimentally induced stress increased susceptibility to infection and viral infection and raised cardiovascular reactivity, such as blood pressure. Several studies found that caregivers of persons with Alzheimer's disease have poorer immune function than age-matched controls. In contrast, cardiovascular functioning differed only between certain subgroups of caregivers and controls, such as men and African Americans, but not in others. Thus caregiving appears to affect physical health more through impaired immune function, and it may affect cardiovascular function in some groups. It also may affect physical health through the effort of caregiving activities among caregivers who are already physically vulnerable. For example, one study found that caregivers who helped with more

ADLs experienced more decline in their own ADLs over a 1-year period than did other caregivers and persons who were not caregivers.

To prevent adverse physical health outcomes among caregivers, primary care clinicians should conduct a complete assessment of the caregiver's current physical health, caregiving tasks performed by the caregiver, whether these tasks are perceived to be physically or psychologically difficult to perform, whether the caregiver receives respite from caregiving, and whether others are available to assist the caregiver (Tables 4-1 through 4-4). Through such evaluation, the clinician may ascertain which caregivers are at risk of physical health decline and other aspects of the caregiving situation that can be modified to prevent health decline among caregivers.

Stress-Related Behaviors

Caregiving is associated with some stress-related behaviors, such as using psychotropic medications, weight change, drinking alcohol, cigarette smoking, and lack of exercise. Caregivers use psychotropic medications more than the general population and persons who are not caregivers. Caregivers of persons with more functional impairment have higher levels of stress and higher rates of use of psychotropic medications.

Caregivers in general report less time for exercise than do persons who are not caregivers. Female caregivers may gain considerably more weight than do persons who are not caregivers. One study found that 19 percent of caregivers gained or lost at least 10 pounds (4.5 kg) when they cared for a person with more disruptive behaviors or more functional limitations and when they reported more stress and burden. Caregivers may cope with the stresses of caregiving through selected behaviors, notably use of psychotropic drugs and behaviors that cause a change in weight. These behaviors may adversely affect the caregiver's physical health.

Primary care clinicians can help prevent physical morbidity among caregivers by assessing

Table 4-1

Methods to Detect Problems Among Caregivers

ASSESSMENT OF ACTIVITIES PERFORMED BY CAREGIVER

Does the caregiver perform (or supervise the care recipient in) the following tasks, and are they difficult to perform?
 Shopping
 Taking medications
 Preparing meals
 Managing money
 Using the telephone
 Mobility-related tasks
   Walking across a room
   Housework
 Basic activities of daily living
   Eating
   Bathing
   Dressing
   Getting in and out of bed
   Toileting
 How many hours a day does the caregiver supervise or perform these tasks for the care recipient?

ASSESSMENT OF SOURCES OF STRESS
Responsibilities in job   Children in household   Other family responsibilities   Relationships with other family members, friends, coworkers   Not enough time to take care of all responsibilities   Unable to get to places on time   Trouble making ends meet financially   No time for self   No vacation in a long time
ASSESSMENT OF SYMPTOMS EXPERIENCED BY CAREGIVER IN THE PAST MONTH
Fatigue   Difficulty sleeping   Loss of appetite   Irritability, tension, anger, stress   Depression   Physical symptoms, such as back pain, headaches, stomach aches

coping behaviors and recommending other methods to cope with the strains of caregiving. Alternative methods include receiving respite from caregiving, hobbies, meditation or yoga, regular walking with a friend, or those suggested by the caregiver.

Table 4-2

Physician Assessment of Detection of Caregiver Stress

ASSESSMENT OF SOURCES OF CAREGIVER STRESS: PHYSICIAN ASKS CAREGIVER

Care recipient's cognitive status
   Care recipient's functional status
   Care recipient's emotional status
   Tasks caregiver performs
   Demands on caregiver's time
   Multiple roles of caregiver
   Interpersonal relationship between caregiver and care recipient
   Other sources of stress in caregiver's life
Assessment of symptoms of caregiver stress
Physical symptoms
   Headaches
   Backaches
   Insomnia
   Fatigue
   Weight gain/weight loss
   Digestion difficulties
   Other physical symptoms
Emotional symptoms
   Anger
   Depression
   Tension/stress
   Guilt/resentment
   Other emotional symptoms
Behavioral symptoms (Does caregiver engage in these behaviors? Have behaviors increased in past month?)
   Use of psychotropic medications
   Cigarettes
   Alcohol
   Decreased social activities
   Other behavioral symptoms

RECOMMENDATIONS REGARDING REDUCTION OF CAREGIVER STRESS

Support groups
   Counseling
   Respite care services
   Information from local organizations
   Adult day center for care recipient
   Elder-care policies at workplace
   Caregiver gets time away from caregiving, time for herself or himself

PHYSICIAN-PATIENT COMMUNICATION

Ask about caregiver's feelings toward caregiving
   Ask caregiver open-ended questions
   Show empathy to caregiver
   Acknowledge caregiver's feelings
   Discuss options with caregiver

Table 4-3

Patient-Caregiver Functional Unit Scale

ADL/IADL TASK	PATIENT IMPAIRED IN ADL/IADL TASK CAN CARE RECIPIENT DO ADL/IADL TASK? 0 = WITHOUT HELP 1 = WITH SOME HELP 2 = UNABLE TO DO TASK	CAREGIVER HELPS WITH ADL/IADL TASK DOES CAREGIVER CURRENTLY HELP CARE RECIPIENT WITH ADL/IADL TASK? 0 = NO 1 = YES	ADL/IADL TASK IS PHYSICALLY DIFFICULT IS IT/WOULD IT BE PHYSICALLY DIFFICULT TO HELP CARE RECIPIENT WITH ADL/IADL TASK? 0 = NO 1 = YES	ADL/IADL TASK IS EMOTIONALLY DIFFICULT IS IT/WOULD IT BE EMOTIONALLY DIFFICULT TO HELP CARE RECIPIENT WITH ADL/IADL TASK? 0 = NO 1 = YES
Use telephone				
Get to places within walking distance				
Shop for groceries				
Prepare meals				
Do housework				
Take medicine				
Handle finances				
Feed self				
Dress self				
Groom self				
Transfer from bed to chair				
Walk across a room				
Bathe self				
Use the toilet				

ABBREVIATIONS: ADL, activities of daily living; IADL, instrumental activities of daily living.
SOURCE: Adapted with permission from Fredman L, Daly M. The Patient-Caregiver Functional Unit Scale (PCFUS): a new instrument to measure the stability of the patient-caregiver dyad. *Fam Med* 29:658, 1997.

Table 4-4

Burden Interview Questions

The following is a list of statements that reflect how people sometimes feel when taking care of another person. After each statement, indicate how often you feel that way: never (0), rarely (1), sometimes (2), quite often (3), or nearly always (4). There are no right or wrong answers.

1. Do you think that your relative asks for more help than he or she needs?
2. Do you feel that because of the time you spend with your relative, you don't have enough time for yourself?
3. Do you feel stressed between caring for your relative and trying to meet other responsibilities for your family or work?
4. Do you feel embarrassed over your relative's behavior?
5. Do you feel angry when you are around your relative?
6. Do you feel that your relative currently affects your relationship with other family members or friends in a negative way?
7. Are you afraid of what the future holds for your relative?
8. Do you feel that your relative is dependent on you?
9. Do you feel strained when you are around your relative?
10. Do you feel your health has suffered because of your involvement with your relative?
11. Do you feel that you don't have as much privacy as you would like because of your relative?
12. Do you feel that your social life has suffered because you are caring for your relative?
13. Do you feel uncomfortable about having friends over because of your relative?
14. Do you feel that your relative seems to expect you to take care of him or her as if you were the only one he or she could depend on?
15. Do you feel that you don't have enough money to care for your relative in addition to your other expenses?
16. Do you feel that you will be unable to take care of your relative much longer?
17. Do you feel that you have lost control of your life since your relative became ill?
18. Do you wish you could just leave the care of your relative to someone else?
19. Do you feel uncertain about what to do about your relative?
20. Do you feel you should be doing more for your relative?
21. Do you feel you could do a better job in caring for your relative?
22. Overall, how often do you feel burdened caring for your relative?

SOURCE: Adapted with permission from Zarit SH, Reever KE, Bach-Peterson J. Relatives of the impaired elderly: correlates of feelings of burden. *Gerontologist* 20:649, 1980.

Poor Self-Care Behaviors

Caregiving also may adversely affect physical health through neglect of self-care and injuries. These behaviors include not receiving regular health examinations, not having time to rest to recuperate from illness, and forgetting to take prescription medications. Caregivers who help with more ADLs have poorer health behaviors. In one study, 67 percent of caregivers had sustained injuries while lifting the care recipient. Thus caregivers may experience adverse health effects through neglect of their own health or attempts at caregiving activities that are too demanding for them.

Finances

Caregivers' lifestyle and psychological health may be affected by increased financial burdens and changes in living arrangements to care for the care recipient. Most insurance policies do not fully pay for home health care or adult day care, which may be necessary to keep the care recipient in the community, and some caregivers must stop or reduce working to care for the care recipient. Daily supplies, such as special food or incontinence pads, may add to the costs of caregiving. The financial expense of caregiving may thus increase a caregiver's sense of stress.

Medicare and Medicaid cover some expenses for persons with Alzheimer's disease, for example, and caregivers may qualify for income tax deductions for some medical care, personal care, and long-term care costs (Table 4-5). A plan of care prescribed by a licensed health care provider, annual certification, and other requirements often are needed to qualify for deductions. A great deal of information is available through Internet sites, the Alzheimer's Association (800-272-3900), and booklets on planning for and managing the financial aspects of caregiving (see Table 4-5).

Living Arrangements

Most caregivers (75 percent) live with the care recipient. Caregivers often arrange for the care

Table 4-5

Web Sites for Information on Caregiver-Related Problems

NAME	WEB SITE	DESCRIPTION
National Institute on Aging (NIA)	www.nih.gov/nia/health	Information on educational materials, specific diseases, research, and resources for health professionals, patients, and family members
NIA Age Pages	www.nih.gov/nia/health	Fact sheets on topics related to aging, such as medications, planning for long-term care, diseases
Eldercare Locator	www.aoa.dhhs.gov	Information on local long-term care resources and programs
Alzheimer's Disease Education and Referral (ADEAR) Center	www.alzheimers.org/adear	Information on Alzheimer's disease and related disorders, including NIA research updates, clinical trials database, information and referral services
Alzheimer's Association	www.alz.org	Information for persons with Alzheimer's disease (what to expect, resources), caregivers (helping care recipient with personal care, legal planning, understanding challenging behavior, stress), and care professionals (programs, end-of-life issues)
Online caregiver support, information, resources	www.caregiving.com	A monthly newsletter for caregivers, caregiver discussion group, information on hospice and other resources
Information for caregivers	www.agenet.com	Information on resources for older adults and caregivers, information on financial planning, drugs, online wills, senior centers

recipient to move in with them, particularly when the patient, usually a parent, declines in ability to perform ADLs and IADLs independently. Unfortunately, many studies find that caregivers who live with the care recipient report more stress and depression than do those who do not. The causes may be the time spent helping the care recipient with ADLs, disruption of sleep, lack of respite from caregiving, or not having enough time to perform caregiving responsibilities in addition to other roles.

Some families prefer that the care recipient alternate living with each adult child for several months at a time. This arrangement gives each child a chance to be the caregiver and to have respite from it. The clinician should be aware of the potential disadvantages of such arrangements. Moving to unfamiliar surroundings may disorient care recipients, especially if they have mild dementia. If the adult children do not live close to each other, there may be discontinuity in health care providers and social settings such as senior centers or church. The previous caregiver may forget to communicate information about medications and other health care when the care recipient moves in with another caregiver.

Summary

Primary care clinicians should be alerted to caregiving activities, coping methods, and general risk factors for stress that might lead to adverse health effects among caregivers. For example, assisting a person with bathing, transferring, toileting, and other ADLs can increase the risk of physical strain and back strain or exacerbate existing health conditions among caregivers. Sleep disruptions, which are common among caregivers of persons with dementia, can increase the risk of injury and may cause declines in immune function. Stress due to caregiving activities or to balancing these activities with other family and employment responsibilities may lead to a lowering of immunologic function. Assessing caregiver-related problems should include asking whether the caregiver

is performing these activities and experiencing symptoms or signs of these conditions (see Tables 4-1 and 4-2).

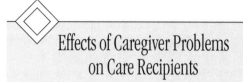

Effects of Caregiver Problems on Care Recipients

Caregiver-related problems can affect the care recipient's well-being. These effects include psychological and psychiatric problems such as anxiety or depression that can lead to neglect or abuse of the care recipient or moving the care recipient to a different environment.

Depression

Care recipients can become depressed or socially isolated if the caregiver is depressed. Among elderly couples, depressive symptoms or poor health in one spouse are strong predictors of depressive symptoms and poor self-rated health in the other spouse. One study found that 40 percent of care recipients felt distressed about receiving care from a caregiver, that the level of distress was higher among those who received more help, and that those who felt distressed were more likely to have depression 1 year after they began to need care. Primary care clinicians should assess whether aspects of the caregiving situation can be altered to improve the psychological well-being of the care recipient.

Abuse and Neglect

An estimated 1.5 to 2 million elderly persons in the United States are abused annually. Elder abuse and neglect includes emotional, physical, and financial abuse and violation of the elderly person's personal rights, such as the right to make decisions for himself or herself. These problems occur among both men and women and across racial and socioeconomic groups. Publications have suggested that clinicians become more involved in detecting and preventing elder abuse and neglect. This begins with knowledge of risk factors of elder abuse or neglect. Among care recipients, risk factors include being frail, having cognitive impairment, having urinary incontinence, being dependent in ADLs, a history of mental illness, alcohol, or drug abuse, and being more socially isolated and dependent on the caregiver.

Aravanis et al suggest that clinicians include routine questions and assessment of elder abuse into their interviews and examinations of elderly patients. They recommend short protocols to detect physical signs of mistreatment of elders that range from bruises, malnutrition, and poor personal hygiene to withdrawal or expression of ambivalent feelings toward the caregiver. Also recommended is asking the care recipient direct questions such as the following: Has anyone at home ever hurt you? Has anyone ever touched you without your consent? Have you ever signed documents that you did not understand? Are you afraid of anyone at home? Are you alone a lot? Has anyone ever failed to help you take care of yourself when you needed help?

Caregivers who are stressed might be more likely to abuse or neglect the care recipient. This might result from anger, inability to cope with a care recipient's disruptive behavior, forgetting to administer the care recipient's medications, overmedicating the care recipient, or neglecting to care for the recipient. Lack of education on how to administer medications, on caring for the psychological and social needs of the care recipient, and on methods to manage caregiver stress may result in elder abuse and neglect. Many studies suggest that a history of psychological abuse between the caregiver and care recipient, not caregiver stress, is a more likely predictor of elder abuse. In any case, primary care clinicians should be aware of the potential for caregiver stress to result in abuse and neglect of the care recipient. Clinicians can help prevent elder abuse by treating the care recipient for correctable problems, such as urinary incon-tinence and dementia-related or drug-induced behavioral problems; educating caregivers about ways to cope with caregiver stress; and referring the caregiver and care recipient to respite and community services.

Changes in Living Arrangements

Caregivers who are stressed are more likely to find other living arrangements for the care recipient, such as living with another relative or placement in a nursing home. Changes in living arrangements may be disorienting for a person with dementia or other cognitive impairments, may disrupt continuity of care and daily routines, and may lead to increased stress and morbidity for the care recipient. Sometimes moving from a detrimental living arrangement may improve the quality of life for the care recipient. Clinicians are best positioned to review living arrangement options with the caregiver and care recipient and help with decisions about the most appropriate arrangement for their needs. Internet sites for organizations such as the National Institute on Aging Age Pages, the Eldercare Locator, and the Alzheimer's Association provide information on alternative living arrangements and planning for long-term care (see Table 4-5).

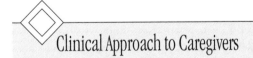

Clinical Approach to Caregivers

Caregiver-related problems often are not detected and necessitate that the primary care clinician maintain suspicion that such problems may exist. Identification of these problems can occur in multiple settings, including office, home, hospital, assisted living, and continuing care retirement communities. It is important to determine whether the problem is due to caregiving or other medical or psychological issues in the caregiver's life; whether the problem is a potential hazard to the caregiver, care recipient, or other family members; and whether the problem can be managed within the current caregiving situation.

An essential question that guides when and how the physician detects caregiver-related problems is, "Who is the patient?" The patient may be viewed as the care recipient, the caregiver, or the caregiver-care recipient dyad. Primary care clinicians can assess caregivers for stress and other problems when the caregiver brings the elderly patient for an office visit or when the caregiver has a medical appointment for himself or herself. Huston recommends that primary care clinicians ask all patients 40 years and older whether they are caregivers. Given that more caregivers are arranging care for a parent from long distance, following this recommendation may identify caregivers who would otherwise be unrecognized.

There are many barriers to the detection of caregiver-related problems. Caregivers may be unfamiliar with the term itself, and therefore may not consider themselves caregivers. Many caregivers consider caregiving part of being married or being a family member. They may not be aware that caregiving responsibilities become unmanageable or that services are available to give them time away from caregiving. Because caregivers may receive strong messages from family members and health professionals that reinforce the caregiving role, they may feel guilty about discussing their problems with caregiving or their desire for a break from it. By complimenting caregivers on their heroic efforts, health professionals may be giving the unintended message that the caregiver should not discuss problems stemming from caregiving.

Caregivers may feel guilty and embarrassed about discussing specific aspects of caregiving that are stressful. These might include tasks such as bathing the care recipient or managing urinary or fecal incontinence. Caregivers may feel guilty about their anger or irritation with the care recipient's behavior or need for constant supervision, not having time for oneself, or, among caregivers of persons with dementia, not understanding the care recipient's outbursts or inappropriate behav-

iors. For these reasons, caregivers may deny feeling stressed or may not identify sources of their anger or stress.

Detection of caregiver-related problems might be difficult when the caregiver is not psychologically able to accept that the care recipient needs more assistance than the caregiver can provide, when other family members do not want changes in the caregiving situation, or when no other informal caregivers are available, as when the caregiver is the only adult child. Caregivers who are stressed often have had a long-lasting, difficult relationship with the care recipient, so the primary care clinician may be addressing not simply current problems arising from caregiving but a history of problems.

Detecting caregiver-related problems necessitates that the physician recognize first that the person is a caregiver and that caregivers may experience psychological and physical consequences of caregiving. Detecting caregiver-related problems is more difficult if the caregiver does not have symptoms of stress, denies symptoms that he or she does have, does not believe that problems can develop, or has relatives, such as other potential caregivers, who deny that there is a problem.

Methods to Detect Problems Among Caregivers

Caregiver-related problems may be detected by means of asking caregivers about their caregiving responsibilities and health symptoms that may be related to caregiving (see Tables 4-1 and 4-2) or with short instruments to assess caregiver stress that are administered by the practitioner or an office assistant or are self-administered by caregivers (see Tables 4-3 and 4-4). The benefit of such instruments is that they have been validated in studies of caregivers and may guide diagnosis and treatment.

Corradetti and Hills reviewed assessment instruments according to types of caregivers for whom they are designed, domains that are evaluated, such as depression and caregiving activities performed, and length of time needed to administer the instrument, among other factors. For example, the burden interview is a 22-item instrument to evaluate the multidimensional aspects of burden among caregivers of persons with dementia (see Table 4-4). An advantage of this scale is questions on the caregiver's feelings of embarrassment and guilt, which validates feelings that caregivers often feel ashamed to admit.

Another scale, the PCFUS was developed to assess the stability of patient-caregiver dyads, regardless of the patient's diagnosis (see Table 4-3). The PCFUS asks caregivers to document whether they help the patient with each of 14 ADL and IADL tasks; whether performing each task is emotionally or physically difficult; and, for tasks that are not currently performed by the caregiver, whether it would be emotionally or physically difficult for the caregiver to help the patient with the task. This focus on tasks of caregiving identifies specific aspects of caregiving that may be stressful and relates directly to interventions to reduce stress. For example, personal care aides can be recommended for caregivers who report physical difficulty in helping with basic ADL tasks, and support groups, adult day care, or respite care can be recommended for caregivers who report emotional difficulty in helping with tasks of ADLs or IADLs.

Treatment

Management of caregiver-related problems depends on the current and predicted health status of the care recipient; at what point during caregiving the primary care clinician becomes involved; and the fit between the caregiver's capability to continue to provide care and the care recipient's predicted need for care. Treatment may focus on patient problems, caregiver problems, and the overall caregiving situation.

The primary care clinician should become involved early in the caregiving process. The general goal is educating the caregiver, care recipient, and other family members about the anticipated disease and long-term care planning and preventing negative health outcomes of caregiving. Early intervention may focus on preparing for caregiving over the course of several years, and discussing long-term care options and perhaps terminal care. This may include recommending resources through local community-based agencies and continuing care facilities; discussing caregiving options with other family members; and assisting in planning for more involved care and in making decisions about long-term care. Discussing advance directives and durable power of attorney is important at this time.

Primary care clinicians may identify caregivers who have been caregiving for a moderate amount of time. In these situations or when the primary care clinician is providing ongoing care to patient-caregiver dyads, the care focus may shift to alleviating short-term problems in the caregiving situation, such as relieving caregiver stress, finding sources to help the caregiver assist the care recipient with daily activities and supervision, and educating the caregiver and care recipient about long-term care options that might be considered in the future. Support groups may help at this point by introducing the caregiver to other caregivers and providing a sympathetic environment to discuss caregiving-related problems. Comprehensive geriatric assessment also may be recommended, especially if the care recipient has not undergone a comprehensive biopsychosocial health assessment, or if the primary care clinician suspects that the care recipient's symptoms might have complex causes.

During the late caregiving experience, the primary care clinician can discuss alternative living situations ranging from in-home assistance by home health aides, to a continuing care community for both the caregiver and care recipient, to a skilled nursing facility or a group home for the care recipient. The caregiver may be stressed and conflicted about whether to obtain additional help or to find alternative placement for the care recipient. The focus may be on changing the caregiving situation and anticipating the end of caregiving, grief, and loss.

Community Resources

Caregivers may benefit from community resources to assist with emotional, legal, and medical aspects of caregiving as well as day care programs for the care recipient (see Table 4-5). Brochures are available from government agencies, such as area agencies on aging, the county office on aging, and from private foundations, such as the Alzheimer's Association. Some caregivers may benefit from support groups or searching the Internet for information and chat rooms. The caregiver's church or religious group may be an excellent source of referral; many churches have volunteers who provide home-based respite care.

Caregivers report anecdotally that respite from caregiving lowers stress and depression, although overall there is little evidence that respite interventions reduce stress in the short term. Many types of respite programs exist. They may include respite workers' coming to the caregiver's home, adult day care programs, and overnight and short-term care provided by nursing homes. These programs allow caregivers to get away for a few hours to several days. Caregivers report that simply having time away from caregiving responsibilities is rejuvenating. The Yellow Pages and Internet sites list national and local organizations, private companies, and nursing homes that provide respite care.

Medical Resources

Caregivers may benefit from referral to medical assessment programs. A comprehensive evaluation of the patient and often the family is tied to specific recommendations for improving or maintaining the patient's physical, functional, and psychological health. Clinicians might recommend comprehensive geriatric assessment programs or dementia assessment programs. For caregivers with limited finances and who qualify, assessment programs at local Veterans Affairs medical centers may be recommended.

Options for Long-Term Care

Many caregivers are unaware of the variety of long-term care options, ranging from in-home to nursing home arrangements. In-home care might help the caregiver to continue to keep the care recipient at home. Decisions about in-home care may address the type of care needed by the care recipient; whether full-time or part-time care is needed; when care is needed, such as at night so that the caregiver can get a full night's sleep; the training and credentials of the care provider; and cost and insurance reimbursement issues. In-home care may provide respite from caregiving, a better quality of nursing and personal care than the caregiver can give, and allow the caregiver to continue to work outside the home. Continuing care facilities may provide the range of housing, medical, and social settings that meet caregivers' and care recipients' needs. Various levels of care and programs offered by nursing homes should be discussed, such as special care units for persons with Alzheimer's disease, and programs that assist caregivers to adjust to placing a spouse or other relative in a nursing home. The National Institute on Aging Age Pages on long-term care provide information on long-term care options, questions to ask when looking for residential care facilities, and addresses of agencies that may help the caregiver choose a long-term care arrangement.

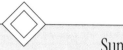

Summary

Growth of the elderly population in general and of the oldest-old population in particular is increasing the number of caregivers in the United States. Primary care clinicians are in an ideal position to educate caregivers and their elderly relatives, detect stress and health problems among caregivers, and make recommendations to prevent physical and psychological health decline among caregivers. Increased awareness of the types of problems caregivers experience, potential sources of caregiver stress, and the impediments to the detection of caregiving-related problems will improve the ability of the primary care clinician to identify and manage caregiver-related problems. These steps should enhance the quality of life of caregivers, care recipients, and other family members.

Bibliography

Aneshensel CS, Pearlin LI, Schuler RH: Stress, role captivity, and the cessation of caregiving. *J Health Soc Behav* 34:54, 1993.

Aravanis SC, Adelman RD, Breckman R, et al: Diagnostic and treatment guidelines on elder abuse and neglect. *Arch Fam Med* 2:371, 1993.

Baumgarten M, Battista RN, Infante-Rivard C, Hanley JA, Becker R, Gauthier S: The psychological and physical health of family members caring for an elderly person with dementia. *J Clin Epidemiol* 45:61, 1992.

Bookwala J, Schulz R: Spousal similarity in subjective well-being: the Cardiovascular Health Study. *Psychol Aging* 11:582, 1996.

Brown AR, Mulley GP: Injuries sustained by caregivers of disabled elderly people. *Age Aging* 26:21, 1997.

Burton LC, Newsom JT, Schulz R, Hirsch CH, German PS: Preventive health behaviors among spousal caregivers. *Prev Med* 26:162, 1997.

Corradetti E, Hills G: Assessing and supporting caregivers of the elderly. *Top Geriatr Rehabil* 14:12, 1998.

Emlet CA: Assessing the informal caregiver: team member or hidden patient? *Home Care Provid* 1:255, 1996.

Fredman L, Daly M: The Patient-Caregiver Functional Unit Scale (PCFUS): a new instrument to measure the stability of the patient-caregiver dyad. *Fam Med* 29:658, 1997.

Fredman L, Daly MP: Weight change: a measure of caregiver stress. *J Aging Health* 9:43, 1997.

Harper S, Lund D: Wives, husbands, and daughters caring for institutionalized and non-institutionalized

dementia patients: toward a model of caregiver burden. *Int J Aging Hum Dev* 30:241, 1990.

Huston P: Family care of the elderly and caregiver stress. *Am Fam Phys* 42:671, 1993.

Kiecolt-Glaser JK, Dura JR, Speicher CE, Trask OJ, Glaser R: Spousal caregivers of dementia victims: longitudinal changes in immunity and health. *Psychosom Med* 53:345, 1991.

Knight BG, Lutzky SM, Macofsky-Urban F: A meta-analytic review of interventions for caregiver distress: recommendations for future research. *Gerontologist* 33:240, 1993.

Lawton MP, Moss M, Kleban MH, Glicksman A, Rovine M: A two-factor model of caregiving appraisal and psychological well-being. *J Gerontol* 46:181, 1991.

Meshefedjian G, McCusker J, Bellavance F, Baumgarten M: Factors associated with symptoms of depression among informal caregivers of demented elders in the community. *Gerontologist* 38:247, 1998.

Mort JR, Gaspar PM, Juffer DI, Kovarna MB: Comparison of psychotropic agent use among rural elderly caregivers and noncaregivers. *Ann Pharmacother* 30:583, 1996.

Newsom JT, Schulz R: Caregiving from the recipient's perspective: negative reactions to being helped. *Health Psychol* 17:172, 1998.

Ory MG, Hoffman RR, Yee JL, Tennstedt S, Schulz R: Prevalence and impact of caregiving: a detailed comparison between dementia and nondementia caregivers. *Gerontologist* 39:177, 1999.

Picot SJ, Zauszniewski JA, Delgado C: Cardiovascular responses of African American female caregivers. *J Natl Black Nurses Assoc* 9:3, 1997.

Riedel S, Fredman L, Langenberg P: Associations among caregiving difficulties, burden, and rewards among caregivers to older post-rehabilitation patients. *J Gerontol B Psychol Sci Soc Sci* 53:165, 1998.

Rosenblatt DE: Elder abuse: what can physicians do? *Arch Fam Med* 5:88, 1996.

Scharlach AE, Midanik LT, Runkle MC, Soghikian K: Health practices of adults with elder care responsibilities. *Prev Med* 26:155, 1997.

Schulz R, AT O'Brien, Bookwala J, Fleissner K: Psychiatric and physical morbidity effects of dementia caregiving: prevalence, correlates, and causes. *Gerontologist* 35:771, 1995.

Shaw W, Patterson T, Semple S, et al: Longitudinal analysis of multiple indicators of health decline among spousal caregivers. *Ann Behav Med* 19:101, 1997.

Stein M, Miller AH: Stress, the immune system, and health and illness. In: Goldberger L, Breznitz S (eds): *Handbook of Stress, Theoretical and Clinical Aspects*, 2nd ed. New York: Free Press; 1993;127.

Suzman R, Willis D, Manton K: *The Oldest Old.* New York: Oxford University Press; 1992.

Tower RB, Kasl SV: Depressive symptoms across older spouses: longitudinal influences. *Psychol Aging* 11:683, 1996.

Uchino BN, Kiecolt-Glaser JK, Cacioppo JT: Age-related changes in cardiovascular response as a function of a chronic stressor and social support. *J Pers Soc Psychol* 63:839, 1992.

Vitaliano PP, Russo J, Niaura R: Plasma lipids and their relationships with psychosocial factors in older adults. *J Gerontol B Psychol Sci Soc Sci* 50:18, 1995.

Vitaliano PP, Russo J, Scanlan JM, Greeno CG: Weight changes in caregivers of Alzheimer's care recipients: psychobehavioral predictors. *Psychol Aging* 11:155, 1996.

Winslow BW: Effects of formal supports on stress outcomes in family caregivers of Alzheimer's patients. *Res Nurs Health* 20:27, 1997.

Chapter 5

Robert J. Michocki

Polypharmacy and Principles of Drug Therapy

Overview

Although persons older than 65 years represent 12.7 percent of the U.S. population, they receive some 700 million, or 28 percent, of all prescriptions per year. It is estimated that 75 percent of the ambulatory elderly take at least one prescription medication daily. About two-thirds of the elderly also use nonprescription drugs, often without discussing drug use with their clinician. One study reported that elderly women took an average of 5.7 prescription drugs and 3.2 over-the-counter (OTC) drugs concurrently. In another study of office visits of persons older than 85 years, 21 percent took one drug; 14 percent, two drugs; and 11 percent, three drugs. Cardiovascular and renal agents, analgesics, endocrine agents, and antibiotics were most frequently prescribed.

Residents of long-term care facilities on average receive eight or more medications each day, much more than the average community-dwelling elderly person. Falls, delirium, depression, and many other conditions, such as incontinence and constipation, are prevalent among elderly persons residing in nursing homes and are frequently caused by or are side effects of medications.

Drug use among the elderly will continue to rise as the population older than 65 years increases and new therapies for Alzheimer's disease, Parkinson's disease, arthritis, and osteoporosis are brought to market. This trend is supported by the fact that industry sales of prescription drugs in 1996 totaled $85.4 billion, an increase of 12 percent from the previous year.

Although Medicare provides for hospital and physician benefits for 38 million persons older than 65 years, it does not include a general prescription drug benefit. Therefore the elderly who are most likely to have multiple chronic medical problems and have the greatest need for long-term drug therapy often are the least likely to be able to afford medications. About 20 percent of persons older than 65 years are currently enrolled in managed care Medicare plans that frequently include drug benefits, potentially offering some relief from the financial burdens of managing chronic illnesses with medications. The number of drugs, cost of medications, compliance, potential for adverse drug effects, drug interactions, and physiologic, pharmacokinetic, and pharmacodynamic changes among the elderly are challenges to those providing pharmaceutical care to this population.

Despite the proven benefits of an optimal medication plan, many patients are not receiving the most appropriate medications, and in many instances, they are being overmedicated. There may be a number of explanations for this phenomenon. First, great advances have been made in pharmacologic research, and many new drugs are continuously being approved, often making it difficult for health care providers to keep abreast of current information. In 1999, more than 40 new medications were approved by the Food and Drug Administration. Second, it is not unusual for elderly patients to see multiple providers, including many subspecialists, who may not be aware of all the medications the patient is receiving. Third, elderly patients may not be compliant with taking their medications as prescribed because of cost, side effects, poor understanding of the importance of taking the medication, and a perception of no or marginal benefit. Fourth, because of patient noncompliance new medications may be added or dosages increased in an attempt to achieve defined therapeutic end points. This may cause toxicity or adverse drug events. Finally, pharmacodynamic and pharmacokinetic changes that occur with aging can affect the expected therapeutic response.

Using many drugs to treat patients with multiple chronic diseases may lead to drug-drug, drug-disease, and drug-nutrient interactions. When deciding to use a pharmacologic intervention in the care of an elderly patient, the provider must perform a comprehensive assessment. The provider should evaluate the presence and severity of concurrent diseases; use of other medications, including prescription and OTC drugs; economic factors that may affect the affordability of the medication to be prescribed; and familiarity with all pharmacologic aspects of the proposed drug.

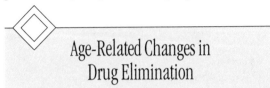

Age-Related Changes in Drug Elimination

Pharmacokinetics is the absorption, distribution, metabolism, and excretion of drugs. The aging process may affect these processes.

Absorption

Few changes in absorption of medications have been demonstrated, and drug absorption generally is complete, although slower, among elderly persons. The time to peak onset of action of certain medications may be delayed. Analgesics are a common medication for which absorption is slowed. The amount of drug that reaches the systemic circulation depends on the bioavailability of the drug after absorption. Some drugs, such as the bisphosphonates (alendronate, etidronate, risedronate, tiludronate), are poorly bioavailable. In the fasting state, less than 1 percent of the administered dose reaches the systemic circulation. Administration of these medications with food decreases absorption and further reduces the amount of drug that reaches the systemic circulation.

Drug-drug and drug-food interactions may influence the absorption of medications. For example, the fluoroquinolones interact with divalent and trivalent cations (antacids, iron, sucralfate) and reduce absorption of these antibiotics. On the other hand, concurrent diseases such as heart failure may increase serum concentrations of drugs such as levodopa, nifedipine, and omeprazole by reducing hepatic blood flow. The reduction in hepatic flow minimizes the hepatic first-pass effect and increases the amount of drug that reaches the systemic circulation. Medications such as levodopa, nifedipine, and omeprazole have been shown to have increased bioavailability in the elderly.

Body Composition

Age-associated changes in body composition, including increased fat mass and a general decline in body weight, account for altered distribution of many medications among older persons. Drug dosage recommendations may have to be altered on the basis of estimations of lean body mass. Loading doses may have to be modified because of decreases in total body water. Fat-soluble drugs (sedative-hypnotic agents) may have to be administered in lower doses because of the potential for accumulation in fatty tissues and therefore a longer duration of action.

Metabolism

Most drug metabolism occurs in the liver. Hepatic metabolism of medications occurs mainly through oxidation, reduction, and hydrolysis, which may decline with advancing years. Normal aging is associated with few changes in metabolic liver capacity, but hepatic blood flow declines as much as 40 percent with advanced age. Thus there is marked variability in hepatic drug metabolism with advancing years.

Biotransformation that occurs through the cytochrome P450 system also may occur more slowly among older persons. This process may affect the metabolism of drugs such as warfarin, phenytoin, and diazepam. Cigarette smoking, alcohol use, and caffeine use also may affect hepatic metabolism of medications.

Distribution

Drug distribution can be affected by serum concentration of binding proteins, such as albumin and α_1-acid glycoprotein. Chronic disease and protein-calorie undernutrition affect serum albumin levels, and α_1-acid glycoprotein levels may be affected by acute illnesses such as infection, cancer, heart failure, stroke, and trauma. Protein binding is especially important for medications with low therapeutic indexes, such as phenytoin, lidocaine, quinidine, and tricyclic antidepressants. Albumin binding also is important for acidic medications such as warfarin and naproxen.

Phenytoin therapy is particularly difficult among the elderly. High protein binding (90 percent) and complex pharmacokinetics necessitate careful dosing and monitoring for this population. Serum concentrations of phenytoin reflect total drug, free and bound phenytoin. In the presence of a low serum albumin level, the free fraction increases while total drug concentration remains unchanged. Toxicity can occur with a "therapeutic" serum concentration.

Elimination

Drug elimination among older persons is most affected by age-related declines in glomerular filtration rate and renal blood flow, which declines approximately 1 percent per year after 50 years of age. Serum creatinine levels do not always reflect accurate estimates of glomerular filtration rate because of age-associated declines in muscle mass. Among patients with protein-calorie undernutrition, results of renal function tests may be normal despite substantial renal impairment. Estimates of creatinine clearance should be carefully considered when establishing dosing levels in treatment of elderly persons. Dosing of medications with narrow therapeutic indices should be based on serum drug levels. Table 5-1 lists some medications that require dosing modifications in the care of patients with reduced renal function.

Other Changes

A final consideration in age-related drug elimination is that older persons may respond to medications differently from younger persons. This may occur because of alterations at a receptor level, such as down-regulation of β-adrenergic receptor activity, or at a tissue or organ level, such as

Table 5-1

Drugs That Require Dosing Modification in the Care of Patients with Reduced Renal Function

Antimicrobial agents
Amantadine
Ciprofloxacin, levofloxacin, ofloxacin,
Sparfloxacin
Ethambutol
Gentamicin, tobramycin, amikacin
Imipenem
Penicillins
Vancomycin
Cardiovascular agents
Atenolol
Digoxin
Enalapril, lisinopril, quinapril, ramipril
Nadolol
Gastrointestinal agents
Cimetidine, famotidine, nizatidine, ranitidine
Oral hypoglycemic agents
Acetohexamide
Chlorpropamide
Glyburide
Tolazamide

enhanced sedation, memory loss with benzodiazepines, or greater pain relief with narcotics. This alteration in receptor sensitivity often is referred to as the *pharmacodynamic changes associated with aging.* There is much interindividual variability in effects of most medications used to treat older persons.

Polypharmacy

Definition

Polypharmacy or polymedicine often is defined as the use of multiple drugs. Other definitions of polypharmacy include prescribing more medications than are clinically indicated, a medical regimen that includes at least one unnecessary medicine, or the empiric use of five or more medications. Recent definitions are that *polymedicine* is the use of multiple medications to treat elderly patients for multiple comorbid conditions, whereas *polypharmacy* is a less-than-desirable state in which duplicative medications are prescribed, drug-drug interactions are likely, and prescribers pay inadequate attention to pharmacokinetic and pharmacodynamic principles. *Polypharmacy* indicates that a particular patient receives too many drugs, drugs for too long a time, or drugs in exceedingly high doses.

Regardless of semantics, polypharmacy is universally condemned, widely practiced, often unnecessary, yet sometimes required. The elderly are particularly sensitive to the effects of drugs, yet multiple drugs often are necessary to manage the numerous medical problems that occur among this population. German and Burton suggested that the following major factors contribute to polypharmacy: multiple chronic medical problems; prescribing by multiple physicians; lack of coordination of care; vague symptoms; patient pressure to prescribe; and use of additional medications to manage drug-related disorders.

Guidelines for Drug Use

Perhaps the best way to approach managing the often complex drug regimens of elderly patients is to adhere to a few simple guidelines (Table 5-2). Patients should be instructed to bring all medications to each visit with the physician for visual inspection and review of directions and indications.

OVER-THE-COUNTER MEDICATIONS

Because there is good evidence that older persons are likely to be taking as many as three OTC drugs at any given time with potentially deleterious consequences, use of these agents, such as vit-

Table 5-2

Guidelines to Follow before Prescribing a Drug

Visually inspect and review all medications and their directions and indications at each visit.

Ask about over-the-counter drugs and vitamin supplements.

For new problems, review whether any of the current medications may be responsible.

Keep the dosing regimen as simple as possible.

Establish a therapeutic goal for each medication.

Establish indexes of toxicity.

Look for potential drug-drug interactions.

Look for drug-disease interactions.

Know how the drug is eliminated.

Start with the lowest dose.

Provide verbal instructions to the patient and caregiver.

Have the patient and caregiver repeat the verbal instructions.

Do not make too many changes in the drug regimen at any one time.

Use medications that have been shown to decrease morbidity and mortality.

amins, cold remedies, analgesics, and antacids, always should be explored. For example, chronic use of phenylpropanolamine, found in many OTC cough and cold preparations and appetite suppressant products, may cause or worsen high blood pressure, nervousness, and restlessness. With the widespread availability of OTC nonsteroidal anti-inflammatory drugs (NSAIDs), patients unknowingly may predispose themselves to toxicity by consuming a prescription NSAID along with an OTC NSAID.

ASSESSING SYMPTOMS

When assessing a new patient's symptoms, physicians should consider whether any of the currently prescribed medications is responsible. All current medications should be reviewed for potential drug-drug interactions. All intercurrent and concurrent diseases must be carefully evaluated to make sure there is no potential for drug-disease interactions.

CONCOMITANT CONDITIONS

It is especially important to review the list of medical problems to identify conditions in which drug therapy has been shown to decrease morbidity and mortality. For example, there is excellent evidence that, among patients with congestive heart failure, therapy with angiotensin-converting enzyme inhibitors improves quality of life and reduces mortality. Among patients who have sustained myocardial infarction the use of β-blockers improves survival and alleviates symptoms.

PHARMACOKINETICS

Physicians must be thoroughly familiar with the pharmacokinetics and pharmacodynamics of each of the medications a patient is currently taking and how these drugs may interact with a new medication to be prescribed. It is important to know how each drug is eliminated, especially drugs that are renally excreted (see Table 5-1) and may require a dosage reduction. When a decision is made to prescribe a new medication, the dosing regimen should be as simple as possible. In general, a low dose should first be prescribed to ensure tolerance. Thereafter dosing should be increased slowly to minimize potential adverse events. Once or twice a day dosing is preferable to other schedules and is likely to improve compliance and adherence.

GOALS OF TREATMENT AND LIKELY SIDE EFFECTS

Before prescribing drugs, physicians should determine a therapeutic goal and specific indexes of toxicity. Patients should be informed of potential usual and unusual adverse effects, how to monitor for occurrence of these effects, and what to do should an effect occur. It often is useful to provide patients and family members with verbal and written instructions regarding the indications for and proper use of prescription medications in the hope that compliance will be ensured. Written instructions are most useful, especially for patients who are taking multiple concurrent medications. For patients with cognitive impairment, it is vital that the caregiver understand the indications and instructions for use of the medication. Compliance often is improved when caregivers set out medications for patients on a daily or weekly basis or when pharmacists provide convenient dose and schedule packaging of medications. Table 5-3 provides a list of compliance aids.

CHANGING MEDICATION

It is important not to attempt to make too many changes in medication regimens at any one time and to recognize that using multiple drugs to manage many comorbid medical conditions often is necessary in the care of older patients. The medication regimen should be reviewed at preset intervals to determine whether components of the regimen can be deleted. It is always easier to start medications but often is difficult to discontinue them. Drugs can be administered safely if appropriate precautions are followed. Patients, physicians, and caregivers must be educated about rational drug use. The necessary monitoring must be conducted in a timely manner to ensure that therapeutic end points have been achieved and that adverse drug events are avoided.

Table 5-3
Compliance Aids

Calendars
Charts
Blister packs
Pill boxes
Programmable alarm devices
Pill dispensers
Caregiver training
Home health aides

Adverse Drug Reactions

Occurrence

Adverse drug reactions (ADRs), unlike medication errors, which are preventable events caused by health care providers, patients, and caregivers, are unexpected, unintended, or excessive responses to medication. In a study of ambulatory veterans taking five or more scheduled medications, 35 percent of the patients reported adverse drug events, and more than 90 percent of the events were classified as predictable. The use of OTC medications in the ambulatory setting also leads to many undocumented ADRs. For example, OTC cold medications that have anticholinergic or α-agonist properties can cause serious toxicity among elderly persons, such as confusion, urinary retention, dry mouth, constipation, and potential exacerbation of closed-angle glaucoma.

ADRs occur in many settings. In a tertiary-care teaching hospital, over a 1-year period, 696 prescribing errors were identified that had the potential for adverse effects. Over a 9-year period, more than 11,000 confirmed medication prescribing errors with the potential for adverse patient consequences were detected.

In long-term care facilities, despite the implementation of federal regulations for comprehensive drug regimen review, ADRs are frequent. In two nursing homes in rural Georgia, more than 50 percent of the residents had probable ADRs. The frequency of those events was greatest among patients taking multiple medications. Cardiovascular drugs, mainly digoxin and diuretics, NSAIDs, and psychotropic agents, because of their high frequency of use by the elderly, have been the largest contributors to ADRs. The most commonly implicated drugs are shown in Table 5-4. One example is the use of the antihistamine diphenhydramine (Benadryl), commonly prescribed as a hypnotic medication in the care of elderly institutionalized patients. It has significant anticholinergic

Table 5-4

Medications Commonly Implicated in Adverse Drug Reactions in Nursing Homes

Antibiotics
Antipsychotics
Anxiolytics
Digoxin
Diuretics
Histamine 2 receptor antagonists
Insulin
Nonsteriodal anti-inflammatory agents
Potassium supplements
Theophylline

properties and potential toxicity, such as sedation, dry mouth, confusion, and urinary retention.

Causes and Risk Factors

Whether age is an independent risk factor of ADRs remains to be determined. In a comprehensive literature review covering articles from 1966 through 1990, Gurwitz and Avorn concluded that most studies neglected to address the issues of whether the increased frequency of ADRs among the elderly is attributable to age alone and whether older patients are more likely to have coexisting illnesses and to be taking more medications. It seems reasonable to conclude that, regardless of age, the more medications prescribed, the greater is the risk of an adverse event.

In a study of ADRs in hospitals, the most common factors associated with errors were those related to knowledge—application of knowledge about drug therapy and knowledge regarding patient factors that affect drug therapy. Dosing errors, prescribing medications to which patients were allergic, and prescribing inappropriate dosage forms were the most common types of errors. The authors suggested that the availability of new drugs and the intensity of medical care were playing a major role in the occurrence of medication prescribing errors.

It is apparent that the use of multiple medications increases the risk of ADRs, drug-drug, and drug-disease interactions in a variety of clinical settings. Health providers who care for the elderly must become more knowledgeable about the drugs they prescribe and be more vigilant in monitoring their effects so that potential adverse drug consequences may be prevented. Stewart and Cooper suggested that methods to reduce polypharmacy should include patient and physician education, including education and feedback systems, and regulatory intervention with continual drug and disease monitoring components.

Cost

Adverse drug events occur frequently among hospitalized patients, often prolonging hospital stays at an increased cost of $2000 to $4600 per hospital stay and a twofold increase in the risk of death than that for aged-matched controls. An analysis by Johnson and Bootman estimated that drug-related morbidity costs $76.6 billion annually in the ambulatory setting; the largest component of this total cost is associated with drug-related hospitalization.

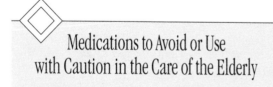

Medications to Avoid or Use with Caution in the Care of the Elderly

Medications to Avoid

Some drugs should be avoided if at all possible in the care of elderly patients because of undocumented efficacy, safety, and cost problems relative to other preferred drug or nondrug modalities for the usual indications. For example, long-acting benzodiazepines should be avoided by the elderly if at all possible. These drugs have been shown to

be associated with a markedly increased risk of falling and hip fracture and risk of motor vehicle crashes among the elderly population. Other drugs to avoid include centrally acting antihypertensive agents (methyldopa, clonidine), propoxyphene combinations, indomethacin because of potential gastrointestinal and renal toxicity, and chlorpropamide. Knapp examined the appropriateness of drug prescribing by U.S. physicians for ambulatory geriatric patients and found that approximately 10 percent of all drugs prescribed were those that should be avoided by the elderly.

Medications to Use with Caution

Medications with a narrow therapeutic index require special attention when used by any age group. The elderly, because of alterations in physiologic reserve and pharmacodynamic and pharmacokinetic changes, may be particularly prone to adverse drug events. For example, digoxin is used frequently for ventricular rate control in the care of patients with atrial fibrillation. Digoxin has a narrow therapeutic index; small changes in serum concentration may produce dramatic changes in clinical effects. Because this drug is excreted by the kidneys, and older persons have an age-associated reduction in creatinine clearance, the dose must be carefully titrated to avoid accumulation and potential digoxin toxicity. Thus digoxin and other medications that have narrow therapeutic indexes (carbamazepine and phenytoin, theophylline, and warfarin) should be used cautiously and monitored appropriately.

NSAIDs are frequently prescribed for the elderly. As a class, these drugs are effective at providing analgesia and reducing signs and symptoms of inflammation. Although these drugs are well-tolerated by most patients, a small percentage of patients may have substantial morbidity and mortality. Use of NSAIDs may be associated with gastrointestinal hemorrhage, and advancing age is a primary risk factor. The introduction of the new selective cyclooxygenase 2 (COX-2) inhibitors may decrease some of the adverse gastrointestinal side effects associated with the use of these drugs. Until more data become available, use of these drugs should continue but with caution in the care of the elderly. The results of postmarketing surveillance will be critical in determining the ultimate benefit and safety profile of COX-2 inhibitors. NSAIDs, including the COX-2 inhibitors, also may worsen renal function, and the elderly are especially at risk. The presence of reduced renal function, volume depletion, and the concurrent use of other nephrotoxic drugs predispose patients to NSAID-induced nephropathy. Elderly patients undergoing long-term NSAID therapy should be carefully monitored to prevent worsening renal function.

Criteria for Appropriate Prescribing

To develop explicit criteria for appropriate prescribing for the elderly, Beers assembled a nationally recognized expert panel in geriatric care and pharmacology. The panel defined criteria for medications that would be inappropriate to prescribe for elderly patients with 15 common medical conditions. Beers' final criteria provide the rationale for a number of medications or drug classes that should not be used by older patients. The medications, independent of diagnosis, are listed in Table 5-5. These medications should be avoided or be used with caution with appropriate monitoring because they lack efficacy, increase toxicity when safer alternatives are available, or increase sensitivity to side effects among the elderly. Beers also provides disease-specific information on drugs to avoid in the care of older persons (Table 5-6).

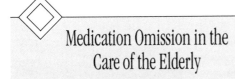

Medication Omission in the Care of the Elderly

Table 5-5

Medications to Avoid or Use with Caution in the Care of the Elderly

Lack of efficacy
  Ergot mesyloids
  Muscle relaxants (methocarbamol,
    chlorzoxazone, carisoprodol)
  Trimethobenzamide
Increased toxicity; safer alternatives are
  available
  Barbiturates, excluding phenobarbital
  Chlordiazepoxide
  Chlorpropamide
  Diazepam
  Digoxin
  Dipyridamole
  Disopyramide
  Doxepin
  Flurazepam
  Meperidine
  Meprobamate
  Methyldopa and combinations
  Propoxyphene and combinations
  Reserpine
  Ticlopidine
Increased sensitivity to side effects
  Amitriptyline and combinations
  Antihistamines with potent anticholinergic
    effects
  Diphenhydramine
  Gastrointestinal antispasmodics
  Indomethacin
  Iron more than 325 mg
  Long-acting benzodiazepine
  Pentazocine
  Phenylbutazone

SOURCE: Modified with permission from Beers M: Explicit criteria for determining potentially inappropriate medication use by the elderly. *Arch Intern Med* 157:1531, 1997.

Health care providers must be careful not to overlook omissions of important medications, that is, those for which there is strong scientific evidence

that a particular therapeutic intervention reduces morbidity and mortality. In one study more than 1 million patients 65 years or older with a chronic

Table 5-6

Disease-Drug Interactions Among the Elderly

DISEASE OR CONDITION	MEDICATIONS TO AVOID
Heart failure	Disopyramide and drugs with high sodium content, such as sodium bicarbonate
Diabetes	β-blockers in the care of patients receiving oral hypoglycemics or insulin
Hypertension	Diet pills, amphetamines
Chronic obstructive pulmonary lung disease	β-blockers, sedative-hypnotic agents
Asthma	β-blockers
Ulcers	NSAIDs, potassium supplements Aspirin >325 mg/d
Seizures, epilepsy	Clozapine, chlorpromazine (Thorazine), thioridazine, chlorprothixene, metoclopramide
Peripheral vascular disease	β-blockers
Blood clotting disorders among patients taking anticoagulants	Aspirin, NSAIDs Dipyridamole, ticlopidine
Benign prostatic hypertrophy	Anticholinergic antihistamines Gastrointestinal antispasmodics Muscle relaxants, narcotic drugs Flavoxate, oxybutynin, bethanechol Anticholinergic antidepressants
Incontinence	α-blockers
Constipation	Anticholinergic drugs, narcotic drugs Tricyclic antidepressants
Syncope or falls	β-blockers Long-acting benzodiazepines
Arrhythmia	Tricyclic antidepressants
Insomnia	Decongestants, theophylline, desipramine, selective serotonin reuptake inhibitors, methylphenidate, monoamine oxidase inhibitors, β-agonists

SOURCE: Adapted with permission from Beers M: Explicit criteria for determining potentially inappropriate medication use by the elderly. *Arch Intern Med* 157:1531, 1997.

disease (diabetes mellitus, pulmonary emphysema, psychotic syndromes) were found to have concurrent unrelated medical disorders for which they frequently were not treated. Estrogen replacement therapy and therapy for hyperlipidemia and arthritis were underprescribed for these groups. Among women in the early postmenopausal period, estrogen replacement therapy may reduce cardiovascu-

lar risk and risk of osteoporosis. Lipid lowering can reduce cardiovascular mortality, especially among elderly persons at high risk. Treating patients for chronic arthritis can improve quality of life. It is important for health care providers to recognize that treating patients for these conditions can improve the quality or duration of life or both, even among those with concomitant chronic illnesses.

β-Blockers after Myocardial Infarction

An example of missing a treatment opportunity that has been shown to prolong survival is failing to prescribe β-blockers after myocardial infarction. Gottlieb et al reported that patients who had sustained acute myocardial infarction and received β-blockers had a 28 to 40 percent lower mortality than those who did not have β-blockers prescribed at the time of discharge from the hospital. However, in the study in which most of the patients were older than 65 years, only one of three heart attack survivors received β-blockers, indicating suboptimal use of this therapy among the elderly.

Angiotensin-Converting Enzyme Inhibitors for Congestive Heart Failure

Because of their beneficial effects on mortality risk and functional status, angiotensin-converting enzyme inhibitors should be prescribed for patients with left-ventricular systolic dysfunction unless a specific contraindication exists (history of intolerance or adverse reaction, renal insufficiency, serum potassium level greater than 5.5 mEq/L, symptomatic hypotension).

Warfarin for Atrial Fibrillation

The beneficial effects of reducing the risk of thromboembolic events among patients with chronic atrial fibrillation deserve attention. Atrial fibrillation is the most common cause of cardioembolic stroke and accounts for more than 50,000 strokes per year. Despite convincing evidence that anticoagulation therapy reduces the risk of stroke among patients with atrial fibrillation, there is still reluctance to initiate anticoagulation therapy in the care of elderly patients. In 1992 and 1993, only 15 percent of patients with atrial fibrillation being observed by general or family practitioners received anticoagulant therapy. Older patients were found to have the lowest rates of anticoagulant use. It is estimated that 40,000 strokes could be prevented each year with appropriate use of anticoagulant therapy. There is convincing evidence that prophylactic use of warfarin reduces the incidence of new cerebrovascular events among patients with chronic atrial fibrillation. The elderly are at high risk of falling; thus it is important to weigh the risk-to-benefit ratio of therapy, the likelihood of compliance with therapy, and the potential for adverse consequences.

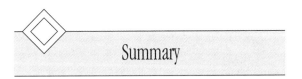

Summary

Drug therapy continues to be one of the most cost-effective methods of management of chronic disease among the elderly. Polypharmacy or polymedicine often is inevitable in the care of elderly patients who have multiple chronic diseases. As health care providers, we should attempt to ensure that our patients receive appropriate pharmacologic interventions and that the regimen is reviewed, evaluated, and monitored in a timely way. Chronic care is constantly changing care and therefore requires timely reevaluation. Health care providers should minimize the number of drugs prescribed but not withhold medications that can improve quality of life and prolong survival. Providers must become familiar with the medications that they prescribe and with the effects of these drugs on an older population. Duplicative therapy should be recognized and avoided. Dosing regimens should be as simple as possible with once- or twice-daily schedules to enhance compliance. Providers must be aware of drug-drug and drug-disease interactions to avoid potential adverse drug events.

Most of the elderly population is ambulatory, and a large percentage of Medicare patients do not have a drug benefit. Therapeutic plans will be successful only if the patient purchases the drugs and complies with treatment. As difficult as it may be, providers must become more aware of the

Table 5-7

Stepwise Approach to Avoiding Polypharmacy

> Step 1. Disclose all medications being used.
> Step 2. Identify medications by generic name and drug class.
> Step 3. Identify the clinical indication for each medication.
> Step 4. Know the side-effect profile of each medication.
> Step 5. Identify risk factors of an adverse reaction.
> Step 6. Eliminate medications with no therapeutic benefit.
> Step 7. Eliminate medications with no clinical indication.
> Step 8. Substitute a safer medication.
> Step 9. Avoid managing an adverse drug reaction with a drug.
> Step 10. Use a single drug with an infrequent dosing schedule.

SOURCE: Adapted with permission from Carlson JH: Perils of polypharmacy: 10 steps to prudent prescribing. *Geriatrics* 51:26, 1996.

costs of pharmaceuticals and the effects of high costs on the cash-paying elderly. Most physicians do not understand the economic implications of the prescriptions they write. Elderly patients with complex medical problems and on fixed incomes may not be able to afford a medication. Alternatives that are less expensive should be evaluated.

Patients play an important role in their health care. Patients should be encouraged to use one pharmacy for their pharmaceutical needs. This can help reduce duplicative therapy, potential drug interactions, and adverse drug events. Patients also should be encouraged to bring all medications to the office at each visit. This ensures that the provider is aware of the medication regimen. It also provides an opportunity for health professionals to reinforce the directions and indications for each medication.

Providers may not be able to reduce the number of medications prescribed, but at least they should insist that the therapeutic regimen be prescribed

rationally so that potential side effects are minimized. Providers should monitor drug therapy and perform timely evaluations. Carlson describes a stepwise approach to polypharmacy (Table 5-7).

In managing chronic medical conditions of the elderly, health care providers should be vigilant in assessing the consequences of their prescribing decisions and be cognizant of the numerous variables that may adversely affect elderly patients. It is important to remember that the goal should be to improve quality of life, prolong survival, and avoid adverse events.

Bibliography

Albers G, Yim J, Belew K, et al: Status of antithrombotic therapy for patients with atrial fibrillation in university hospitals. *Arch Intern Med* 156:2311, 1996.

Bates DW, Spell N, Cullen DJ, et al: The costs of adverse drug events in hospitalized patients. *JAMA* 277:307, 1997.

Beers MH: Explicit criteria for determining potentially inappropriate medication use by the elderly. *Arch Intern Med* 157:1531, 1997.

Carlson JH: Perils of polypharmacy: 10 steps to prudent prescribing. *Geriatrics* 51:26, 1996.

Classen DC, Pestotnik SL, Evans RS, et al: Adverse drug events in hospitalized patients: excess length of stay, extra costs, and attributable mortality. *JAMA* 277:301, 1997.

Cooper JW: Probable adverse drug reactions in a rural geriatric nursing home population: a four year study. *J Am Geriatr Soc* 44:194, 1996.

Cummings SR, Nevitt MC, Browner WS, et al: Risk factors for hip fracture in white women. *N Engl J Med* 332:767, 1995.

Double-digit growth for industry in 1997. *US Pharmacist* 23:129, 1998.

Everitt DE, Avorn J: Drug prescribing for the elderly. *Arch Intern Med* 146:2393,1986.

German PS, Burton LC: Medications and the elderly: issues of prescription use. *J Aging Health* 1:4,1989.

Glickman L, Bruce EA, Caro FG, et al: Physician's knowledge of drug costs for the elderly. *J Am Geriatr Soc* 42:992, 1994.

Gottlieb SS, McCarter RJ, Vogel RA: Effect of beta blockade on mortality among high-risk and low-risk patients after myocardial infarction. *N Engl J Med* 339:489, 1998.

Gurwitz JH, Avorn J: The ambiguous relation between aging and adverse drug reactions. *Ann Intern Med* 114:956, 1991.

Hanlon JJ, Schmader KE, Koronkowski MJ, et al: Adverse drug events in high risk older outpatients. *J Am Geriatr Soc* 45:945, 1997.

Hemmelgarn B, Suissa S, Huang A, et al: Benzodiazepine use and the risk of motor vehicle crash in the elderly. *JAMA* 278:27, 1997.

Johnson JA, Bootman JL: Drug-related morbidity and mortality: a cost-of-illness model. *Arch Intern Med* 155:1949, 1995.

Knapp D, Michocki R: Drug prescribing for very elderly ambulatory patients: 1985. *J Am Geriatr Soc* 35:1036, 1987.

Knapp DA: National ambulatory prescribing of 'do not use' drug products for patients >60 years. *J Geriatr Drug Ther* 9:47, 1995.

Lesar T, Lomaestro BM, Pohl H: Medication prescribing errors in a teaching hospital: a 9 year experience. *Arch Intern Med* 157:1569, 1997.

Lesar TS, Briceland L, Stein DS: Factors related to errors in medication prescribing. *JAMA* 277:312, 1997.

Michocki R, Lamy P, Hooper F, et al: Drug prescribing for the elderly. *Arch Fam Med* 2:441, 1993.

Monane M, Monane S, Semla T: Optimal medication use in elders: key to successful aging. *West J Med* 167:233, 1997.

Ray WA, Griffin MR, Downey W: Benzodiazepines of long and short elimination half-life and the risk of hip fracture. *JAMA* 262:3303, 1989.

Redelmeier DA, Tan SH, Booth GL: The treatment of unrelated disorders in patients with chronic medical problems. *N Engl J Med* 338:1516, 1998.

Stafford RS, Singer DE: National patterns of warfarin use in atrial fibrillation. *Arch Intern Med* 156:2537, 1996.

Stewart RB, Cooper JW: Polypharmacy in the aged: practical solutions. *Drugs Aging* 4:449, 1994.

US Department of Commerce, Bureau of Census. *Projections of the Population of the United States by Age, Sex, and Race: 1988 to 2080*. Washington, DC: US Government Printing Office; 1989.

US National Center for Health Statistics. *Health, United States, 1993*. DHHS Publication no. (PHS) 94-1232. Hyattsville, MD: US National Center for Health Statistics, 1994.

Wolfe M, Lichtenstein DR, Singh G: Gastrointestinal toxicity of nonsteroidal anti-inflammatory drugs. *N Engl J Med* 340:1888, 1999.

Part 2

Genitourinary Problems

Barry D. Weiss

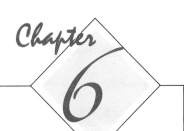

Chapter 6

Urinary Incontinence

Overview: How Common Is Incontinence in Office Practice?

Urinary incontinence can occur at any age. It is normal among newborns, occurs as enuresis among young children, and may develop as stress incontinence among women of childbearing age. Urinary incontinence is most common, however, among older persons—so common that it is considered a classic syndrome in geriatric medicine.

Definition

The precise prevalence of incontinence is difficult to determine, because published studies on the frequency of incontinence have used different subject populations, different methods for questioning subjects about incontinence, and different definitions of what constitutes incontinence. In clinical practice, perhaps the most practical and patient-centered definition is an uncontrollable loss of urine at inappropriate or unwanted times, regardless of the specific frequency or amount of urine lost, that the patient perceives to be a social or hygienic problem. This definition is rarely used in epidemiologic research.

Definitions of incontinence in prevalence surveys vary widely in terms of both the frequency and volume of episodes of incontinence (Table 6-1). The prevalence of incontinence has been studied by means of questioning patients in clinicians' offices, hospitals, day-care centers, and long-term care facilities. Other studies have focused on patients enrolled in a practice or specific segments of a community or on national samples. Questioning methods also vary. They

Table 6-1

Definitions of Urinary Incontinence Used in Prevalence Studies

Urine-loss definitions
  Difficulty holding urine until you get to a
    toilet
  Unexpected or uncontrolled loss of urine
  Loss of control of urine
  Wet underpants
Severity definitions
  Once or more
  Twice or more
  Three times or more
  Bad enough to cause social or hygienic
    problems
Frequency definitions
  Ever
  Past year
  Past month
  Past week
  Per day

SOURCE: Data reproduced from Thom D: Variations in estimates of urinary incontinence prevalence in the community: effects of differences in definition, population characteristics, and study type. *J Am Geriatr Soc* 46:473, 1998.

have included in-person interviews, telephone interviews, and mailed surveys, each of which likely elicits a different response from subjects.

Prevalence

The approximate prevalence of incontinence in community-based populations of older persons can be estimated by averaging the results of the many studies and focusing on studies with the most representative sampling methods. About one-half of older persons who are homebound or in long-term care facilities have some degree of urinary incontinence. Among persons living in the community who are not homebound, some degree of incontinence occurs among about one-third of women and just fewer than one-fourth of men older than 60 years. The prevalence increases with age. A

smaller percentage of community-dwelling older persons have continuous or daily incontinence with no appreciable urinary control (Table 6-2).

Unrecognized Incontinence

Although incontinence is common, it is frequently not identified by clinicians. Few clinicians report rates of incontinence among their office patients equal to the rate of incontinence in the general population.

Underrecognition of incontinence occurs partly because clinicians do not routinely ask patients about incontinence. A study involving geriatric-aged simulated patients (i.e., actors) sent to primary care clinicians' offices found that only one-third of physician assistants and only 11 percent of physicians and nurse practitioners asked these patients about incontinence, even though the simulated patients would have responded "yes" had they had been asked whether they had incontinence.

Underrecognition also occurs because patients do not seek care for or volunteer information about incontinence. Fewer than one-third of older persons with urinary incontinence have ever

Table 6-2

Prevalence of Incontinence Among Geriatric-Aged Populations

DEMOGRAPHIC GROUP	PREVALENCE MEAN PERCENTAGE (RANGE)
Community-dwelling older women	
Any frequency of incontinence	35 (17–55)
Daily incontinence	14 (3–17)
Community-dwelling older men	
Any frequency of incontinence	22 (11–34)
Daily incontinence	4 (2–11)

SOURCE: Data reproduced from Thom D: Variations in estimates of urinary incontinence prevalence in the community: effects of differences in definition, population characteristics, and study type. *J Am Geriatr Soc* 46:473, 1998.

sought care for the problem. Patients tend to avoid discussing the problem because of embarrassment, because they believe incontinence is a normal aspect of aging for which no treatment is available, or because they do not want to undergo surgery and they believe surgery is the only available treatment.

If incontinence is to be detected, therefore, it is important to include specific questions about incontinence when taking a medical history from any older patient. The data in Table 6-2 provide evidence that such questioning will yield many positive responses.

Principal Diagnoses

For practical purposes, it is useful to consider three basic pathophysiologic mechanisms, or common pathways, that lead to urinary incontinence. The three basic mechanisms are overactivity of the bladder detrusor muscle (urge incontinence), malfunction of the urinary sphincters (stress incontinence), and overflow bladder (urinary retention). Each of the three mechanisms can have transient or irreversible causes. Transient causes are those that can be resolved with removal of or therapy for a potentially transient factor, such as a medication or an infection. Irreversible causes cannot be eliminated and necessitate therapy aimed at restoration of urinary control. Although a great number of conditions can cause urinary incontinence among older persons, all of these conditions can be categorized under one of the three major mechanisms of incontinence. Within each category, the conditions are classified as being either transient or irreversible.

Detrusor Overactivity (Urge Incontinence)

Detrusor overactivity (urge incontinence) occurs when patients lack the ability to control or inhibit

contractions of the bladder detrusor muscle, the principal contractile structure of the urinary bladder. When the bladder fills with urine, stretch receptors in the bladder wall transmit neural signals through the sacral plexus and spinal cord to a micturition center in the brainstem. The brainstem micturition center then transmits neural impulses back through the spinal cord and sacral plexus to the detrusor muscle. This reflex loop produces detrusor muscle contractions and voiding. Innervation of the detrusor muscle is primarily cholinergic.

Stimulation of detrusor contractions by the brainstem micturition center is inhibited by neural centers in the frontal cortex, basal ganglia, and cerebellum. Inhibitory activity from these centers keeps the bladder relaxed during filling and allows voluntarily postponement of urination when the urge to void occurs.

Incontinence occurs when the detrusor muscle is overactive in relation to the ability of the inhibitory centers to prevent it from contracting. Detrusor muscle overactivity can occur because function of the inhibitory centers is impaired from a variety of causes, such as neurologic disease, sedating drugs, or hypoxia. Detrusor overactivity also can be caused by inflammation or irritation within the bladder that increases stimulation of detrusor contractions. This occurs with conditions such as acute urinary tract infection, bladder calculi or neoplasms, or postmenopausal atrophic inflammation of the genitourinary tract. It also occurs when patients have particularly rapid urine production that leads to a high flow of urine into the bladder. This situation can occur when patients take diuretic medications or have a condition such as glycosuria or hypercalciuria that causes endogenous osmotic diuresis.

POTENTIALLY TRANSIENT CAUSES OF DETRUSOR OVERACTIVITY

A variety of potentially transient conditions can cause urinary incontinence caused by detrusor overactivity (Table 6-3). Each can be detected, or at least suspected, with a medical history, physical

Table 6-3

Potentially Transient Causes of Urge Incontinence

CAUSE	MECHANISM
Drug Effects	
Diuretics	Rapid bladder filling overrides ability to delay micturition
Caffeine	Diuretic effect
Sedatives	Depressed function of brain centers that inhibit micturition
Alcohol	Diuretic effect; sedative effect
Metabolic and neurologic effects	
Hypoxemia	Depressed function of brain centers that inhibit micturition
Delirium	Depressed function of brain centers that inhibit micturition
Hyperglycemia	Diuretic effect of accompanying glycosuria
Hypercalcemia	Diuretic effect of accompanying hypercalciuria
Excess fluid consumption	Rapid bladder filling overrides ability to delay micturition
Bladder inflammation	
Acute urinary tract infection	Inflammation leads to uninhibited bladder contractions
Atrophic vaginitis	Inflamed atrophic tissue extends into urethra and bladder, leading to uninhibited bladder contractions

examination, and urinalysis. Such transient causes occur among as many as one-third of older patients with urinary incontinence. Although no good data document the relative frequency of these transient causes, drug effects are likely the most common cause. In addition to drug effects and the other causes shown in Table 6-3, some persons have impairments of walking, such as severe arthritis, which prevent them from reaching toilet facilities with sufficient speed when they feel the urge to void. These persons have relative detrusor overactivity in which they are unable to inhibit micturition for a sufficient length of time. Improvement in mobility may improve or resolve incontinence.

IRREVERSIBLE CAUSES OF DETRUSOR OVERACTIVITY

Irreversible detrusor overactivity can occur when function of the cerebral inhibitory centers is diminished or interrupted by a degenerative neurologic disorder. When detrusor overactivity is caused by such neurologic conditions, the patient is said to have *detrusor hyperreflexia*. The most common degenerative conditions causing detrusor hyperreflexia are dementia, Parkinson's disease, and stroke, but it can occur with any neurodegenerative conditions, ranging from normal-pressure hydrocephalus to cerebral neoplasms.

Impairment of the inhibitory centers can also be idiopathic, in which case it is presumed to be caused by aged-related neuronal degeneration. This situation, often called *detrusor instability*, is even more common than incontinence caused by neurodegenerative disorders. Differentiating detrusor hyperreflexia and detrusor instability, however, has limited value in primary care because both conditions manifest as urge incontinence and the treatments are the same.

Patients with lesions that interrupt the spinal cord lose all cerebral inhibitory input to the detrusor. Among such patients, bladder filling leads to automatic bladder emptying and is mediated by a simple reflex loop through the sacral plexus. This condition often is called *automatic bladder* or *neurogenic bladder*.

Sphincter Malfunction (Stress Incontinence)

Normal urinary sphincter function requires integrity and normal function of the sacral nerves that innervate the sphincter muscles. The function and innervation of the sphincter are complex, but from a clinical point of view, it is useful to consider the sphincter as having voluntary and involuntary components. The voluntary sphincter muscles are the periurethral skeletal muscles of the pelvic floor. The involuntary sphincter muscles are urethral smooth muscles that receive α-adrenergic and β-adrenergic innervation. α-Adrenergic innervation causes constriction of the sphincter and β-adrenergic innervation relaxes the sphincter.

Normal sphincter function also requires appropriate urethral positioning and coaptation (closure of the urethral walls against themselves). The normal position of the urethra is such that it is exposed to intraabdominal pressure. When intraabdominal pressure increases, as from coughing or sneezing, the pressure is transmitted not only to the bladder but also to the urethra. Simultaneous transmission of pressure to both the bladder and urethra prevents establishment of a pressure gradient between the bladder and the urethra and thereby prevents the bladder from emptying.

POTENTIALLY TRANSIENT CAUSES OF SPHINCTER MALFUNCTION

Side effects of medications are the most important transient causes of sphincter malfunction. In particular, α-adrenergic blocking agents used to control hypertension, such as doxazosin, prazosin, and terazosin, reduce the sphincter-constricting influence of α-adrenergic innervation on the sphincter, leading to leakage of urine. β-Adrenergic agonist medication can have a similar effect by augmenting β-adrenergic-mediated urethral relaxation.

IRREVERSIBLE CAUSES OF SPHINCTER MALFUNCTION

The most common nontransient cause of urethral malfunction among older women is hyper-mobility of the urethra (urethral prolapse) that causes the classic syndrome of stress incontinence. In classic stress incontinence, the bladder leaks urine each time intraabdominal pressure increases, because the hypermobile urethra is positioned such that increases in intraabdominal pressure are not transmitted to it. When intraabdominal pressure increases, pressure on the bladder increases without a concomitant increase in urethral pressure, leading to a pressure gradient and leakage of urine.

Sphincter malfunction with stress incontinence also occurs in a syndrome known as *intrinsic urethral deficiency* (ISD), in which the urethral sphincter is unable to generate enough closing pressure to retain urine in the bladder. Among persons of geriatric age, ISD is most often caused by sphincter denervation after prostatectomy, trauma, radiation therapy, malignant disease, or sacral spinal cord lesions. Irreversible sphincter malfunction sometimes occurs among men who have sustained damage to the urethra itself from prostatectomy. Among women, ISD often is associated with multiple previous surgical procedures for incontinence. Patients with ISD leak urine when intraabdominal pressure increases, but some also leak continuously.

Overflow Bladder (Urinary Retention)

Two general mechanisms cause overflow bladder. One is obstruction of urinary outflow. The other is failure of the detrusor to contract effectively and empty the bladder. Regardless of the cause, urinary retention occurs, and the bladder distends until maximum bladder capacity is reached, at which point urine leaks from the bladder by means of overflow.

POTENTIALLY TRANSIENT CAUSES OF OVERFLOW BLADDER

A variety of side effects of medications can cause urinary retention, and retention may be reversed when the medication is discontinued (Table 6-4). Some of these medications, such as those with anticholinergic, calcium channel blocking, or prostaglandin-inhibiting activity, interfere with innervation or contractile function of the detrusor muscle. Those with α-adrenergic agonist and β-adrenergic antagonist actions cause outflow obstruction by enhancing contraction of the urinary sphincter.

Fecal impaction is a common and potentially reversible cause of overflow bladder. In fecal impaction, impacted stool in the rectum puts pressure on the urethra or distal bladder, obstructs urinary outflow, and causes overflow incontinence. Removal of the fecal mass frequently eliminates incontinence.

IRREVERSIBLE CAUSES OF OVERFLOW BLADDER

Among older men, obstruction of bladder outflow caused by prostate enlargement is a frequent nontransient cause of urinary retention. Among women, outflow obstruction can be caused by strictures from previous incontinence surgery or by advanced or inoperable vulvar or cervical cancer.

Irreversible overflow bladder also can be caused by neuropathic, neoplastic, or traumatic injury to the cholinergic pelvic nerves that innervate the detrusor muscle. The result is failure of detrusor contractions and subsequent urinary retention. This scenario is most commonly caused by diabetic neuropathy. Less common neuropathic causes include multiple sclerosis, amyloidosis, syphilis, and heavy metal poisoning.

Mixed Incontinence

Many patients have incontinence of multiple causes, so-called mixed incontinence. Thus some patients have both stress incontinence and urge incontinence, and others have stress or urge incontinence

Table 6-4

Medications That Can Cause Urinary Retention

MEDICATION	MECHANISM

Anticholinergics
   Tricyclic antidepressants
   Phenothiazine antipsychotics
   Antihistamines
   Atropine analogues (e.g., scopolamine)
	Interference with cholinergic innervation of detrusor, decreasing force of detrusor contraction

Calcium channel blocking agents	Smooth-muscle relaxation, which decreases force of detrusor contraction
Nonsteroidal anti-inflammatory drugs	Blockade of prostaglandin receptors in bladder smooth muscle, which decreases force of detrusor contraction
α-Adrenergic agonists	Stimulation of contraction (constriction) of urethral sphincter
β-Adrenergic antagonists	Blockade of β-adrenergic–mediated relaxation of urethral sphincter, which leaves unopposed α-adrenergic-mediated contraction of the sphincter

Nervous system depressants
   Narcotics
   Sedatives-hypnotics
	Nonspecific inhibition of detrusor contraction

along with a transient cause of incontinence. Mixed causes of incontinence are more common among older than among younger persons, who most often have single-cause incontinence.

Typical Presentation

The patient's symptoms and a review of the basic medical history provide useful information about (1) the nature of the incontinence, (2) whether the incontinence is likely to be transient, and (3) referrals or special diagnostic tests that may be appropriate. The history also can provide an estimation of the frequency and timing of incontinence, which can be used as a baseline measure to judge the effectiveness of treatment. Some experts recommend that patients keep a diary of incontinence episodes to enhance the accuracy of such information.

Symptoms Indicating the Nature of Incontinence

The history is useful for identifying the nature of a patient's incontinence—that is, whether the incontinence is caused by detrusor overactivity or sphincter malfunction. It is less useful for identifying overflow bladder. As described later, for all patients with incontinence, overflow bladder is detected by means of measurement of postvoid residual urine volume.

SYMPTOMS OF DETRUSOR OVERACTIVITY (URGE INCONTINENCE)

Symptoms of detrusor overactivity, whether caused by transient or irreversible causes, are similar. They are characterized by urge incontinence, an intense urge to urinate that develops suddenly and that does not allow the person sufficient time to reach bathroom facilities. Other symptoms of

urge incontinence include nocturia, the need to urinate frequently, and a feeling that the bladder has not emptied completely after voiding.

SYMPTOMS OF SPHINCTER MALFUNCTION (STRESS INCONTINENCE)

Symptoms of stress incontinence are highly predictive of sphincter malfunction. The classic symptom of stress incontinence is loss of urine during activities that increase intraabdominal pressure, such as coughing, sneezing, or straining. The urine loss occurs simultaneously with the increase in intraabdominal pressure and ceases when pressure returns to normal. It rarely occurs at night. With the typical physical examination findings of stress incontinence, the positive predictive value of these symptoms for true stress incontinence exceeds 95 percent.

Delayed onset of urine loss, or continued urine loss after intraabdominal pressure returns to normal, are not typical of stress incontinence. These symptoms indicate detrusor overactivity, in which urine loss occurs when repetitive coughing or sneezing stimulates the overactive detrusor muscle to contract. This scenario, in which manifestations of detrusor overactivity mimic the symptoms of stress incontinence, is sometimes called *pseudo-stress incontinence*.

Symptoms Suggesting That Incontinence May Be Transient

No symptoms indicate with certainty that incontinence is transient. However, responses to several items in the medical history, especially questions about medications, can raise the possibility of transient incontinence.

In the presence of symptoms of urge incontinence, using any of the medications listed in Table 6-3 suggests that incontinence may be transient and may resolve when the medication is discontinued. Incontinence also may be transient if symptoms are compatible with any of the potentially treatable medical conditions recorded in Table 6-3.

The possibility of transient sphincter malfunction is suggested by use of medications that affect the urethral sphincters. These are typically α-adrenergic antagonists or β-adrenergic agonists.

If overflow incontinence is present, use of medications listed in Table 6-4 suggests that incontinence may resolve when the medication is discontinued. Constipation, with or without incontinence of liquid stool, suggests the possibility of fecal impaction; incontinence may resolve with disimpaction.

Symptoms Suggesting the Need for Special Evaluation

Several symptoms or findings in the medical history suggest that management of incontinence will not be straightforward or that incontinence may be a manifestation of a serious underlying medical or surgical disorder. Patients who report having undergone anti-incontinence surgery or radical pelvic surgery are unlikely to have successful treatment with simple nonsurgical measures, and they generally should be referred to a urogynecologist. Patients who report onset of urge incontinence within the past 2 months may have a bladder neoplasm or stone and should undergo cystoscopy for diagnosis. Patients who report hematuria or recurrent symptomatic urinary infections may have structural or neoplastic abnormalities in the urinary tract and should undergo imaging studies such as ultrasonography or intravenous pyelography. If the results do not provide enough information to confirm a diagnosis, cystoscopy should be performed.

Physical Examination

As with the history, physical examination is directed at providing information about (1) the nature of the incontinence, (2) whether incontinence might be transient, and (3) referrals or special diagnostic tests that might be appropriate.

Findings Suggesting the Nature of Incontinence

No physical examination findings specifically indicate that detrusor overactivity is present. However, patients with incontinence with examination findings compatible with Parkinson's disease or another degenerative neurologic disorder frequently have uninhibited detrusor contractions. Signs of these disorders found at examination indicate the likely presence of urge incontinence.

The presence of pelvic prolapse suggests that the urine loss may be caused by stress incontinence. Patients with stress incontinence may have marked abnormalities found at physical examination, such as gross prolapse of the cervix through the vaginal introitus. Prolapse also may be less marked and be found only as a cystocele or rectocele that becomes apparent when intraabdominal pressure is forcibly increased. The presence and severity of pelvic prolapse can be demonstrated by having the patient perform a maximal Valsalva maneuver in the supine (dorsal lithotomy) position. It is not necessary to test patients in the standing position to detect pelvic prolapse.

Overflow incontinence is suggested by palpation of a distended bladder in the suprapubic area or abdomen. This finding usually is more apparent in examinations of thin persons and may be confused with uterine enlargement in examinations of others. The presence of an enlarged prostate gland palpable during rectal examination also suggests overflow incontinence. This is not a specific finding because prostate enlargement is common among older men who have no incontinence. Patients who have overflow bladder caused by neuropathic disorders may have a variety of abnormalities detectable at neurologic examination of the lower extremities.

Findings Suggesting Transient Incontinence

The physical examination can reveal evidence of transient causes of either overflow incontinence or detrusor overactivity. The finding that suggests transient overflow incontinence is fecal impaction during a rectal examination.

A finding suggestive of transient detrusor over-activity is atrophic vaginitis. The basis for the association between atrophic vaginitis and incontinence is that, in some women, estrogen-sensitive epithelium is present not only in the vagina but also in the urethra and bladder trigone. The presence of atrophic vaginitis suggests the possibility that atrophic trigonitis is present with trigonal inflammation that causes bladder irritability and detrusor contractions.

Findings Suggesting the Need for Special Evaluation

Three specific findings at physical examination indicate the need for specialized evaluation or treatment. The first is a prostate examination that reveals a nodule or asymmetry. This finding suggests prostate cancer, and evaluation and therapy for cancer should take precedence over evaluation and therapy for incontinence. The second finding is gross pelvic prolapse (prolapse of the cervix beyond the hymen). Treatment of patients with incontinence and gross pelvic prolapse rarely is straightforward and usually necessitates referral to a urogynecologist. The third finding is any abnormality suggesting a neurologic disorder, such as a spinal cord lesion; evaluation of the neurologic problem should be undertaken to detect transient or manageable neurologic conditions.

Ancillary Tests

All patients being evaluated for urinary incontinence should undergo urinalysis and measurement of postvoid residual urine volume (PVR). Simple bladder function tests, described later, also are useful. Other tests, such as renal function tests, cystoscopy, urine cytology, formal cystometrography, and imaging tests, are not needed in the routine evaluation of urinary incontinence but may be appropriate for selected patients.

Urinalysis

Urinalysis is performed primarily to detect acute urinary tract infection, which is a common transient cause of incontinence. If appropriate, a urine culture specimen should also be obtained. Urine dipstick testing also is used to detect hyperglycemia, a potentially transient cause of detrusor overactivity (Table 6-3). Urinalysis may reveal proteinuria or hematuria, both of which necessitate further evaluation to determine a cause.

Postvoid Residual Urine Volume

PVR is defined as the quantity of urine remaining in the bladder after someone urinates. Two methods can be used to measure PVR. The first is in-and-out urethral catheterization immediately after a patient voids with recording of the quantity of urine retrieved. In-and-out catheterization frequently is used to measure the PVR of women.

PVR also can be measured with a portable ultrasound device. Ultrasound often is the preferred technique for measuring the PVR of men because urethral catheterization may be difficult or traumatic for men with enlargement of the prostate.

A normal value for PVR is less than 50 mL. PVR volumes more than 200 mL are considered high. Values between 50 mL and 200 mL are equivocal. Clinical judgment must be used to interpret the result. It may be helpful to repeat the measurement of PVR to clarify the initial findings.

Simple Bladder Function Tests

If the PVR is normal, and history and physical findings do not allow the clinician to differentiate symptoms of urge incontinence and those of stress incontinence, simple bladder function tests may be useful for defining the diagnosis. These tests include simple cystometry, bladder stress testing, and urine flowmetry.

SIMPLE CYSTOMETRY

Simple cystometry is used to detect urge incontinence. To perform simple cystometry, the clinician inserts a 12F to 14F urinary catheter into the patient's bladder. The catheter typically is the same one used to measure PVR, and it is simply left in place after PVR is measured. After the bladder is emptied with the catheter, a 50-cc bayonet tipped catheter with the plunger removed is inserted into the open end of the catheter and positioned about 15 cm above the symphysis pubis (Fig. 6-1).

The examiner slowly pours 50 mL sterile water into the open end of the syringe and allows it to drain into the bladder. Recording the volume instilled, the examiner adds 50-mL aliquots through the syringe until the patient reports the first urge to void. From that point, 25-mL aliquots are slowly poured into the syringe until either the patient experiences severe urgency or bladder contractions are detected in the syringe. Severe urgency is manifested as extreme discomfort from bladder distention and the sensation of being unable to control urination. Bladder contractions appear as up-and-down movements of the fluid level within the syringe.

Severe urgency and bladder contractions occurring at total instilled volumes of less than 300 mL indicate detrusor overactivity. Simple cystometry has a 75 to 100 percent sensitivity, 69 to 89 percent specificity, and a 74 to 91 percent positive predictive value for diagnosis of detrusor overactivity. Formal multichannel cystometrography is the reference standard.

STRESS TESTING

Stress testing is an adjunct to physical examination that can be useful for identifying stress incontinence among women. It includes the pad test and the Marshall test.

In the pad test, patients are initially examined in the supine position when their bladder is full. If simple cystometry has been performed, the pad test can be performed immediately afterward while the bladder is full and after the catheter has

Figure 6-1

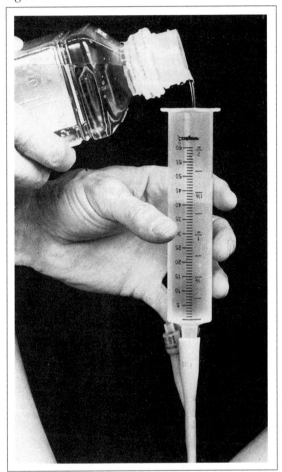

Simple cystometry. A 50-cc syringe with the plunger removed is positioned about 15 cm above the symphysis pubis. Sterile water is poured into the syringe. A catheter without a balloon is best used to avoid balloon-induced detrusor contractions. A ballooned Foley catheter can be used, if necessary, if the balloon is not inflated.

been removed. The examiner holds a dry 4 cm by 4 cm gauze pad on the patient's introitus and asks the patient to cough forcibly. Leakage of urine onto the gauze pad indicates the presence of stress incontinence. If no urine leaks during pad testing in the supine position, the test should be repeated with the patient standing up.

If incontinence is detected with the pad test, the clinician can perform a Marshall test. The

Marshall test involves insertion of the examiner's fingers on either side of the urethra. The examiner's fingers then elevate the urethra, and the patient is asked to cough forcibly. If a patient who leaked urine during the pad test has no leakage while the urethra is elevated, it is likely that incontinence can be improved with incontinence surgery.

URINE FLOWMETRY

The flow of urine can be observed visually or measured quantitatively with a disposable urine flow meter (Fig. 6-2). The normal rate of urine flow varies with age and with the amount of urine in the bladder. It decreases with age and increases with higher voided volumes. In general, flow rates of geriatric-aged men are normally higher than about 20 mL/s, rates slower than 10 to 15 mL/s are abnormal. Measuring the rate of urine flow is useful in evaluating men for suspected outflow obstruction caused by prostate enlargement. However, it cannot help differentiate decreased flow caused by outflow obstruction from decreased flow caused by detrusor weakness unless simultaneous measurement of detrusor function is performed. Urine flowmetry is not useful in evaluating women with urinary incontinence.

Other Tests

In 1996, the U.S. Agency for Health Care Policy and Research (AHCPR) convened a panel of experts to review available research about the diagnosis and management of urinary incontinence. After review of several hundred published articles, the panel issued a report stating that formal multichannel cystometrography, renal function tests, cystoscopy, urine cytology, and urinary tract imaging are not needed in the routine evaluation of the patients with incontinence. These studies are indicated only in special situations.

CYSTOMETROGRAPHY

Formal multichannel cystometrography involves insertion of a multilumen urethral catheter through which sterile water or carbon dioxide gas is

Figure 6-2

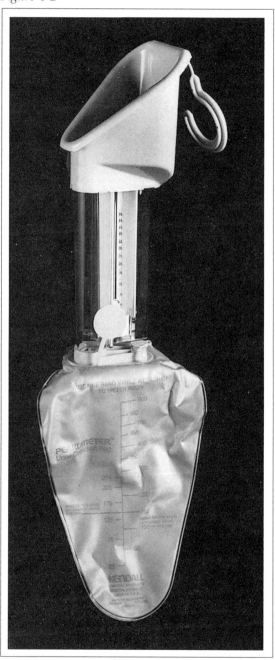

Urine flow meter. Used to measure urine flow rates of male patients.

instilled into the bladder. Pressure measurements from within the bladder are recorded as the bladder is filled. A rectal probe also is inserted and used to measure intraabdominal pressure. Subtraction of intraabdominal pressure from measured bladder pressure facilitates measurement of true intravesical pressure. Other data can be recorded during the examination, such as urethral pressure, pelvic muscle electromyographic findings, leak-point pressure, and urethral flow rate.

Cystometrographic data can be used to diagnose detrusor overactivity, urethral sphincter malfunction, and combinations of detrusor overactivity and sphincter malfunction and to confirm the absence of detrusor contraction among patients with urinary retention. Cystometrography often is performed during the preoperative evaluations of women being considered for stress incontinence surgery to ensure that the patient has evidence of sphincter malfunction and that she does not have incontinence due to detrusor overactivity.

Although formal cystometrography provides reasonably accurate diagnostic information about bladder function and the basis of incontinence, it is generally unnecessary in the routine evaluation of patients with incontinence. This is because, as described earlier, reasonably accurate diagnostic information can be obtained with history, physical examination, measurement of PVR, and, if needed, simple bladder function tests. In addition, the sheer number of persons who have urinary incontinence makes it logistically impossible to consider performing a cystometrography for every patient with the problem. The AHCPR panel recommended that multichannel cystometrography be reserved for patients for whom a presumptive diagnosis cannot be made with simpler diagnostic modalities and for patients with incontinence not controlled after therapy for the presumptive diagnosis.

RENAL FUNCTION TESTS

Renal function tests, such as measurement of creatinine, blood urea nitrogen, and creatinine clearance, rarely are helpful in the evaluation of urinary incontinence. Such tests are useful, however, to patients with overflow incontinence, because urinary retention among these patients

can cause hydronephrosis and impaired renal function. Renal function tests also are appropriate when evaluation of incontinence reveals other abnormalities, such as hematuria, that indicate renal disease.

CYSTOSCOPY

Routine performance of cystoscopy for patients with incontinence helps identify serious abnormalities among fewer than 1 percent of older patients. In evaluations of patients with urinary incontinence, cystoscopy is only needed when there are specific indications for the procedure. Among geriatric-aged patients, these indications often include, but are not limited to, problems such as hematuria not explained by infection, urolithiasis, or upper urinary tract disease; symptoms of urgency that have developed within the past 2 months; or other suspicion of bladder neoplasia.

URINE CYTOLOGY

Urine cytology may be appropriate in the evaluation of patients with suspected bladder neoplasms. It has no role, however, in the routine evaluation of patients with urinary incontinence.

URINARY TRACT IMAGING

Urinary tract imaging tests, such as renal ultrasonography, intravenous pyelography, contrast cystometrography, and radionuclide studies should be performed only if there are specific indications for the tests. They are not appropriate as routine diagnostic procedures for patients with urinary incontinence.

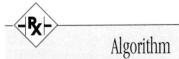

Algorithm

The approach to the diagnosis of urinary incontinence is summarized in the algorithm (Fig. 6-3). The first step is to perform a history, physical

Figure 6-3

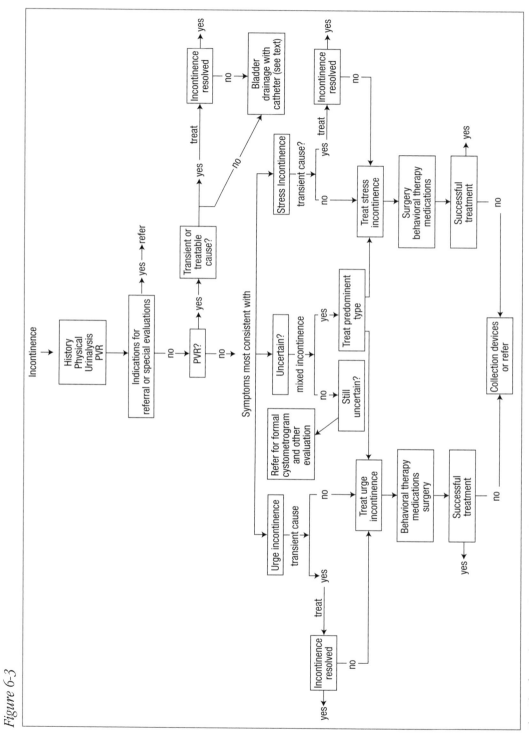

Algorithm for evaluation and management of urinary incontinence. PVR, postvoid residual urine volume.

examination, and basic laboratory tests, including measurement of PVR, to make a presumptive diagnosis of urge, stress, or overflow incontinence and evaluate whether the cause of incontinence might be transient. If there is evidence of a transient cause, diagnostic tests should be undertaken to confirm or exclude that a transient condition exists, and appropriate treatment should be administered. If no transient cause is detected, treatment can be based on the type of incontinence identified: urge, stress, or overflow. If the patient has symptoms of multiple forms of incontinence (mixed incontinence), treatment should be directed first at the form of incontinence that has the predominating symptoms.

If treatment results are satisfactory, nothing further has to be done. If the results of treatment are not satisfactory, more sophisticated tests of bladder function, such as multichannel cystometrography, can be performed to better clarify the nature of the incontinence. If incontinence persists despite diagnostic and treatment efforts, the patient is said to have *intractable incontinence*. Patients with intractable incontinence usually are treated with devices to collect urine and maintain hygiene (see later).

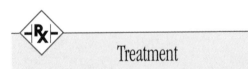

Treatment

There are a variety of therapies for incontinence. Some are administered by patients themselves before they seek medical attention. Some treatments are directed at transient causes of incontinence. Others are directed at irreversible incontinence and are intended to reduce or control symptoms. Some treatments are used simply to collect urine and maintain hygiene.

Self-Treatment

Patients with urinary incontinence use a variety of self-treatments in an attempt to control their symptoms. Some approaches to self-treatment are simple, such as changing patterns of fluid intake or being sure to identify the location of the toilet when arriving at an unfamiliar place. Other methods of self-treatment involve the use of absorbent pads and herbal medications.

ABSORBENT PADS

Numerous types of absorbent pads and underpants are used widely by patients for self-treatment of incontinent urine. Little research has been conducted to measure the effectiveness of absorbent pads and garments, but more than $500 million is spent on these products each year in the United States.

These absorbent products are safe unless wet pads remain in contact with the skin for prolonged periods, in which case there is a risk of skin maceration and infection. The main concern about use of these products for self-treatment is that many persons rely on absorbent pads instead of seeking medical evaluation. They are denying themselves the opportunity to undergo appropriate diagnostic tests for detection of reversible or controllable causes of incontinence. For patients with urinary retention, absorbent products do nothing to drain the bladder and prevent hydronephrosis and renal damage.

HERBAL MEDICATIONS

Some patients attempt to control urinary incontinence with herbal remedies. The most common is saw palmetto, made from an extract of the berries of a Caribbean palm tree, *Serenoa repens*. Saw palmetto works primarily by blocking the binding of dihydrotestosterone in prostate tissue, thus reducing the size of the prostate and symptoms of prostatic hypertrophy. Evidence from double-blind, placebo-controlled trials indicates that symptoms of prostatism and residual urine are reduced by 40 to 50 percent. The specific role and benefit of saw palmetto in the management of urinary incontinence have not been defined.

Management of Transient Causes of Incontinence

If a potentially transient cause of incontinence is identified, the patient should be treated. The usual therapies for the common causes of transient urinary incontinence are shown in Table 6-5. Most of these treatments are straightforward, but a few warrant specific comment: management of urinary tract infection and management of atrophic vaginitis.

MANAGEMENT OF URINARY TRACT INFECTION

Acute urinary tract infection causes incontinence because inflammation in the bladder irritates the mucosa and stimulates the detrusor muscle to contract. In general, only acute infection causes incontinence through this mechanism. Chronic asymptomatic bacteriuria, which is common among older persons, does not usually inflame the bladder mucosa and therefore is not a frequent cause of uncontrolled bladder contractions. If a patient has no symptoms of dysuria or other recent-onset urinary symptoms, and if incontinence is long standing, the absence of white blood cells in an infected urine specimen suggests that inflammation is not present. For such patients, antibiotics are unlikely to resolve urinary incontinence.

MANAGEMENT OF ATROPHIC VAGINITIS

If atrophic vaginitis is detected at physical examination and the patient has symptoms of urge incontinence, it is appropriate to institute therapy for atrophic vaginitis. The usual treatment is estrogen, administered orally, vaginally, or transdermally. In most cases, the route of administration is not important. Patients with severe atrophy, however, may have impairment of the capillary and arteriolar circulation to the estrogen-sensitive mucosa, and systemically administered estrogen may not reach the mucosa in sufficient concentration. For this reason, it often is advisable to begin therapy with topically administered estrogen until mucosal circulatory function improves. After several weeks, topical estrogen can be discontinued, if the patient desires, and replaced with systemic estrogen therapy.

Management of Urge Incontinence

If evaluation indicates that a patient has urge incontinence (detrusor overactivity) and no tran-

Table 6-5

Management of Potentially Transient Conditions Causing or Contributing to Urinary Incontinence

CONDITION	TREATMENT
Transient causes of urge-type incontinence	
Acute urinary tract infection	Antibiotic therapy
Atrophic vaginitis	Estrogen therapy
Delirium or hypoxia	Control underlying cause
Excessive fluid intake	Reduction in fluid intake
Glycosuria	Control diabetes
Hypercalcemia, Hypercalciuria	Treat hypercalcemia
Impaired mobility	Therapy for mobility problem or environmental changes
Medication effects	Discontinue or change medication, if possible
Transient causes of sphincter malfunction	
Medication effects	Discontinue or change medication, if possible
Transient causes of overflow bladder	
Drug side effects	Discontinue or change, if possible
Fecal impaction	Disimpaction, stool softeners

sient causes have been identified, the clinician should institute therapy for urge incontinence. Treatment consists of behavioral therapy, medication, and in rare instances surgery.

BEHAVIORAL THERAPY

The most common form of behavioral therapy to manage urge incontinence is bladder training, sometimes called *bladder retraining*. Bladder training involves having a patient resist or postpone urination for progressively longer periods of time according to a predetermined schedule. The typical starting interval is 2 to 3 h, and the time is increased as tolerated by the patient. The schedule is not usually enforced at night.

This surprisingly simple approach is the most effective therapy for urge incontinence. Most of the research on bladder training involves middle-aged and older women with urge incontinence, and these studies show that the technique controls urge incontinence more effectively than medication and more effectively than no treatment. More recent research indicates that pelvic muscle exercises (Kegels) are also effective in reducing episodes of urge incontinence. Various studies report that between 15 and 90 percent of middle-aged and older women with detrusor overactivity achieve continence with bladder training or pelvic

muscle exercise. Most studies indicate cure rates greater than 50 percent. Even when incontinence is not fully controlled, bladder training reduces the number of incontinence episodes for most patients.

Successful bladder training usually takes several months. Limitations are that bladder training is not useful for patients with marked cognitive impairment and is probably less effective for frail elderly persons.

MEDICATIONS

Pharmacologic management of urge incontinence involves medications that decrease contractions of the detrusor muscles. These medications have anticholinergic or smooth-muscle relaxing properties, or both. All of these medications have potential side effects, including systemic effects and the possibility of inhibiting bladder contraction to the point that patients have drug-induced urinary retention. When medications are used to manage urge incontinence, therapy should begin with small doses, usually administered before bed. The dose is carefully titrated upward as needed to improve urinary control but not cause untoward side effects. Dose recommendations are shown in Table 6-6.

ANTICHOLINERGICS The drug most widely used to treat older persons for urge incontinence is

Table 6-6
Common Medications Used for Management of Urge Incontinence

MEDICATION	STARTING DOSE	USUAL MAXIMUM DOSAGE
First-line therapy		
Oxybutynin	2.5–5 mg before bed	5 mg qid
Tolterodine	0.5 mg before bed	2 mg bid
Second-line therapy		
Propantheline	7.5–30 mg before bed	60 mg qid
Imipramine	10–25 mg before bed	100–150 mg/d
Other medications		
Dicyclomine	10 mg before bed	20 mg tid
Calcium channel blockers	Dosage based on concomitant medical conditions	
Nonsteroidal anti-inflammatory drugs	Dosage based on concomitant medical conditions	

oxybutynin, a drug with both anticholinergic and smooth-muscle relaxant properties. Multiple randomized, controlled trials comparing oxybutynin to placebo have shown that 15 to 60 percent of patients have a reduction in incontinence episodes. In some studies, half or more of patients became fully continent. Most patients taking oxybutynin have anticholinergic side effects, including dry mouth, constipation, blurred vision, and changes in mental status.

Tolterodine is a new anticholinergic medication that has effects on the detrusor muscle similar to those of oxybutynin but less activity on muscarinic receptors in the salivary glands. In controlled trials comparing tolterodine with oxybutynin in the management of detrusor overactivity, the two drugs had similar benefit in reducing the frequency of incontinence episodes, but tolterodine caused fewer anticholinergic side effects.

Other anticholinergic medications have been used to manage urge incontinence. There is extensive clinical experience with propantheline. Dicyclomine also is sometimes used. These drugs are effective at reducing incontinence, but many patients have undesirable anticholinergic effects.

CALCIUM CHANNEL BLOCKING AGENTS   Calcium channel blocking agents have smooth-muscle relaxant properties and may reduce the frequency of uninhibited detrusor contractions. Although not recommended as first-line therapy for urge incontinence, calcium channel blocking agents may have a role in controlling urge incontinence when patients also have other indications for treatment with calcium channel blockers.

TRICYCLIC ANTIDEPRESSANTS   Tricyclic antidepressants, because of their anticholinergic activity, can be used to reduce bladder contractions. Imipramine is the tricyclic most widely used for management of incontinence. Although not first-line treatment, it may be a reasonable choice in the care of patients with concomitant depression.

OTHER DRUGS   Flavoxate is a smooth-muscle relaxant marketed for management of urge incontinence. The AHCPR panel could find no evidence that this agent is effective. Nonsteroidal anti-inflam-matory drugs may have a role in the management of urge incontinence because their action interferes with prostaglandin-mediated bladder contractions. At least one placebo-controlled trial showed benefit to using these drugs. However, because research and experience are limited, nonsteroidal anti-inflammatory agents are not recommended as primary therapy for urinary incontinence.

SURGERY

In rare instances, surgical procedures can be used to treat patients with urge incontinence. These procedures are intended only for patients with severe, intractable, urge incontinence. The most commonly recommended procedures are augmentation cystoplasty, urinary diversion, and bladder denervation.

Augmentation cystoplasty is a procedure in which a patch of intestine is surgically interposed into the bladder wall. In effect, the procedure weakens the bladder wall and decreases the force of contractions. About one-third of patients become continent with spontaneous voiding after augmentation cystoplasty. It is considered the procedure of choice for surgical treatment of urge incontinence, particularly when detrusor overactivity is accompanied by poor bladder compliance. Urinary diversion with an ileal pouch or urostomy can be performed and results in a somewhat higher rate of continence than augmentation cystoplasty. It is considered a second-choice procedure because of a higher rate of serious complications.

Bladder denervation can be accomplished with subtrigonal phenol injections, sacral rhizotomy, transvaginal denervation, sacral dorsal root ganglionectomy, and a variety of other procedures. Bladder denervation procedures rarely are used because cure rates are low, making the risk-to-benefit ratio of these procedures unacceptable.

Treatment of Women for Stress Incontinence

Many treatments are available for patients with stress incontinence. Surgery is the most effective.

For patients with mild stress incontinence, those unwilling to undergo surgery, or those judged to be at poor surgical risk, other treatments are appropriate. The other treatments include behavioral therapy, medications, and devices.

SURGERY

The AHCPR panel reviewed studies involving more than 6000 patients and found that continence was restored completely for an average of 75 to 79 percent of patients who underwent surgical therapy for stress incontinence. This far exceeds the cure rates with other forms of therapy. Patients with stress incontinence who are at low risk for adverse surgical outcomes should be advised to consider surgical repair.

PROCEDURES FOR URETHRAL HYPERMOBILITY The recommended procedures for stress incontinence caused by urethral hypermobility are retropubic suspension (average cure rate 79 percent) and needle bladder neck suspension (average cure rate 74 percent). Anterior vaginal repair also is performed, but is less effective than retropubic or needle suspension; continence is restored to only approximately 65 percent of patients.

PROCEDURES FOR INTRINSIC URETHRAL DEFICIENCY Surgical treatment of women with ISD is best accomplished with a sling procedure. A sling, typically made of synthetic material or autologous tissue (fascia or vaginal wall), is anchored in the retropubic area and placed around the urethra. New procedures permit sling surgery to be performed in a minimally invasive fashion. Cure rates in several studies are 80 to 90 percent. This is remarkable given that these procedures often are performed on women who have undergone unsuccessful incontinence surgery.

ISD also can be managed with periurethral bulking injections and artificial urinary sphincters. Periurethral bulking injections involve injection of materials such as collagen, polytetrafluoroethylene, or autologous fat into an area of incompetent urethra. For women, these injections are performed with local anesthesia. Published cure rates vary widely, but on average, about one-half to two-thirds of women achieve continence after the procedure, although urinary control diminishes over time.

An additional, though not often used, surgical procedure for ISD among women is implantation of an artificial urinary sphincter. Published data on operations on several hundred women with ISD indicate that continence can be achieved by about three-fourths of patients with an artificial sphincter.

BEHAVIORAL THERAPY

Behavioral therapies are useful to women with mild stress incontinence for whom surgery is not being considered and women who refuse or are not candidates for surgery. Behavioral therapy also may have benefit in the postoperative rehabilitation of women who undergo incontinence surgery.

PELVIC MUSCLE EXERCISES Also known as Kegel exercises or pelvic floor exercises, pelvic muscle exercises are used to strengthen the periurethral and perivaginal muscles that make up the voluntary component of the urethral sphincter. For younger women, a common routine is to contract the muscles for at least 10 s and relax the muscles for 10 s and to do this 30 to 80 times a day for at least 8 weeks. Older patients, however, often need more than 8 weeks to benefit from pelvic muscle exercises. Pelvic muscle exercises result in total resolution of incontinence for only 10 to 15 percent of patients. Improvement in symptoms, however, is common and occurs among as many as 75 to 85 percent of patients, including older women. To sustain cure or improvement, exercises often must be continued indefinitely.

Patients with mild stress incontinence who successfully master pelvic muscle contraction also can be taught to contract their pelvic muscles when about to cough or sneeze, thereby limiting the frequency and quantity of urine loss. With this technique, the volume of leaked urine can be reduced an average of 98 percent with moderate coughing and 73 percent with deep coughing.

BIOFEEDBACK   The effectiveness of pelvic muscle exercises can probably be enhanced by combining them with other nonpharmacologic treatments. One of the most common approaches is to use biofeedback techniques. Pressure gauges placed in the vagina provide patients with an auditory or visual display of pelvic muscle contractions, thereby teaching them to better identify and gain control of the pelvic floor muscles. There is some evidence that biofeedback enhances the effect of pelvic muscle exercises. Biofeedback also appears to enhance the speed with which improvement occurs. Because of the intensive counseling involved, biofeedback enhancement of pelvic muscle exercises tends to be expensive. In addition, it is appropriate only for patients who have good cognitive function.

VAGINAL WEIGHTS   Another method for enhancing the effect of pelvic floor muscles is to use vaginal weights. These weights are typically cone-shaped and vary in weight from 20 to 100 g. The patient places a weight in the vagina, with the base of the cone inside and the tip at the introitus. She attempts to retain the weight in the vagina for up to 15 min using pelvic muscle contractions. As success is achieved with the lighter weights, progressively heavier weights are used. Some research on the use of vaginal weights by younger women suggests that the weights may enhance the benefit of pelvic floor exercises. Experience is limited among older women. Because of problems such as vaginal mucosal atrophy and pelvic prolapse, which may be predispositions to vaginal injury, the benefit of use of vaginal weights by geriatric-aged women is unclear.

MEDICATIONS

Several medications can be used to manage stress incontinence. The most widely used are α-adrenergic agonists and estrogen. These medications can be used either alone or in combination.

α-ADRENERGIC AGONISTS   α-Adrenergic agonists are used to manage stress incontinence because they stimulate contraction of the involuntary urethral sphincters. Most research on α-agonists has involved phenylpropanolamine in sustained-release form. The usual dosage is 75 mg by mouth twice a day. Pseudoephedrine, a nonprescription α-agonist commonly used to manage nasal congestion, also is widely used to control stress incontinence. Its effects are similar to those of phenylpropanolamine. The dosage of pseudoephedrine is 15 to 30 mg by mouth three times per day. No more than about 15 percent of patients treated with α-agonists become fully continent, but one-half or more experience improvement in the symptoms. Because α-agonists are vasoconstrictors, neither of these medications is suitable as long-term treatment of patients with hypertension.

ESTROGEN   Estrogen is an effective therapy for stress incontinence. The mechanism of action is unclear, but estrogen probably improves the response of urethral tissues to α-adrenergic stimulation and enhances urethral muscular tone. The usual oral dosage is 0.3 to 1.25 mg/d conjugated estrogen; the typical vaginal dose is 2 g/d. The results of treatment are similar to those with α-adrenergic agonists. No more than 15 percent of patients become continent, whereas more than half experience a reduction in incontinence episodes. Some research indicates that estrogen may be of no value at all.

COMBINED ESTROGEN AND α-AGONISTS   Combination therapy with an α-adrenergic agonist and estrogen supplementation has been recommended for managing stress incontinence that is not responsive to either agent individually. Although results of a few small studies have suggested that combined therapy is more effective than either treatment alone, the evidence is limited, and the role and benefit of combined therapy are not clear.

DEVICES

Several nonpharmacologic modalities, including pessaries and occlusive devices, have been used to manage stress incontinence. All have some benefit, particularly for patients who do not want to undergo or are not suitable candidates for incontinence surgery and who have not responded to behavioral therapy and medications.

PESSARIES Modern pessaries usually are made of rubber, plastic, or silicone, and some have a malleable metal skeleton to maintain shape and support. Pessaries are available in a variety of sizes and shapes (Fig. 6-4), and different incontinence conditions require different types of pessaries (Table 6-7).

Fitting a pessary involves estimating the vaginal width with the fingers and selecting an appropriately sized device. The pessary is compressed between the fingers and inserted into the vagina in such a position that the pelvic organs are elevated out of the vagina. If the pessary is properly fitted, a patient should be able to move about and assume a variety of positions without discomfort.

Patients should remove and inspect the pessary at least once a week. Leaving pessaries in place for prolonged periods increases the risk of infection, vaginal ulceration, and impaction within the vagina. Impaction can cause serious complications, including abscesses and fistula formation, and it sometimes necessitates surgical removal of the device.

OCCLUSIVE DEVICES Several devices that block the outflow of urine can be used by women with

Figure 6-4

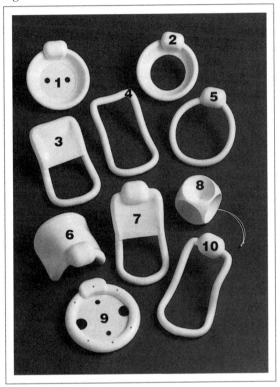

Pessaries used to control stress urinary incontinence. 1. Incontinence dish with support. 2. Incontinence dish. 3. Hodge with support. 4. Hodge. 5. Incontinence ring. 6. Gehrung with knob. 7. Hodge with support and knob. 8. Cube. 9. Ring with support and knob. 10. Hodge with knob. *(Courtesy of Milex Products, Inc.)*

Table 6-7

Indications for Different Types of Pessaries for Stress Incontinence

INDICATION	PESSARY TYPE
Stress incontinence without prolapse	Ring incontinence pessary
	Hodge pessary
	Cube pessary
Stress incontinence with mild prolapse	Incontinence dish pessary
Stress incontinence with mild prolapse and cystocele	Incontinence dish pessary
	Hodge with support pessary

SOURCE: Reproduced from Milex Products, Inc., Chicago, www.milexproducts.com/pessaries.html.

stress incontinence. These include suction devices, urethral inserts, adhesive patches, and others.

Suction devices adhere to the perineum by means of suction and block urine flow through the urethra (Fig. 6-5). These devices are effective at reducing incontinence. Approximately 40 percent of users report restoration of continence. Adverse effects are infrequent; they include urinary infection, bruising, and reversible urethral prolapse into the device. In preliminary studies, these complications each occur among fewer than 2 percent of users.

Another type of occlusive device for women is the intraurethral insert. This device is inserted through the urethra in such a way that part of the device is in the bladder and the rest protrudes through the urethra onto the perineum. The portion within the bladder contains a small inflatable balloon that is expanded within the bladder to prevent the device from being spontaneously expelled. When voiding is desired, the balloon is deflated, and the device is removed. The principal complications of use of this device are urinary tract infection and gross hematuria, which occur among about one-third and one-fourth of users, respectively.

EXTRACORPOREAL MAGNETIC INNERVATION   The FDA recently approved use of a "magnetic chair" for treatment of stress incontinence. The patient sits in a chair, the seat of which generates a magnetic field intended to exercise the pelvic floor muscles. Treatment consists of twice-weekly sessions for 8 weeks. Published data are limited, but three-fourths of women are reportedly improved and one-third are dry after treatment.

Treatment of Men for Stress Incontinence

Stress incontinence among men is most often ISD from surgical trauma, radiation, or another disease that damages the urethra or the nerves that innervate the urethra. Attempts at treatment with behavioral therapy and medication are appropriate, but definitive treatment often is surgical. For patients

Figure 6-5

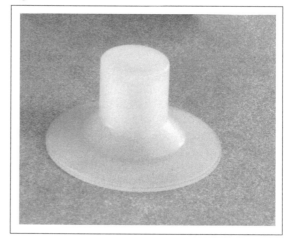

Suction occlusion device. The FemAssist device is one of several for management of urinary stress incontinence. *(Courtesy of Insight Medical.)*

with incontinence immediately after prostatectomy, most experts recommend waiting at least 6 months before undertaking surgical intervention. Behavioral and pharmacologic treatments are used in the interim. Behavioral therapy is the same as that described earlier for women. Pharmacotherapy involves α-adrenergic agonists but not estrogen.

If behavioral and pharmacologic therapy fails to control incontinence and surgery is to be used, the two most widely recommended surgical procedures are periurethral bulking injections and placement of an artificial sphincter.

Periurethral bulking injections are the first-choice surgical treatment of men with ISD, but the injections are not as effective as they are for women. The AHCPR review of studies involving more than 1000 men found that continence is restored to only approximately 20 percent of men treated for ISD with periurethral injections.

Surgical implantation of an artificial urinary sphincter is effective treatment of men with ISD after prostatectomy. Before periurethral bulking procedures were developed, placement of an artificial sphincter was the principal surgical procedure for ISD among men. Placement of an artificial sphincter resolves incontinence for approximately

60 percent of patients. A wide range of results are reported in the literature. Complications such as skin breakdown and infection are not uncommon.

Management of Overflow Incontinence

When no transient or reversible causes of urinary retention can be identified, the objective of therapy becomes drainage of the bladder to prevent hydronephrosis and renal damage. Treatments that do not result in bladder drainage are inappropriate.

If urinary retention is caused by prostate enlargement, surgical treatment (transurethral prostatectomy) is almost always the appropriate therapy. Drugs commonly used to manage prostate enlargement, such as α-adrenergic receptor blockers and 5-α-reductase inhibitors, have a delayed onset of action that makes them unsuitable therapy for urinary retention. The role of other new technologies for managing incontinence caused by urinary retention, such as balloon dilation, lasers, coils, stents, thermal therapy, and hyperthermia, has not been defined.

Long-term drainage of the bladder can be achieved only with catheterization. Three options for catheterization are available: intermittent catheterization, indwelling urethral catheterization, and placement of a suprapubic catheter. In exceptional circumstances, as when advanced neoplasia blocks bladder outflow and precludes catheterization, diverting ileourostomy can be considered.

INTERMITTENT CATHETERIZATION

Intermittent catheterization is standard therapy for all forms of urinary retention caused by inadequate detrusor contractions. It usually is preferable to chronic indwelling urethral catheterization. It cannot, however, be used to treat patients with total or severe bladder outlet obstruction because of difficulty involved in passing the catheter through an obstructed urethra.

Intermittent catheterization is performed by either the patient (self-catheterization) or a caretaker. Persons using self-catheterization must have sufficient cognitive ability and manual dexterity to perform the procedure correctly.

Although some clinicians recommend the use of sterile catheters, use of a clean catheter is sufficient and does not increase the rate of infection, which is one to four episodes per 100 days of intermittent catheterization. Use of sterile catheters frequently is recommended for intermittent catheterization of patients who have a compromised immune system and of frail, elderly patients, but there is no research evidence to support this recommendation.

The usual frequency of catheterization is every 3 to 6 h. However, many patients are catheterized only three times per day with no apparent adverse effects. Chronic suppressive antibiotic therapy is not recommended for patients undergoing intermittent catheterization. Complications of intermittent catheterization include urethritis, urethral trauma and stricture, and urinary tract infection.

INDWELLING URETHRAL CATHETERIZATION

Indwelling urethral (Foley) catheterization is appropriate therapy for irreversible urinary retention among patients for whom intermittent catheterization is impractical or cannot be performed (see later).

SUPRAPUBIC CATHETERIZATION

Suprapubic catheterization involves placing a catheter into the bladder through a surgically created defect in the abdominal wall. It often is the preferred treatment when bladder outlet obstruction prevents passage of a urethral catheter (see "Controversies").

Management of Intractable Incontinence

When incontinence cannot be controlled with measures other than catheterization, the patient is said to have *intractable incontinence*. If intractable incontinence is caused by urinary retention, catheter drainage is essential to prevent hydronephrotic renal damage. For other forms of incontinence, catheterization is appropriate only when no other treatment results in adequate control or collection of urine. A variety of environmental modifications, behavioral approaches, and collection methods should be considered before catheterization is performed.

ENVIRONMENTAL MODIFICATIONS

For some patients, improving physical access to bathroom facilities can decrease the frequency of episodes of incontinence. This is particularly true of persons with intractable urge incontinence who need rapid access to a toilet when they feel the urge to void. Providing ready access to a bedside commode, or locating bathrooms or bedrooms so that patients do not need to climb stairs or walk long distances, can sometimes substantially improve the ability to reach and use a toilet. Similar benefits can be achieved with improvements in lighting, removal of furniture that blocks access to the bathroom, and installation of grab rails to facilitate getting on and off the toilet. Toilet seats should be at least 17 in. (43 cm) from the ground and have bars or arms about 10 in. (25 cm) above the seat.

Avoiding or eliminating dietary diuretics, such as caffeine in coffee, tea, colas, and chocolate, may decrease the frequency of urination and therefore the frequency of episodes of incontinence. Although it may be appropriate to limit

fluid ingestion immediately before bed, patients should not be instructed to reduce total fluid intake or to avoid drinking when thirsty. Older persons, especially those who are frail, often have altered thirst sensation and are at risk of dehydration.

DEVICES AND COLLECTION SYSTEMS

Various nonpharmacologic devices and collection systems are available to control or collect urine for patients with intractable incontinence. These include absorbent pads and garments, male condom catheters, female pouch devices, and penile clamps. None of these methods is suitable for use by patients with urinary retention because these products do not drain the bladder.

ABSORBENT PADS   Numerous absorbent pads and garments can be used to collect urine for patients with intractable incontinence (Table 6-8). There are few data on which to judge which type of absorbent product is most absorbent, has the lowest rate of adverse effects, and is most effective in maintaining hygiene and preventing odor.

MALE CONDOM CATHETERS   Condom catheters are urinary catheters that attach to the penis with a condom-like device made of latex, polyvinyl, or silicone. The condom is secured to the penis with tape, straps, or an inflatable latex cuff. Although effective for collecting urine, use of condom

Table 6-8

Absorbent Pads and Garments

TYPE	DESCRIPTION
Shields	Small absorbent perineal inserts
Guards	Close-fitting products designed for light incontinence
Undergarments	Full-length pads held in place by waist straps
Combination pad–pants systems	Underpants with front pocket to hold absorbent pad
Adult diapers	Similar to large-sized disposable baby diapers
Bed pads	Absorbent pads incorporated into bed coverings

SOURCE: Reproduced from Fantl JA, Newman DK, Colling J, et al: *Urinary Incontinence in Adults: Acute and Chronic Management*. Clinical Practice Guideline No 2, 1996 update. AHCPR publication no. 96-0682. Rockville, MD: US Department of Health and Human Services, Public Health Service, Agency for Health Care Policy and Research, 1996.

catheters is associated with a variety of complications that often make them unsuitable for long-term use. These complications include dermatitis, skin maceration, skin infection; urinary tract infection, and penile edema and ischemia from the apparatus used to secure the condom to the penis.

FEMALE POUCH DEVICES Although not widely used, several external urine-collection devices have been designed for women with incontinence. The typical design of these devices is a plastic pouch that is positioned over the urethra with adhesive, suction, or belts. Limited research suggests that these devices are safe and effective. As many as 80 percent of bedbound women are leak-free during short-term (24 h) use. Leakage of urine is more likely to occur when patients are ambulatory, and there is no information available about long-term use of these devices. Urinary tract infections occur among a small percentage of patients, and some women experience itching or irritation of the perineal skin.

URETHRAL CATHETERS In addition to a role in the treatment of patients with urinary retention, intermittent and indwelling urethral catheterization can be used in the management of intractable urge and stress incontinence that cannot be controlled with other measures. Urethral catheterization also is useful as short-term intervention in the care of patients who have skin ulceration because of incontinence. Temporary use of a catheter keeps the skin dry to facilitate healing of the ulcer.

Intermittent catheterization was discussed earlier. For indwelling catheterization, a Foley catheter with a 5-mL balloon is inserted into the bladder, and the balloon is filled with 10 mL of sterile water. The choice of catheter size is arbitrary and is based largely on the clinician's assessment of the patient's overall body size. The usual size is 14F, 16F, or 18F.

Chronic indwelling catheterization is associated with a variety of complications, including infection, encrustation, urethral trauma, urethritis, and urethral stricture. Two of these that are particularly common are infection and encrustation.

Infection. Chronic indwelling catheterization causes bacteriuria, which is almost universal after 1 month of catheterization. Bacteriuria and complicating infection and sepsis contribute to the increased rate of death among persons who have an indwelling urethral catheter. Long-term catheterization for management of incontinence should not be instituted unless satisfactory hygiene or continence control cannot be achieved with another method. An exception to this general rule applies to patients with terminal illnesses or severely impaired cognition; for these patients other methods of control may be impractical or inappropriate.

Antibiotic therapy for asymptomatic bacteriuria in catheterized patients is not recommended because it results in selection of resistant microorganisms. Antibiotic treatment should be reserved for patients with fever or other signs and symptoms of infection.

Encrustation. Another common problem associated with long-term catheterization is encrustation and obstruction of the catheter lumen with calcified proteinaceous debris. Obstruction of the lumen causes leakage of urine around the sides of the catheter. This development often leads health care providers to replace the catheter with one of larger diameter in the mistaken belief that the catheter is leaking because it is too small. In most cases, however, the correct response to catheter leakage is to replace the catheter with one of similar size and schedule future catheter changes more often, before encrustation develops to the point of obstruction and leakage. Catheters usually are changed once a month, but if leakage occurs sooner than 1 month after a catheter is inserted, the catheter can be changed more often.

Use of silver-coated, antimicrobial, lubricous-coat catheters may decrease the rate of accumulation of encrusted debris, but further research is necessary to clarify the ideal material from which to manufacture catheters. Irrigation of catheters to remove obstructing debris is not recommended.

PENILE CLAMPS Penile clamps are appropriate only for temporary use, as by patients awaiting definitive surgical treatment. They are mentioned here only to emphasize that these devices are not suitable for long-term use by patients with intractable incontinence. Little research has been conducted on the safety of these devices. There are reports of complications such as penile ischemia and cutaneous erosion, including erosion into the urethra. The clamp must be removed every 3 h to allow bladder drainage and assure good circulatory function.

Controversies

The current recommendations for diagnosis and management of incontinence are based largely on expert opinion rather than on evidence from research. Clinicians in different specialties tend to take different approaches to evaluating and managing incontinence. Thus there are many unanswered questions about how to best approach the care of patients with incontinence. Several of the most controversial issues are discussed here.

Diagnostic Evaluation

Considerable controversy exists about the role of certain ancillary tests, specifically cystometrography and cystoscopy, in the routine evaluation of patients with urinary incontinence. When the AHCPR panel reviewed the medical literature seeking evidence of the benefit of performing such tests, none was found. Therefore, the AHCPR guideline on urinary incontinence is not to perform these tests routinely. Nevertheless, many urologists and urogynecologists recommend cystometrography, cystoscopy, or both as part of the routine evaluation of incontinence. They argue that these tests enhance diagnostic accuracy and that diagnoses based on historical and physical findings are not sufficiently specific. This argument may or may not be valid, because the research data cited earlier show that the predictive value of diagnosis made without cystoscopy and cystometrography is quite good.

Cystometrography sometimes provides misleading information. For example, cystometrograms of patients who have no incontinence or symptoms of urgency sometimes demonstrate bladder contractions at low urine volumes, a finding that would be expected only for patients who have detrusor overactivity. Likewise, cystometrography can be falsely negative when performed on patients with known detrusor overactivity. The controversy about the role of these tests in the evaluation of incontinence is likely to persist until better evidence becomes available about their value.

Evaluation before Surgery for Stress Incontinence

When surgery for stress incontinence fails to restore urinary control, the reason is sometimes that the patient had detrusor overactivity, either instead of or in addition to stress incontinence. Many surgeons recommend performance of cystometrography and related urodynamic tests to document sphincter laxity and exclude detrusor overactivity before proceeding with surgery for stress incontinence. It is not clear, however, that cystometrographic testing is appropriate in this situation. Cystometrography may not show detrusor contractions in some patients who have them. For some women, cystometrographic testing may reveal evidence of stress incontinence, thereby seeming to confirm the need for stress incontinence surgery, yet the cause of the symptomatic incontinence may be detrusor overactivity. Furthermore, even if urge incontinence is present with stress incontinence, the urge incontinence often resolves when stress incontinence is corrected. More study is needed to determine the role of cystometrographic testing for patients being considered for stress incontinence surgery.

Use of Suprapubic Catheters

Some experts believe that suprapubic catheters are an acceptable alternative, if not preferable, to urethral catheters for patients who need long-term catheterization, because suprapubic catheterization avoids the complications associated with urethral catheters (urethral stricture, urethritis, and trauma, among others). However, suprapubic catheters present their own problems, such as surgical injury during placement, leakage around the catheter or through the urethra, skin erosion, and difficulty changing and reinserting the catheter. Suprapubic catheterization is not suitable for patients with incontinence caused by severe uncontrolled detrusor contractions or an incompetent sphincter, because leakage of urine still may occur through the urethra while the suprapubic catheter is in place. Many clinicians are unfamiliar with use and care of suprapubic catheters, creating potential problems for management. Despite these concerns, suprapubic catheters are an alternative approach to control of urine for patients who have intractable urinary incontinence that cannot be managed with other methods. However, the advantages and disadvantages relative to urethral catheters have not been clarified. Further study is needed to define the role of these catheters in the management of intractable urinary incontinence.

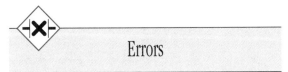

Errors

Geriatricians and primary care clinicians make a variety of errors in the evaluation and treatment of patients with incontinence. Some pitfalls in managing incontinence have already been discussed. They include the fact that chronic asymptomatic bacteriuria is not usually the cause of incontinence and the need to use topical, rather than systemic, estrogens in the initial treatment of patients with severe atrophic vaginitis. The following are other common errors.

Failure to Detect Urinary Incontinence

Most instances of urinary incontinence are not identified as such by the clinicians. This failure to detect incontinence results from a failure to ask

patients about symptoms of incontinence. This error can easily be avoided by asking all geriatric-aged patients about symptoms of incontinence.

Failure to Exclude Urinary Retention

A serious and unfortunately common error in evaluating patients with urinary incontinence is failure to measure PVR. Clinicians often mistake overflow incontinence for stress incontinence, because patients with overflow incontinence often leak urine when they cough, sneeze, or even walk. Clinicians who misinterpret this incontinence as stress incontinence may prescribe Kegel exercises or α-agonists. Worse still, they may mistakenly consider the symptoms to indicate urge incontinence because the patient reports the sensation of incomplete bladder emptying. They then prescribe oxybutynin, a medication that is contraindicated for patients with urinary retention. This error can be avoided by always measuring PVR in the initial evaluation of patients with incontinence.

Failure to Use Nonpharmacologic Therapy

Another common error is prescribing oxybutynin or similar medications as a first-line approach to treatment of all patients with urinary incontinence or all patients with urge incontinence. Although these medications are effective for controlling urge incontinence, bladder training is more effective than medications, and it has no side effects. For these reasons bladder training is considered the initial treatment of choice. This error can be avoided by beginning therapy for urge incontinence with behavioral therapy rather than medications.

Failure to Start Medications for Urge Incontinence at a Low Dose

Many clinicians prescribe medications for urge incontinence starting at a full therapeutic dose. This can and does lead to development of acute urinary retention, which necessitates temporary insertion of a urethral catheter. Older persons, especially frail older persons, are particularly sensitive to the anticholinergic effects of drugs used to manage urge incontinence. This error can be avoided by beginning therapy with the lowest available dose and increasing the dose only if a satisfactory response is not achieved, and then only if the patient experiences no adverse effects.

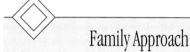

Family Approach

When geriatric-aged persons have urinary incontinence, there can be several important effects on family function. First, persons with incontinence may experience a loss of self-esteem and sometimes depression, which affects their relationships with other members of the family. Second, embarrassment or concerns about odor and wetness may lead persons with incontinence to avoid social interactions with friends and family or even to avoid leaving the home, further disturbing normal family activities and relationships. Later, if incontinence cannot be adequately controlled or is accompanied by deterioration of health, family members may be called on to provide care and assistance to persons with incontinence. Most family members find dealing with incontinence one of the more difficult and time-consuming aspects of caregiving. Difficulty dealing with incontinence in the home often is a contributing factor, though rarely the primary factor, in the decision to place a family member in a nursing home.

The clinician's responsibility in dealing with patients with incontinence and their family members includes being aware of the effect of incontinence on the patient and on family dynamics. Questionnaires are available with which to measure these effects.

Clinicians should provide patients and families with education about the nature of and prognosis for urinary incontinence (see "Patient Education").

Family members should be assured that reversible causes of incontinence will be sought and controlled if present. The wide array of therapies for incontinence should be discussed. Patients and families need some optimism that the problem can be controlled to a degree sufficient to allow the patient to continue usual activities.

Referral to appropriate support groups may be helpful to patients and their families. Information about support groups can be obtained from the organizations listed in Table 6-9. For patients with advanced or intractable incontinence accompanied by a general decline in the ability to function independently, clinicians must provide appropriate support through community and home assistance programs.

Patient Education

Many persons with urinary incontinence consider the condition to be a normal consequence of

Table 6-9

Organizations with Support Groups and Information for Patients

Bladder Health Council of the American Foundation for Urologic Disease 300 W. Pratt St., Suite 401 Baltimore, MD 21201 (800) 242-2383
Continence Restored, Inc. 407 Strawberry Hill Ave., Stanford, CT 06902 (914) 493-1470
National Association for Continence PO Box 8310 Spartanburg, SC 29305-8310 (800) 252-3337
The Simon Foundation for Continence PO Box 835 Wilmette, IL 60091 (800) 237-4666

aging for which no good treatments are available or for which the only treatment is surgery. This causes many patients not to seek medical evaluation of incontinence. When they do seek care, expectations for cure often are low.

This pessimistic outlook is not warranted. Clinicians must provide patients and their families with an explanation of the range of therapies for incontinence. They must give them an honest but optimistic estimate of the likelihood that the problem can be brought under control. Approximately one-third of patients with incontinence have transient, fully reversible causes of incontinence. For patients without a transient cause, the treatment options, including behavioral treatment, medication, and surgery, offer most patients a reasonable expectation that incontinence can be eliminated or at least reduced.

In addition to providing information about support groups, the organizations listed in Table 6-9 produce patient education materials for the general public. Similar organizations provide the same service in other countries, such as the Continence Foundation in the United Kingdom.

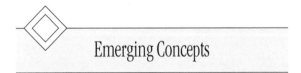

Emerging Concepts

Electrical Stimulation

Electrical stimulation is a relatively new therapeutic modality that has been widely used in research settings to manage both stress incontinence and urge incontinence. When used to mange stress incontinence, electrical stimulation of electrodes placed on the periurethral skin or in the vagina causes contraction of the urethral sphincters. The electrical stimulation is of low voltage, and patients report minimal or no discomfort. Most studies show that resolution or improvement in incontinence occurs among 25 to 50 percent of patients. However, in one study involving nursing home patients with cognitive impairment,

electrical stimulation produced no improvement in urinary control. Although this form of treatment may be used widely in the future, its ultimate role is unclear. Electrical stimulation therapy also has been used to treat patients with urge incontinence and mixed incontinence. Electrodes are placed in the vagina or surgically implanted in the spinal cord. The recently approved Inter-Stim implanted sacral stimulator is one such device. Results from preliminary studies show some benefit, and such therapies may have potential for management of incontinence.

New Drugs and Devices

Just as tolterodine was developed to retain the bladder-relaxing action of oxybutynin while reducing anticholinergic action on other organs, the future is likely to bring development of other medications designed to work specifically on the detrusor muscle or urethral sphincters while limiting action on receptors in other organs. The development of several incontinence devices, including urethral plugs and suction–occlusion devices, suggests the likelihood that other such devices will be developed. Problems with skin reactivity and urinary infection have occurred with all such devices, but developments in biomaterials may solve these problems.

Bibliography

Abrams P, Freeman R, Anderstrom C, Mattiawsson A: Tolterodine, a new antimuscarinic agent: as effective but better tolerated than oxybutynin in patients with an overactive bladder. *Br J Urol* 81:801, 1998.

Burgio KL, Locher JL, Goode PS, et al: Behavioral vs. drug treatment for urge urinary incontinence in older women: a randomized controlled trial. *JAMA* 280:1995, 1998.

Coombes GM, Millard RJ: The accuracy of portable ultrasound scanning in the measurement of residual urine volume. *J Urol* 152:2083, 1994.

Fantl JA, Bump RC, Robinson D: Efficacy of estrogen supplementation in the treatment of urinary incontinence. *Obstet Gynecol* 88:745, 1996.

Fantl JA, Newman DK, Colling J, et al: *Urinary Incontinence in Adults: Acute and Chronic Management.* Clinical Practice Guideline No. 2, 1996 update. AHCPR publication no. 96-0682. Rockville, MD: US Department of Health and Human Services, Public Health Service, Agency for Health Care Policy and Research, 1996.

Fantl JA, Wyman JF, McLish DK: Efficacy of bladder training in older women with urinary incontinence. *JAMA* 265:609, 1991.

Finlay OE, Bayles TB, Rosen C, et al: Effects of chair design, age and cognitive status on mobility. *Age Aging* 12:329, 1983.

Flaherty JH, Miller DK, Col RM: Impact on caregivers of supporting urinary function in noninstitutionalized chronically ill seniors. *Gerontologist* 32:541, 1992.

Flynn L, Cell P, Luisi E: Effectiveness of pelvic exercises in reducing urge incontinence. *J Gerontol Nurs* 20:23, 1994.

Fonda D, Brimage PJ, D'Astoli M: Simple screening for urinary incontinence in the elderly: comparison of simple and multichannel cystometry. *Urology* 42:536, 1993.

Johnson DE, Muncie HL, O'Reilly JL, Warren JW: An external urine collection device for incontinent women: evaluation of long-term use. *J Am Geriatr Soc* 138:1016, 1990.

Jones TV, Bunner SH: Approaches to urinary incontinence in a rural population: a comparison of physician assistants, nurse practitioners, and family physicians. *J Fam Pract* 11:207, 1998.

Kadar N: The value of bladder filling in the clinical detection of urine loss and selection of patients for urodynamic testing. *Br J Obstet Gynaecol* 95:698, 1988.

Koelbl H, Doerfler D, Guenther H, et al: Transurethral injection of silicone microimplants for intrinsic urethral sphincter deficiency. *Obstet Gynecol* 92:332, 1998.

Lamhut P, Jackson TW, Wall LL: The treatment of urinary incontinence with electrical stimulation in nursing home patients: a pilot study. *J Am Geriatr Soc* 40:48, 1992.

McDowell BJ, Engberg S, Weber E, et al: Successful treatment using behavioral interventions of urinary incontinence in homebound older adults. *Geriatr Nurs* 15:303, 1994.

Miller JL, Bavendam T: Treatment with the Reliance control insert: one-year experience. *J Endourol* 10:287, 1996.

Miller JM, Ashton-Miller JA, DeLancey JOL: A pelvic muscle precontraction can reduce cough-related urine loss in selected women with mild SUI. *J Am Geriatr Soc* 46:870, 1998.

Muller JL, Clauson KA: Pharmaceutical considerations of common herbal medicine. *Am J Manag Care* 3:1753, 1997.

Ouslander JG, Hepps K, Raz S, Su HL: Genitourinary dysfunction in a geriatric outpatient population. *J Am Geriatr Soc* 34:507, 1986.

Ouslander JG, Leach GE, Staskin DR: Simplified tests of lower urinary tract function in the evaluation of geriatric urinary incontinence. *J Am Geriatr Soc* 37:706, 1989.

Palmer MH: A health promotion perspective of urinary continence. *Nurs Outlook* 42:163, 1994.

Roberts RO, Jacobsen SJ, Rhodes T: Urinary incontinence in a community-based cohort: prevalence and healthcare-seeking. *J Am Geriatr Soc* 46:467, 1998.

Sand PK, Richardson DA, Staskin DR, et al: Pelvic floor electrical stimulation in the treatment of genuine stress incontinence: a multicenter, placebo-controlled trial. *Am J Obstet Gynecol* 173:72, 1995.

Santarosa RP, Blaivas JG: Periurethral injection of autologous fat for the treatment of sphincteric incompetence. *J Urol* 151:607, 1994.

Shumaker SA, Wyman JF, Uebersax JS, et al: Health-related quality-of-life measures for women with urinary incontinence: the incontinence impact questionnaire and the urogenital distress inventory. *Qual Life Res* 3:291, 1994.

Swift SE, Herring M: Comparison of pelvic organ prolapse in the dorsal lithotomy compared with the standing position. *Obstet Gynecol* 91:961, 1998.

Terpenning SM, Allada R, Kauffman CA: Intermittent urethral catheterization in the elderly. *J Am Geriatr Soc* 37:411, 1989.

Thom D: Variations in estimates of urinary incontinence prevalence in the community: effects of differences in definition, population characteristics, and study type. *J Am Geriatr Soc* 46:473, 1998.

Versi E, Griffiths DJ, Harvey MA: A new external urethral occlusive device for female urinary incontinence. *Obstet Gynecol* 92:286, 1998.

Videla FLG, Wall L: Stress incontinence diagnoses without multichannel urodynamic studies. *Obstet Gynecol* 91:965, 1998

Weiss BD: Nonpharmacologic treatment of urinary incontinence. *Am Fam Physician* 44:579, 1991.

Weiss BD: The diagnostic evaluation of urinary incontinence in geriatric patients. *Am Fam Physician* 57:2675, 1998.

Yamanishi T, Yashuda K, Suda S, et al: Effects of functional continuous magnetic stimulation for urinary incontinence. *J Urol* 163:456, 2000.

Zeitlin MP, Lebherz TB: Pessaries in the geriatric patient. *J Am Geriatr Soc* 40:635, 1992.

Noel H. Ballentine

Chapter

7

Prostate Disorders

Overview: How Common Are Prostate Problems in the Office Practice?

Principal Diagnoses

Prostate disorders are extremely common among elderly men. They were once the almost exclusive domain of urologists. Now primary care physicians are becoming more involved in the diagnosis and management of these disorders. There is a broadening awareness among physicians, payers, and patients that the treatment of patients with prostate disorders is controversial. There are widely varying opinions about the best treatment. There also is increasing awareness that treatment options can greatly affect quality of life, both adversely and positively. The management of prostate disorders highlights the need to involve patients in decision making. Decisions have to take into account patient preference and quality of life, both central concepts in the treatment of elderly patients.

This chapter focuses on two common prostate disorders—benign prostatic hyperplasia (BPH) and prostate cancer. The controversy surrounding screening for prostate cancer also is discussed. Prostatitis and its management are discussed in Chap. 17.

The diagnosis and management of BPH accounts for at least 1.7 million visits to physicians each year. The number of visits to primary care physicians has increased steadily because the diagnosis and management of BPH have become a primary care concern rather than the exclusive province of urologists. If one adds counseling of men older than 50 years about screening for prostate cancer, then prostate problems are a very common topic of discussion for primary care providers.

Benign Prostatic Hyperplasia

EPIDEMIOLOGY

The prevalence of BPH is difficult to determine from the medical literature, largely because the definition is not standard. Histologic changes are not apparent in microscopic specimens from men before the third or fourth decade of life, whereas 80 to 90 percent of specimens have microscopic changes by the eighth decade. Symptoms of prostatism occur among approximately half of these patients, and the prevalence increases after 50 years of age. Estimates from the era before pharmacologic management suggest that approximately 25 percent of men need prostatectomy during their lifetimes. The effect of drug therapy on this statistic is unclear. Only 50 percent of men with observable symptoms of prostatism experience worsening. The condition of the others stabilizes or improves.

Morbidity associated with BPH is caused by complications including acute urinary retention, bladder stones, and infection. Before prostate resection was developed, mortality from BPH was caused by renal failure due to obstructive uropathy and sepsis due to urinary stasis. With current therapies, mortality is rarely an issue; symptoms and quality of life are now the major concerns.

PATHOPHYSIOLOGY

Among infants and preadolescents the prostate is rudimentary. In adolescence it begins to grow to its adult size of approximately 20 cm^3, the size of a walnut. The gland remains about this size until the fourth decade of life, when it begins to enlarge in nearly all men.

The cause of BPH is unknown. Prostate gland metabolism is under hormonal control by dihydrotestosterone (DHT). Hyperplasia involves both the stromal fibrous elements of the gland and the glandular tissue. Because the glandular tissue is concentrated around the intraprostatic urethra (glandular transitional zone), the glandular tissue appears to be more important in terms of the development of symptoms of urethral obstruction. These hyperplastic nodules enlarge in size and increase in number and begin to obstruct and irritate the intraprostatic urethra, causing symptoms that begin in the fifth or sixth decade of life.

In the prostate testosterone is converted to DHT by the enzyme 5α-reductase, which is the active intracellular androgen of the prostate. This androgen is responsible for other changes in male humans, including the increase in ear, eyebrow, and nasal hair among men. DHT is important in the development of male pattern baldness, which among affected men occurs at the same time the prostate begins hyperplastic enlargement.

Prostate Cancer

EPIDEMIOLOGY

Apart from skin cancer, carcinoma of the prostate is the leading cancer among men. In recent years the number of cases reported each year in the United States has climbed steadily to more than 300,000 cases in 1997. The increase can be attributed in part to the aging of the population but mostly to increased detection because of the widespread use of prostate-specific antigen (PSA) testing. Mortality rates from prostate cancer have remained remarkably stable since the mid 1970s despite the availability of PSA screening and new therapies. Approximately one in five men are found to have prostate cancer in their lifetime. Autopsy studies confirm that the prevalence of the disease increases with age from approximately 12 percent in the fifth decade to more than 40 percent among men in their eighties.

Few risk factors are known for prostate cancer. The incidence of prostate cancer is higher among African Americans than among other racial or ethnic groups, and the disease usually is more advanced at the time of diagnosis and is associated with higher mortality. Asians have a lower incidence of prostate cancer; however, the incidence among naturalized Asian men approximates that of U.S.-born men, suggesting that an environmental risk factor, possibly dietary, may be more important than a genetic predisposition. High intake of dietary fat and low vitamin D levels have been implicated as risk factors. Family history is a major risk factor. Men who have multiple close relatives with the disease are at twice the risk of prostate cancer as men who do not. There is evidence that a familial form of prostate cancer may account for approximately 10 percent of cases.

Mortality rates for prostate cancer depend on the patient's age, the histologic characteristics, and the stage of the tumor at the time of diagnosis. There are four stages: Stage A is prostate cancer that is not palpable at digital rectal examination (DRE). Stage B is palpable at DRE, but the cancer is confined to the gland. Stage C describes disease that has spread beyond the prostate capsule to the periprostatic area but is nonmetastatic. Stage D is metastatic disease. Younger patients, those with poorly differentiated tumor, and those with extracapsular spread have shorter life expectancies than do older patients and patients with small, localized, well-differentiated tumors.

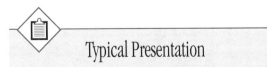

Typical Presentation

Benign Prostatic Hyperplasia

The history is the most important element in the diagnosis of BPH. Most men are at least 50 years of age and have symptoms referable to the lower urinary tract. The range and severity of symptoms is broad. Most men have symptoms that suggest obstruction or irritation, such as slow urinary stream or nocturia. Some patients have already had urinary tract infections or undergone catheterization because of urinary retention.

Patients should be asked about symptoms related to lower urinary tract or prostate diseases that could cause the symptoms or exist concomitantly. Other known causes of prostatism include urinary tract infection, urethral stricture, prostate cancer, drug side effects, and neurologic conditions that cause bladder dysfunction.

SYMPTOMS

Symptoms of BPH, often called *prostatism*, are attributable to two basic mechanisms and are outlined in Table 7-1. Obstructive symptoms are caused by direct pressure on the intraprostatic urethra from hyperplastic prostate tissue. Irritative symptoms may be caused by bladder irritability due to overdistention and instability of the detrusor muscle or urinary tract infection due to chronic retention of urine. Most patients have a combination of obstructive and irritative symptoms, although often one or two symptoms predominate. Irritative symptoms have been described as *dynamic obstruction* because they are mediated by stimulation of α-adrenergic receptors concentrated in the bladder outlet, prostate, and intraprostatic urethra. Symptoms of BPH often fluctuate over time.

MEDICATION HISTORY

Many medications can affect symptoms of prostatism. α-Adrenergic agonists are commonly available in prescription and over-the-counter preparations, such as cold remedies, nasal decongestants, and allergy medications. The effects of this class of agents are to increase the tone of the urethral sphincter and worsen the obstructive symptoms of BPH. Medications with anticholinergic properties, including antihistamines, tricyclic antidepressants, sedative-hypnotic agents, narcotics, and alcohol can decrease the tone and strength of contraction of the bladder muscles. These effects may be reversible. If the medication is withdrawn, the adverse effects diminish, and therapy may be avoided. The anticholinergic effect also may contribute to symptoms such as overflow incontinence and dribbling. Many over-the-counter cold remedies contain both a decongestant and an antihistamine. The net effect of both the α-adrenergic agonist and antihistamine can be urinary retention.

SYMPTOM CHECKLIST

Several scoring systems have been developed and validated to quantify symptoms of prostatism. The American Urological Association (AUA) symptom index (Table 7-2) is well accepted. This tool is increasingly being referred to in the literature as the International Prostate Symptom Score. The instrument contains seven questions and can be easily completed by patients. This semiquantitative record of symptoms can be used to monitor symptom severity or response to therapy over time.

Table 7-1

Symptoms of Benign Prostatic Hyperplasia

OBSTRUCTIVE SYMPTOMS	IRRITATIVE SYMPTOMS
Hesitancy to initiate voiding	Urinary frequency
Decreased urinary stream force or caliber	Nocturia
Straining to void	Dysuria
Dribbling after voiding	Urinary urgency
Urinary retention, incomplete emptying	Urge incontinence
Interruption of urine flow (intermittency)	Suprapubic discomfort

Prostate Cancer

Symptoms of prostate cancer often are absent or nonspecific. Patients may have obstructive or irritative symptoms as in BPH. Some patients have hematuria, infection due to urinary retention, or vague suprapubic discomfort. Metastatic disease may be present at the time of diagnosis with symptoms that depend on the site of metastasis. Disease metastatic to the spine usually causes back pain or symptoms of cord compression such as lower extremity weakness, paresthesia, or bowel or bladder incontinence.

Table 7-2

American Urological Association Symptom Index

URINARY SYMPTOMS	NOT AT ALL	LESS THAN 20%	LESS THAN 50%	ABOUT 50%	MORE THAN 50%	ALMOST ALWAYS
1. During the past month or so, how often have you had a sensation of not emptying your bladder completely after you finished urinating?	0	1	2	3	4	5
2. During the past month or so, how often have you had to urinate again less than 2 hours after you finished urinating?	0	1	2	3	4	5
3. During the past month or so, how often have you found you stopped and started several times when you urinated?	0	1	2	3	4	5
4. During the past month or so, how often have you found it difficult to postpone urination?	0	1	2	3	4	5
5. During the past month or so, how often have you had a weak urinary stream?	0	1	2	3	4	5
6. During the past month or so, how often have you had to push or strain to begin urination?	0	1	2	3	4	5

7. During the past month or so, how many times did you most typically get up to urinate from the time you went to bed at night until the time you got up in the morning?

| 0 Times | 1 Time | 2 Times | 3 Times | 4 Times | 5 Times |

Total AUA Symptom Score = sum of questions 1 to 7 = _____

Interpretation of AUA Symptom Index
  Mild prostatic disease ≤ 7
  Moderate prostatic disease = 8 to 18
  Severe prostatic disease > 18
Highest possible score = 35

ABBREVIATION: AUA, American Urological Association.
SOURCE: Adapted from McConnell JD, Barry MJ, Bruskewitz RC, et al: *Benign Prostatic Hyperplasia: Diagnosis and Treatment*. Clinical Practice Guideline no. 8. AHCPR publication no. 94-0582. Rockville, MD, U.S. Department of Health and Human Services, 1994. Agency for Health Care Policy and Research, 1994.

Physical Examination

Symptoms of prostatism do not necessarily correlate with the size of the prostate as determined at DRE. Hyperplastic nodules that form in the periurethral area of the prostate are likely to cause obstruction because of proximity to the urethra, even if they are small. Nodules that grow in the peripheral zone of the prostate may not impinge on the urethra or affect urine flow despite attaining large size. Hyperplastic prostatic tissue may grow outward and cause little obstruction despite a large prostate. Inward growth may result in static obstruction, which can be quite severe even though the prostate is small. Nodules tend to first grow in the periurethral area of the prostate but then may grow throughout the gland. It is not unusual to find men with symptoms of prostatic disease in their fifth decade who have little or no enlargement of the prostate at DRE or to find elderly men with few or no symptoms and a large or occasionally very large prostate gland.

Benign Prostatic Hyperplasia

In a patient with BPH, the DRE commonly reveals an enlarged prostate. This is more a correlate of the patient's age than an indicator of the degree of obstruction. At examination, a normal, benign gland is firm and elastic. Enlargement with multiple nodules may cause irregularity of the surface of the gland that may be difficult to differentiate from induration or nodules suggestive of cancer. Hard nodules within the prostate or on the surface may represent prostate cancer; however, prostate cancer also may manifest more subtly as areas of induration rather than as a definite nodule. The finding of a soft, so-called boggy, tender prostate suggests chronic prostatitis. When questioned specifically, patients usually can discriminate between *uncomfortable*, the normal feeling at DRE, and *tender*, associated with a boggy area

suggestive of chronic prostatitis. The rest of the physical examination includes evaluation of the rectum for sphincter tone, abnormal masses or polyps, and hemorrhoids. Examination of the abdomen may reveal an enlarged bladder due to chronic urinary obstruction and retention.

Prostate Cancer

The DRE has been used widely to screen for prostate cancer. Tumors often cannot be palpated or may be palpable only when they are large and are already nonlocalized. Some clinicians rely on DRE alone for diagnosis with the thought that only clinically important tumors are found. PSA testing is now widely available as a screening and diagnostic test for prostate cancer and is more sensitive and specific than DRE. Clinicians who advise PSA testing generally believe that the addition of DRE increases the diagnostic yield. DRE can yield other important information about the prostate and rectal vault. Examination of the back for spinous process tenderness and the lower extremities for abnormal neurologic findings occasionally reveals signs suggestive of metastatic prostate cancer.

Ancillary Tests

Prostate-Specific Antigen

PSA is a protease glycoprotein secreted by prostatic epithelial cells. Its function is to liquefy the seminal coagulum. PSA was discovered in the mid 1970s and initially was used in rape cases. Next it was used to monitor the effectiveness of treatment interventions for prostate cancer. PSA is prostate-specific, not prostate cancer–specific. It has a half-life of approximately 3 days. The normal serum level varies with age from approximately 2 ng/mL in 40-year-old men to 6 to 7 ng/mL in 70- to 80-year-old men. Normal PSA levels increase as men age; a PSA level of 4.5 ng/mL in a 49-year-old man might warrant a biopsy but not such a level in a 65-year-old man. Refinements in age-specific norms are now taking into account race-related variations.

Elevations in PSA level not caused by prostate cancer are caused by any injury or inflammation of the prostate, including acute or chronic prostatitis, urinary retention, BPH, infarction or trauma, prostatic biopsy, and urethral calculi. Performance of DRE raises PSA level slightly but not enough to be clinically significant. Therefore it is not necessary to delay PSA measurement after DRE. Finasteride, used in therapy for BPH, halves PSA level. For accurate interpretation when a patient is taking this drug, the measured PSA level should be doubled. When this is taken into account, finasteride does not seem to interfere with the ability to use PSA assays in the diagnosis of prostate cancer.

PSA screening has not been tested in any large prospective trial. Therefore the true sensitivity and specificity of the test are not known. Gann et al reported results of a retrospective study in which they examined the development of prostate cancer within 4 years of PSA measurement. Seventy-three percent of men who had a PSA level greater than 4.0 ng/mL had prostate cancer. When the PSA level was less than 4.0 ng/mL, 91 percent of the men did not have clinically significant prostate cancer. In a different study, Richie et al showed a specificity of 78 percent for men in their seventies. One of every five to eight men in their sixties or seventies have normal biopsy findings after a falsely elevated PSA. The positive predictive value (the proportion of persons with positive tests who have prostate cancer) for a PSA level between 4 and 10 ng/mL is approximately 20 percent.

Because of the relatively low sensitivity and specificity of current PSA assays found in many studies, several attempts at improving the operating characteristics have been suggested. PSA velocity (change in PSA value over time with serial reevaluation) can be used for early detection. Carter et al showed that a rate of increase greater than 0.8 ng/mL per year is more likely to be associated with cancer. A potentially important use of PSA velocity is to aid diagnosis when PSA levels are elevated and the biopsy result is negative. A rapidly rising PSA level at repeated annual measurements may suggest the increase is caused by prostate cancer and may suggest that prostate biopsy be repeated. PSA density (PSA level divided by the volume of the prostate from transrectal ultrasound measurement) may have diagnostic usefulness. Because of expense and difficulty, this approach has not gained widespread popularity.

Another development is measurement of free PSA. PSA circulates in the bloodstream bound to a number of different proteins, but it also can circulate unbound in a free form. The percentage of free PSA is lower (less than 25 percent) among men with prostate cancer than among other men. The percentage of free PSA may be used to determine which patients require further evaluation with prostate biopsy. Catalona et al predicted that among men with a PSA between 4.0 and 10.0 mg/mL and normal findings at DRE, using a free PSA value less than 25 percent as a criterion for biopsy would miss only 5 percent of cancers and avoid 20 percent of unnecessary biopsies. The positive predictive value was 24 percent.

Transrectal Ultrasonography and Biopsy

Transrectal ultrasonography (TRUS) is a poor tool for screening and diagnosing prostate cancer. The sensitivity of TRUS is 35 to 98 percent, and the specificity is 30 to 94 percent. The positive predictive value ranges between 9 percent and 59 percent, depending on the population studied. The sensitivity of TRUS in the detection of prostate cancer is low, particularly for smaller-volume tumors. The examination also is relatively expensive and uncomfortable.

The main use of TRUS is to guide needle biopsy either of palpable nodules or for systematic sampling when a patient has elevated PSA levels. The procedure has low morbidity. Desmond et al conducted a study that focused on patients undergoing biopsy with contemporary techniques (prophylactic antibiotics, 18-gauge needle with automated biopsy device, under TRUS guidance, and no prebiopsy enema). The investigators found a 2.1 percent total complication rate. Complications included fever or prostatitis, gross hematuria, vasovagal reactions, and hematospermia. Only 0.6 percent of patients needed hospitalization. Prophylactic antibiotics are recommended because the rectal wall is transgressed multiple times during the procedure. Studies of procedures performed with no prophylactic antibiotics, larger-bore needles, or preprocedure enemas show higher postprocedure complication rates. Most reports state that the procedure is mildly uncomfortable; however, the discomfort is quite variable. Finally, a potential problem with systematic biopsy may be the finding of low-risk, clinically insignificant cancer that results in patient anxiety and unnecessary treatment.

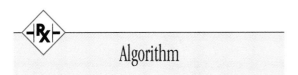

Algorithm

There are multiple ways to approach BPH. Any approach must take into account patient preference and comfort with both symptoms and therapy. Figure 7-1 shows an approach to the treatment of patients with BPH. When a patient has symptoms of prostatism (see Table 7-1), the history and physical examination should be concentrated on the potential causes of the symptoms. If drug side effects are suspected, discontinuation of the offending agent alone may result in resolution of the symptoms. Therapy for a urinary tract infection or prostatitis also can alleviate the symptoms. Therapy for obstructive symptoms caused by prostate cancer is discussed later.

Once a diagnosis of BPH is suspected, the clinician should evaluate the severity of symptoms using the AUA or other symptom checklist. Patients with high symptom checklist scores or an indication for surgical therapy, such as complete obstruction, should be referred for appropriate

surgical intervention. A patient with mild symptoms may want to monitor the symptoms and consider therapy only if symptoms worsen. Pharmacologic therapy is appropriate for men with moderate symptoms.

As described later, there are many options for pharmacologic treatment. The algorithm in Fig. 7-1 shows that when pharmacologic therapy is considered, an α-adrenergic blocker is the treatment of choice because of its rapid onset of action. Saw palmetto also may be considered. Finasteride may be indicated for treatment of men with larger prostate glands because of its mechanism of action, but this therapy has not been proved effective in randomized trials. For patients who also have hypertension, an α-adrenergic blocker can be chosen for both its antihypertensive and anti-BPH effects. If blood pressure is well controlled and there is concern about orthostatic side effects of an α-adrenergic blocker, finasteride or the more selective α-adrenergic blocking agent tamsulosin may be considered. If therapy is ineffective after an adequate trial in terms of both duration of therapy and dosage of an agent, switching to another class of agent should be considered. Adding a drug of another class makes most sense for patients with a partial response who want additional symptom relief. If symptoms progress or the patient is not responding, surgery should be considered.

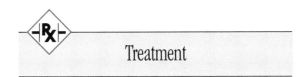

Treatment

Benign Prostatic Hyperplasia

Treatment options have changed dramatically with the development of new pharmacologic approaches. Transurethral resection of the prostate (TURP) was without question the therapy of choice in the 1980s. Patients and physicians now are more reluctant to pursue surgical intervention without first considering nonsurgical options. New approaches, so-called minimally invasive therapies, are being

Figure 7-1

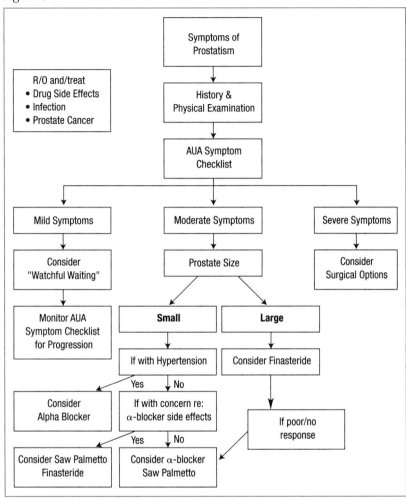

Treatment algorithm for patients with benign prostatic hyperplasia.

developed and tested. If they prove effective, they will add choices to the management of BPH (see "Emerging Concepts").

The decision to treat a patient for BPH must be individualized and based on the patient's concern over the symptoms. Many patients seek medical advice because of symptoms, but once reassured that the cause is benign and that many treatment options are available, they often decide to live with the symptoms without treatment. Many men with mild symptoms accept a plan of watchful waiting. The AUA symptom index can be useful in this setting to monitor changes in symptoms over time. Among men with moderate symptoms of prostatism, approximately 40 percent improve, 45 percent have no change in symptoms, and only 15 percent worsen after 5 years. Symptoms of prostatism often fluctuate over time.

Only a small percentage of patients have complications. The average incidence of acute urinary retention among untreated men with BPH is 6.8 per 1000 person-years. Men who have more severe symptoms when they seek medical attention have as much as a fourfold higher risk of acute retention than men with milder symptoms. Other complications include recurrent urinary tract infection, acute urinary retention, bladder calculi, incontinence, and renal compromise from hydronephrosis.

Most men choose therapy when the symptoms become intolerable, but there is a wide spectrum as to what patients find intolerable. For one patient getting up four or five times a night is no problem; for another it is enough to necessitate treatment. Some men are not disturbed by dribbling; others see it as an indication for treatment.

Once a patient decides the symptoms are intolerable, the clinician needs to counsel him on the treatment options. Not enough studies have been performed comparing one therapy with another to make valid conclusions regarding superiority of one over another. The follow-up periods with all therapies except TURP and open prostatectomy are relatively short. Watchful waiting has emerged as an important option for many if not most patients and must not be overlooked. TURP and open prostatectomy have retained an important place in the treatment of patients with severe symptoms and complications of BPH such as acute urinary retention. Mild symptoms generally do not warrant therapy other than watchful waiting. Therapeutic decisions mostly apply to patients with moderate symptoms.

PHARMACOLOGIC MANAGEMENT

Some patients with mild to moderate symptoms and those who cannot tolerate surgery or refuse surgery are candidates for drug therapy. Currently two classes of drugs are available— α-adrenergic blockers and 5α-reductase inhibitors. These drugs have been shown effective, safe, and well tolerated. Whether drug therapy can prevent or delay surgical intervention or improve quality of life for the long term is not clear.

α-ADRENERGIC BLOCKERS   This class of drugs reduces smooth muscle tone through an effect on the α-adrenergic nerves in the neck of the bladder and the prostatic urethra. The result is decreased resistance to urine flow and improvement in symptoms of prostatism. Three α-adrenergic blockers have been approved by the U.S. Food and Drug Administration (FDA)—terazosin (Hytrin), doxazosin (Cardura), and tamsulosin (Flomax). Terazosin and doxazosin have been shown effective in multiple randomized, controlled trials. Tamsulosin has been found in open-label trials to have similar efficacy as terazosin and doxazosin. Use of α-adrenergic blockers has been associated with 50 percent improvement in measured urinary flow rate, 60 to 70 percent improvement in obstructive symptoms, and approximately 35 percent improvement in irritative symptoms. The side effects of terazosin and doxazosin are listed in Table 7-3. Side effects for tamsulosin appear to be uncommon, possibly because it is more specific for the α_{1A} subtype adrenergic receptor.

One clinical advantage of use of terazosin or doxazosin is that a large number of patients with hypertension and BPH can use one drug to control both conditions.

Terazosin and doxazosin must be started in small doses and increased gradually in a stepwise manner to avoid the phenomenon of first-dose syncope caused by sudden vasodilatation and

Table 7-3

Common Side Effects of Terazosin and Doxazosin

SIDE EFFECT	PERCENTAGE OF PATIENTS REPORTING
Dizziness	9–15
Headache	10
Fatigue, asthenia	8
Postural hypotension	2–8
Impotence	4
Decreased libido	<1
Syncope	<1

hypotension. Terazosin should be started at 1 mg and taken for several days, then increased to 2 mg for several more days, then 5 mg for about a week, then 10 mg. Some patients need the maximum dose of 20 mg. Symptoms should be monitored. Some patients, particularly elderly patients and those being treated for hypertension with other agents, may need to have postural blood pressure checked before each dose increase. Doxazosin is dosed similarly, starting at 1 mg, then 2 mg, 4 mg, and occasionally 8 mg. Many patients do not notice improvement until the higher dosage is reached (10 mg for terazosin and 4 to 8 mg for doxazosin). It is recommended that these drugs be taken at bedtime because the maximum vasodilatory effect occurs in the first several hours, when presumably the patient is sleeping. If the drug is withdrawn, held, or missed for more than 1 day, receptors become unblocked and again sensitive to the first-dose phenomenon. Patients need to be counseled how to restart these medications, starting at the lowest dose and gradually increasing the dose.

Tamsulosin can be started at its full dose of 0.4 mg at the same time each day. It is not necessary to take it at night. Postural hypotension and syncope are less of a problem with tamsulosin. A few patients may need 0.8 mg to control the symptoms. It may turn out that the ease of dosing and the apparent lack of side effects offer patients an advantage, but clinical experience with tamsulosin is limited at this time.

The onset of action of α-adrenergic blockers is rapid. Patients respond within weeks. Therapy must be continued, or symptoms will recur. The annual cost of the drugs alone is $300 to $400.

5α-REDUCTASE INHIBITORS   The other pharmacologic treatment available is 5α-reductase inhibition. Finasteride (Proscar) is the only drug in this class approved by the FDA for management of BPH. The drug works by blocking the conversion of testosterone to DHT. DHT is the active androgen within the prostate responsible for hyperplasia of the gland. Treatment with finasteride markedly decreases intraprostatic levels of DHT and shrinks the prostate. This shrinks periurethral nodules and decreases obstruction of the intraprostatic urethra. The drug does not affect serum testosterone levels and therefore has no effect on nonprostatic effects of testosterone, such as bone mass.

Finasteride shrinks the prostate an average of 25 percent, which results in improvement in symptoms and urine flow for approximately 35 percent of men with BPH. Finasteride therapy may reduce serum PSA level approximately 50 percent, but it may take as long as 6 months before the maximum effect occurs. If the drug is discontinued, symptoms return. Symptoms after discontinuation may be slightly worse because of normal progression of the disease. This is not a rebound effect.

Finasteride is generally well tolerated. Studies show a 3 percent incidence of impotence, diminished libido, or decreased volume of ejaculate. Side effects are reversible with discontinuation of therapy. Although no teratogenic effects have been reported, women who want to bear children should not be exposed to the drug directly or through contact with semen of men taking finasteride. Finasteride can cause feminization of the genitalia of male fetuses. The annual cost of the drug alone is approximately $600.

TRANSURETHRAL RESECTION OF THE PROSTATE

The indications for TURP have changed dramatically because of the development of pharmacologic therapies (Table 7-4). In the 1980s, this operation was the tenth most common surgical procedure performed in the United States. A high morbidity rate and variable results led to reevaluation of the procedure and interest in other therapies.

Despite the problems, TURP is the procedure of choice when surgery is needed for BPH. TURP improves urine flow with rates higher than those obtained with any other therapy, generally 15 to 20 mL/s. Most patients have marked improvement in symptoms. TURP is effective and has good long-term results for most patients. Seventy-five percent of patients are satisfied with the results.

Table 7-4

Relative Indications for Surgical Management
of Benign Prostatic Hyperplasia

Significant symptoms of prostatism (patient quality of life)
Acute urinary retention
Urinary tract infection, including urosepsis
Azotemia, renal failure, obstructive uropathy
Recurrent gross hematuria
Urinary incontinence (overflow or urge)

Graversen et al reported that approximately 20 percent of patients need reoperations 8 years after the original procedure, a rate of 2 to 2.5 percent per year in several studies. The procedure costs approximately $7000.

TURP is performed with spinal or light general anesthesia. A scope is inserted into the intraprostatic portion of the urethra, and a diathermy loop is used to remove chips of hyperplastic tissue through the scope. A relatively large cavity is produced in the prostate to relieve the obstruction. The denuded tissue epithelializes after several weeks. After the operation a catheter must be placed for several days to allow irrigation of the lower urinary system to prevent thrombus occlusion.

Complications of TURP are uncommon. Although most patients who undergo TURP are elderly and 70 percent have underlying medical problems, the mortality is low (0.2 percent). Morbidity usually is caused by sepsis (rare), hemorrhage (2.5 percent), urinary retention (3 to 5 percent), infection (2 percent), and transurethral syndrome (dilutional hyponatremia, confusion, nausea, vomiting, hypertension). Erectile dysfunction (10 to 20 percent) and retrograde ejaculation (70 to 90 percent) are more common and troublesome complications. Because there is no physiologic explanation for the erectile dysfunction, some clinicians speculate that many of these men had erectile dysfunction before the operation. The most troublesome complication of TURP is incontinence, occurring among fewer than 1 percent of patients.

Only occasionally do patients have permanent urinary incontinence.

Prostate Cancer

There are three initial approaches to the treatment of patients with nonmetastatic prostate cancer—watchful waiting, surgery, and radiation therapy. The choice among the three is difficult because prostate cancer is a relatively common disease (lifetime risk 8.7 percent) but not a common cause of death (2.6 percent). There are patient and tumor characteristics that are associated with a more aggressive course. Because aggressive treatment with either radical prostatectomy or radiation therapy has risk, tumors that are not expected to become clinically relevant or would not respond to surgical therapy ideally should be managed conservatively. Willet Whitmore articulated the dilemma regarding prostate cancer eloquently when he said,

> Is cure necessary in those for whom it is possible?
> Is cure possible in those for whom it is necessary?

PREDICTING WHO NEEDS TREATMENT

One approach to solving this dilemma is attempting to predict which tumors carry the greatest risk. Albertsen reviewed known tumor characteristics and risk factors to help determine when watchful waiting is appropriate. The histologic features of the tumor, rated with the Gleason score, are an important factor in determining tumor aggression. Using this system, the pathologist grades the two predominant histologic patterns from 1 to 5 and sums these to give a score between 2 and 10. Well-differentiated tumors have Gleason scores from 2 to 4, moderately differentiated 5 or 6, more aggressive but not poorly differentiated 7, poorly differentiated 8 to 10. The less well-differentiated the tumor, the higher is the Gleason score and the greater is the chance the tumor has invaded the prostatic capsule or metastasized. Aggressive surgical therapy usually fails. The more well-differentiated the tumor, the greater the chance for a benign tumor course. Watchful waiting may be more appropriate in this case. Tumors that are moderately differentiated have a better chance of necessitating and responding to surgical or radiation therapy.

Other factors that predict survival and tumor course have been examined. DNA analysis by means of flow cytometry can determine the percentage of aneuploid versus diploid versus tetraploid cells in samples of prostate tissue. Patients with tumors that have higher percentages of diploid cells have better survival rates. Small tumor volume also is associated with better outcomes. Most of the clinically irrelevant tumors found in autopsy specimens from older men are less than 0.5 cm^3 in volume. Tumors that are larger than 3 cm^3 usually have metastasized. The doubling time for prostate cancer appears to be more than 5 years. It may be that tumor volume can be estimated from the amount of neoplastic tissue present in needle biopsy specimens. Thus older men with small-volume tumors have a better survival rate and may not need aggressive therapy.

Aggressive tumors have a higher absolute PSA level than incidental tumors, and the rate of increase (PSA velocity) is a steeper curve. More than 50 percent of men with a PSA greater than 10 ng/mL no longer have localized disease. The percentage of free PSA in patients with prostate cancer may predict outcome.

Other risk factors to consider when deciding which patients should be aggressively treated include age and presence of coexisting disease. Because prostate cancer tends to be relatively slow in progression, patients often do not have clinically relevant disease for 5 to 15 years. Thus patients who have a life expectancy shorter than this, because of their age or the presence of other disease, are not candidates for aggressive intervention and should be treated conservatively. Albertsen showed that 40 percent of men found to have localized prostate cancer were dead of other causes within 10 years.

TREATMENT OPTIONS

Management of prostate cancer varies from region to region. The three main options are prostatectomy, radiation, and watchful waiting. In the United States attempts at curative therapy with radical prostatectomy or radiation therapy are much more common than in Europe and Asia, where observational therapy or watchful waiting with delayed hormonal manipulation is preferred. However, in one study investigators found that even in the United States most cases of localized prostate cancer are managed expectantly. In 1990 more than 65 percent of patients with stage A and 17 percent with stage B disease were treated with observational therapy. Within the United States there are great regional differences in choice of the two main curative therapies.

PROSTATECTOMY The benefit of curative therapy is that patients may be spared the burden of advanced disease. However, curative surgery is not always effective. A prostatectomy follow-up study showed that 35 percent of men treated with radical prostatectomy needed additional therapy. The risk of erectile dysfunction, even with nerve-sparing surgery, is high and is a function of the age of the patient. For men older than 65 years, the rate of erectile dysfunction is approximately 90 percent. A rate of 20 to 50 percent is found among younger men. Incontinence necessitating use of pads or a penile clamp affects 6 to 26 percent of men who undergo a radical prostatectomy. This causes emotional distress and restriction of activities. Other complications of radical prostatectomy include a 1 percent surgical mortality, approximately 15 percent risk of urethral stricture, and a 3 percent risk of rectal injury.

RADIATION THERAPY The other potentially curative therapy, radiation therapy, also carries risk of complications—radiation cystitis and proctitis. As many as 10 percent of men who undergo radiation therapy sustain rectal injury. There also is an approximately 5 percent risk of urinary incontinence after radiation therapy. Erectile dysfunction also may become a problem, affecting about one-half of patients treated.

MONITORING AFTER SURGERY OR RADIATION THERAPY

After curative therapy, patients can be observed with PSA measurements. After radical prostatectomy, PSA should be undetectable. After radiation therapy, PSA levels are low, but PSA is detectable. An increase in PSA level after either procedure is indicative of residual disease. Many clinicians measure PSA every 6 months. Patients with residual disease after radical surgical intervention can undergo radiation therapy. When curative treatment fails, hormonal manipulation can be attempted. Some patients have residual disease 10 to 15 years after initial treatment.

MANAGEMENT OF METASTATIC DISEASE

The major benefit of observational therapy is that the patient's quality of life is not affected by complications. However, once disease spreads beyond the prostatic capsule, the chance for cure is lost. Hormonal manipulation resulting in androgen ablation is based on the observation that growth of prostatic cells, including prostate cancer, is stimulated by androgen. Circulating testosterone is converted to DHT in the prostate. Deprivation of testosterone by means of castration or therapy with estrogen or nonsteroidal antiandrogens is not curative but has been shown to prolong survival. Therapy usually is started when metastatic disease is first diagnosed, usually with a bone scan. Conventional chemotherapy has not been shown to be useful, but several new agents are under investigation and show promising results. In terminal disease, pain management, particularly of pain from bone metastasis, is important. Opiate analgesics usually are needed. Radiation therapy to affected sites is also of great benefit.

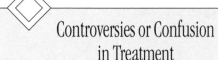

Controversies or Confusion in Treatment

Screening for Prostate Cancer

Screening for prostate cancer remains a controversial issue. Many organizations give differing recommendations. The American College of Physicians, the National Cancer Institute, and the United States Preventive Services Task force have stated that there is insufficient evidence to support the use of PSA measurement for screening for prostate cancer. Both the American Urological Association and the American Cancer Society recommend starting screening with PSA measurement at 50 years of age. The AUA recommends starting screening at 40 years of age for men at high risk of prostate cancer.

When considering screening for prostate cancer it is useful to recall criteria for a valid screening test. The controversy regarding screening for prostate cancer centers on two questions. First, is PSA measurement a good screening test for prostate cancer? Second, is there effective therapy once the cancer is detected early?

SCREENING TEST

The test characteristics of DRE, PSA measurement, and TRUS are described earlier. Although it can be argued whether these are good screening tests, there is no controversy that prostate cancer diagnosed as the result of PSA screening is more likely to be in an earlier stage. Brett summarized the situation aptly when he said that "In advising these patients, clinicians face the task of balancing their own views, their patient's expectations, and conflicting guidelines issued by professional organizations."

If clinician and patient elect to screen for prostate cancer, most advocates of screening use a strategy of combining DRE and PSA measurement.

This approach essentially doubles the number of cases found. Patients with localized prostate cancer have a normal finding at DRE 45 percent of the time and a normal PSA level 35 percent of the time. In screening situations DRE has a cancer detection rate of 1.3 to 1.7 percent; PSA measurement has a rate of 2.2 to 4.0 percent. When prostate cancer is diagnosed through DRE it is still confined to the organ in 50 percent of cases. When it is detected because of an abnormal PSA level it is localized in 75 percent of patients at diagnosis. If either test result is abnormal, further evaluation with TRUS and biopsy is the next step.

There are problems with this approach. Studies of this strategy found that approximately one of every four or five men has an abnormality and undergoes the expense and risk of biopsy. Yet the cancer detection rate with this approach is approximately one case of cancer among 25 patients. Therefore, a relatively large number of patients undergo a moderately invasive and expensive test to find relatively few cases of cancer. This approach raises another question: What follow-up treatment should be given when the biopsy results are normal? This question was fueled by a study in which patients were evaluated serially with biopsies. The investigators found that 25 percent of men who had mildly elevated PSA results (4 to 9 ng/mL) later had cancer. Two tests have been proposed to help guide this decision. First, an abnormal PSA velocity (a normal increase is approximately 0.75 ng/mL per year) may help ascertain which patients need repeated biopsies. An alternative is to determine percentage of free PSA to direct who needs another biopsy. Patients with a percentage of free PSA less than 25 percent have a higher likelihood that the elevation is caused by prostate cancer.

IS TREATMENT EFFECTIVE?

The second question concerning screening is whether early treatment prolongs life or increases longevity. Using a favorable set of assumptions regarding the effectiveness of therapy and side effects, Fleming et al concluded that screening for prostate cancer with DRE and PSA measurement among men 50 to 69 years of age may increase the average life span approximately 2 weeks. Among older men, or if a less favorable set of assumptions is used, the benefits are less, and more harm than good may result. No large randomized, controlled trials have shown any benefit from early detection of prostate cancer. The current best evidence is from a prospective, population-based study by Johansson et al in Sweden. Watchful waiting was compared with radiation therapy of men with an average age of 72 years and with localized disease. If the disease progressed, the men were treated with hormonal therapy. After follow-up study for 15 years, the outcomes were similar. The authors concluded that an aggressive approach to the care of patients with early disease would result in substantial overtreatment.

RESOLVING THE DILEMMA

The controversy in the literature over screening for prostate cancer places both the primary care physician and the patient in a dilemma. The Prostate Cancer Intervention versus Observation Trial (PIVOT) is enrolling patients with clinically localized prostate cancer of all histologic grades. Participants have been randomized to receive expectant management with palliative therapy for metastatic or symptomatic disease or to undergo radical prostatectomy with early intervention for persistent or recurrent disease. Randomization was completed in 1997, and patients will be observed a minimum of 12 years. This study should answer the question. Until the results are available, physicians and patients have to base decisions on limited information.

There has been increasing interest in following the principle of informed consent when helping a patient choose a course of action. The American College of Physicians in its clinical guidelines on prostate cancer screening states, "Routine PSA testing without frank discussion of the issues involved is inappropriate." Current thinking aimed at making the best decisions possible is focused on two concepts. One is informed consent and how physicians need to inform patients about the important benefits and risks of screening or treating them for prostate cancer. The second concept involves decision analysis to determine who specifically may benefit from screening and possible treatment so that physicians can approach the care of the individual patient and help that patient make the best decision. Although decision analysis models are far from perfect, and there continues to be controversy and disagreement, the second approach should help patients decide more rationally.

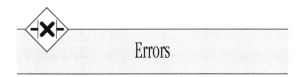

Errors

Benign Prostatic Hyperplasia

There are a number of errors, misconceptions, and misunderstandings involved in the management of BPH.

DIAGNOSING BENIGN PROSTATIC HYPERPLASIA

BPH is a clinical diagnosis based on symptoms; several other entities, such as medication use, prostate cancer, and urinary tract infection, must be excluded. A common error is that in taking histories regarding drugs that can cause urinary obstruction, physicians do not ask directly, or patients may not think to tell, about the use of medications that contain an α-agonist. These compounds are frequent ingredients in over-the-counter cold remedies that contain drugs such as pseudoephedrine or phenylpropanolamine. They can cause complete obstruction or lesser degrees of prostatism. When these drugs are withdrawn, considerable improvement occurs. Many herbal medications contain drugs that can adversely affect the prostate. *Ma huang* and *guarana* contain ephedrine. Patients may not be inclined to tell physicians they are using alternative medications,

or they may simply assume that because these agents are "natural," they cannot cause harm.

Some patients with uncontrolled diabetes and glycosuria or uncompensated congestive heart failure who experience redistribution of peripheral edema fluid when supine at night have nocturia that may suggest the presence of BPH.

Some patients who have underlying urge incontinence caused by detrusor hyperactivity or instability are protected from wetting by an obstructing prostate gland. Physicians may recommend TURP to these patients because of the symptoms of prostatism; however, after the operation, the patient's quality of life is far worse because the underlying urge incontinence may become fully expressed. Patients who are at risk of urge incontinence are those who have central nervous system diseases such as stroke, multi-infarct dementia, multiple sclerosis, spinal cord injury, or Parkinson's disease. Bladder irritation from stones, tumors, or BPH also may cause urge incontinence. Patients with diabetes mellitus perceive the urge to void and are unable to arrest emptying the bladder. They usually pass larger volumes of urine when they become incontinent, although this too can be mitigated by prostatic hyperplasia. These patients should undergo urodynamic testing before TURP is considered.

RELATION BETWEEN PROSTATE SIZE AND SEVERITY OF SYMPTOMS

Another common error is failing to recognize that there is no relation between the size of the prostate and the degree of obstructive or irritative symptoms. A patient with a small prostate can have severe symptoms, and an elderly man with no symptoms at all can have a huge prostate. The possibility of BPH should not be excluded simply because the prostate gland does not feel enlarged at physical examination.

THERAPY FOR BENIGN PROSTATIC HYPERPLASIA

To avoid first-dose syncope associated with some α-blockers, this side effect should be discussed with patients. Patients also should be instructed to take the pill at bedtime because the hypotensive effect is most prominent in the first few hours after dosing. Patients, especially those taking higher doses of α-blockers, need to be told not to miss their pills for more than a day, or they will have to retitrate from small doses just as when they started.

Clinicians should keep in mind that PSA levels can be affected by finasteride. PSA level can decrease by one-half in patients who have been treated for more than 6 months. A PSA level that does not decline suggests either the patient is not taking the medication or there may be another cause of increased PSA level, such as prostate cancer.

Although patients with symptoms of BPH deserve to have attempts at treatment, practitioners should avoid overzealous treatment with drug therapy or another modality if the patient is not greatly bothered by the symptoms. Therapy for BPH should be instituted only when the symptoms interfere with what the patient would like to be doing or when quality of life is compromised.

Symptoms of prostatism can wax and wane dramatically. Studies of BPH consistently show that 35 percent of patients in the placebo group routinely improve. Basing conclusions about any one patient's likelihood of improving on the therapy provided therefore is difficult. Results of any study that does not have a placebo group, even if it shows a significant improvement over the pretreatment condition, must be viewed with great suspicion.

Prostate Cancer

Many clinicians fail to perform a rectal examination properly. Performing a careful DRE is an important first step in diagnosing early prostate cancer. The entire gland should be swept over with firm, gentle pressure at least two or three times to identify asymmetries that manifest as firm nodules or areas of induration. The sensitivity and specificity of DRE are variable and often depend on the level of experience and expertise of the examiner.

PSA testing for screening and diagnosis of prostate cancer must take into consideration that the specificity of this test in the diagnosis of prostate cancer is 40 to 60 percent. An elevated PSA level has a differential diagnosis that includes prostate cancer but also less serious disorders such as BPH, kidney stone (passage), and prostatitis. PSA elevations need to be taken in clinical context, and some patients may not need a biopsy immediately. In the correct clinical context, such as therapy for prostatitis, some patients may be observed carefully. If the examination findings and PSA level normalize, biopsy may be avoided.

Family Approach

Family implications of prostate disease are informed decision making and social isolation. Prostate disease is a common occurrence in old age, and decisions regarding care and treatment may have to be shared with a spouse or children because the patient has limited decision-making ability. Family members need to understand diagnoses, implications, and concepts of prostate disease, the value of therapies, and prognosis.

Aggressive therapy for prostate cancer in the form of radical surgical or radiation therapy often produces side effects that are disturbing to patients. Urinary incontinence is a problem that leads many elders to progressive social isolation. Erectile dysfunction is common among the elderly, and therapy for prostate cancer may cause or aggravate the problem. Erectile dysfunction may directly affect the spouse, who may wish to continue sexual intercourse. This can put considerable strain on a marriage, even one long established. It is the responsibility of the clinician to explore issues of sexuality with all patients, particularly in the context of prostate cancer. Simple, frank discussion of issues of sexual desire or alternative forms of intimacy may be all that is necessary. Various therapies exist to help with erectile dysfunction if this is what the couple, or patient, wants.

Androgen ablation for advanced prostate cancer may include castration, which for some patients causes a loss of masculine identity. If a spouse is present, counseling about how to restore the patient's identity may prove relatively simple and effective.

Although it is often said "patients die with prostate cancer, not of prostate cancer," this is not always true. Terminal care may become an issue for some families. As with any other terminal disease, palliative care consisting of social support and medical care for symptom relief, including pain relief and nutrition, requires interaction with families. Physicians are in an excellent position to help direct care and to help patients dying of prostate cancer appreciate the time they have left.

Patient Education

Men Considering Prostate-Specific Antigen Testing

Several fact sheets are available to aid in instructing men about the benefits and limitations of PSA testing. Hahn and Roberts published a truth in advertising sheet that reviewed options for men. Although the sheet was published in 1993, the issues remain unchanged. The National Health Service Center for Reviews and Dissemination has published "Screening for prostate cancer: Information for men considering or asking for PSA tests" on its Web site (http://www.york.ac.uk/inst/crd/em22b.htm). This document, intended for patients, reviews a variety of topics, including prostate cancer, issues regarding screening for prostate cancer, PSA testing, and therapy for prostate cancer.

Treatment Choices for Prostate Cancer

Most of the time, patients are counseled regarding treatment options by a urologist or radiation oncologist. However, men frequently consult their primary care provider in the hope of obtaining an "unbiased" viewpoint. Explaining the options for management of prostate cancer can be a difficult and time-consuming task. The Foundation for Informed Medical Decision Making* produces an hour-long videotape that outlines what prostate cancer is and the treatment options. The consequences of treatment, including erectile dysfunction, urinary and fecal incontinence, and diarrhea also are presented. A balanced presentation is given for surgery, radiation therapy, and watchful waiting. Interviews with men who have undergone the treatments and their consequences help make this an interesting and informative way to present this material.

Emerging Concepts

Alternative Therapy

In the United States, alternative therapy for BPH has drawn wide attention and is frequently used by men. Phytotherapy, the use of plant extracts, for BPH is well accepted in Europe. In Italy phytotherapy accounts for half the medications prescribed for BPH. In Germany it accounts for an even greater percentage. Multiple preparations are available, but the two that have drawn the most attention is saw palmetto extract (*Serenoa repens*) and *Pygeum africanum*, an evergreen native to Africa. Saw palmetto extract is derived from the fruit of the American dwarf saw palmetto plant. A meta-analysis showed the effectiveness of saw palmetto extract. Eighteen randomized clinical trials were examined. Saw palmetto extract was as effective as finasteride in the management of mild to moderate symptoms. No trials

---

*The videotape *Treatment Choices for Prostate Cancer* was produced in 1995 and can be obtained by writing Shared Decision Making Programs, Foundation for Informed Medical Decision Making, PO Box 5457, Hanover, NH 03755-5457. The telephone number is 603-650-1107.

compared saw palmetto with α-adrenergic blocking agents. Side effects were minimal. All trials were of short duration, so the long-term effectiveness of saw palmetto is still not known. Saw palmetto extract is much less expensive than finasteride or α-blockers. There is a similar literature for *Pygeum* showing its effectiveness. A 90-day supply costs $10 to $50, whereas finasteride costs approximately $200 and terazosin approximately $120. Because the FDA does not regulate herbal medications, the purity and effectiveness of saw palmetto extract or *Pygeum* can vary from product to product.

Minimally Invasive Surgical Procedures

Table 7-5 lists the minimally invasive surgical procedures now performed for BPH. So far the results are disappointing. The only results available are from studies with short follow-up periods. No long-term follow-up studies have been completed. Most of the reported studies have small samples and represent local experience. For this reason, most patients should choose more conventional therapy. There may be reasons to consider alternative techniques in the care of patients who have not had success with pharma-

Table 7-5

Partial List of Minimally Invasive Therapies for Benign Prostatic Hyperplasia

Transurethral incision
Balloon dilation of the prostate
Prostatic stents (permanent, temporary)
Transrectal high-intensity focused ultrasound
Transurethral microwave thermotherapy
Transrectal hyperthermia
Transurethral hyperthermia
Laser ablation (transurethral incision, endoscopic, interstitial)
Transurethral needle ablation
Transurethral electrosurgical vaporization

ceuticals and are not candidates for TURP. Patients need to look to their primary care providers to help them determine whether involvement in local research is appropriate for them.

Bibliography

Albertsen PC: Early stage prostate cancer. when is observation appropriate? *Hematol Oncol Clin North Am* 10:611, 1996.

American College of Physicians: Clinical guideline III: screening for prostate cancer. *Ann Intern Med* 126: 480, 1997.

Andro MC, Riffaud JP: *Pygeum africanum* extract for the treatment of patients with benign prostatic hyperplasia: a review of 25 years of published experience. *Curr Ther Res Clin Exp* 56:796, 1995.

Berry SJ, Coffey DS, Walsh PC, et al: The development of human benign prostatic hyperplasia with age. *J Urol* 132:474, 1984.

Brett AS: The mammography and prostate specific antigen controversies: implication for patient-physician encounters and public policy. *J Gen Intern Med* 10:266, 1995.

Carter HB, Pearson JD, Metter EJ, et al: Longitudinal evaluation of prostate specific antigen levels in men with and without prostate disease. *JAMA* 267:2215, 1992.

Catalona WJ, Patin AW, Slawin KM, et al: Use of the percentage of free prostate-specific antigen to enhance differentiation of prostate cancer from benign prostatic disease. *JAMA* 279:1542, 1998.

Coley CM, Barry MJ, Fleming C, et al: Early detection of prostate cancer: clinical guidelines part II. *Ann Intern Med* 126:468, 1997.

Desmond PM, Clark J, Thompson IM, et al: Morbidity with contemporary prostate biopsy. *J Urol* 150:1425, 1993.

Fleming C, Wasson JH, Albertsen PC, et al: A decision analysis of alternative treatment strategies for clinically localized prostate cancer. *JAMA* 269:2650, 1993.

Fowler FJ, Barry MJ, Lu-Yao G, et al: Patient reported complications and follow-up treatment after radical prostatectomy. *Urology* 42:622, 1993.

Gann PH, Hennekens CH, Stampfer MJ: A prospective evaluation of plasma prostate-specific antigen for detection of prostate cancer. *JAMA* 273:289, 1995.

Gormley GJ, Stoner E, Bruskewitz RC, et al for the Finasteride Study Group: The effect of finasteride in men with benign prostatic hyperplasia. *N Engl J Med* 327:1185, 1992.

Graversen PH, Gassner TC, Wasson JH, et al: Controversies about indications for transurethral resection of the prostate. *J Urol* 141:475,1989.

Guess HA: Benign prostatic hyperplasia antecedents and natural history. *Epidemiol Rev* 14:131, 1992.

Hahn DL, Roberts RG: PSA screening for asymptomatic prostate cancer: truth in advertising (editorial). *J Fam Pract* 37:432, 1993.

Hulka BS: Cancer screening: degrees of proof and practical application. *Cancer* 62:1776, 1988.

Jacobsen SJ, Jacobsen DJ, Girman CJ, et al: Natural history of prostatism: risk factors for acute urinary retention. *J Urol* 158:481, 1997.

Johansson JE, Holmberg L, Johansson S, et al: Fifteen-year survival in prostate cancer: a prospective, population-based study in Sweden. *JAMA* 277:467, 1997.

Keetch DW, Catalona WJ, Smith DS: Serial prostatic biopsies in men with persistently elevated serum prostate specific antigen values. *J Urol* 151:1571,1994.

Lepor H: The emerging role of α-antagonists in the therapy of benign prostatic hyperplasia. *J Androl* 12:389, 1991.

Lu-Yao GL, Potosky AL, Albertsen PC: Follow-up prostate cancer treatments after radical prostatectomy: a population-based study. *J Natl Cancer Inst* 88:166, 1996.

McConnell JD, Barry MJ, Bruskewitz RC, et al: *Benign Prostatic Hyperplasia: Diagnosis and Treatment.* Clinical Practice Guideline no. 8. AHCPR publications no. 94-0582. Rockville, MD, Department of Health and Human Services, Public Health Service, Agency for Health Care Policy and Research Public Health Services, 1994.

Mebust WK, Holtgrewe HL, Cockett ATK, et al: Transurethral prostatectomy: immediate and post-operative complications: a cooperative study of 13 participating institutions evaluating 3,885 patients. *J Urol* 141:243, 1989.

Mettlin C, Jones GW, Murphy GP: Trends in prostate cancer care in the United States, 1974–1990: observations from the patient care evaluation studies of the American College of Surgeons Commission on Cancer. *CA Cancer J Clin* 43:83, 1993.

Monda JM, Oesterling JE: Medical treatment of benign prostatic hyperplasia: 5α-reductase inhibitors and α-adrenergic antagonists. *Mayo Clin Proc* 68:670, 1993.

National Health Service Center for Reviews and Dissemination, The University of York, February 1997. Available at http://www.york.ac.uk/inst/crd/em22b.htm. Accessed 3/20/00.

Oesterling JE: Benign prostatic hyperplasia: medical and minimally invasive treatment options. *N Engl J Med* 332:99, 1995.

Oesterling JE, Jacobson SJ, Chute CG, et al: Serum prostate-specific antigen in a community-based population of healthy men: establishment of age-specific reference ranges. *JAMA* 270:860, 1993.

Richie JP, Catalona WJ, Hudson MA, et al: Effect of patient age on early detection of prostate cancer with serum prostate-specific antigen to digital rectal examination. *J Urol* 42:365, 1993.

Schatzl G, Madersbacher S, Lang T, et al: The early postoperative morbidity of transurethral resection of the prostate and of 4 minimally invasive treatment alternatives. *J Urol* 158:105, 1997.

Schmid HP, McNeal JE, Stamey TA: Observation on the doubling time of prostate cancer. The use of serial prostate-specific antigen in patients with untreated disease as a measure of increasing cancer volume. *Cancer* 71:2031, 1993.

Selly S, Donovan J, Faulkner A, et al: Diagnosis management and screening of early localised prostate cancer. *Health Technol Assess* 1:1, 1997.

Smith JR, Freije D, Carpten JD, et al: Major susceptibility locus for prostate cancer on chromosome 1 suggested by a genome-wide search. *Science* 274:1371, 1996.

Vashi AR, Oesterling JE: Percent free prostate-specific antigen: entering a new era in the detection of prostate cancer. *Mayo Clin Proc* 72:337, 1997.

Wasson JH, Cushman CC, Bruskewitz RC et al for the Prostate Disease Patient Outcomes Research Team: a structured literature review of treatment for localized prostate cancer. *Arch Fam Med* 2:487, 1993.

Whitmore WF Jr: Consensus development conference on the management of clinically localized prostate cancer: overview—historical and contemporary. *NCI Monogr* no 7:7, 1988.

Wilt TJ, Ishani A, Stark G, et al: Saw palmetto extracts for treatment of benign prostatic hyperplasia: a systematic review. *JAMA* 280:1604, 1998.

Wingo PA, Tong T, Bolden S: Cancer statistics, 1995. *CA Cancer J Clin* 45:8, 1995. [Published erratum appears in *CA Cancer J Clin* 45:127, 1995].

Part 3

Aches and Pains

Luanne Thorndyke

Osteoporosis

Overview: How Common Is This Problem in the Office Practice?

Osteoporosis is the most common skeletal disorder worldwide. Approximately 25 million persons in the United States are affected, 80 percent of whom are women. The economic impact of the disease on the health care system is impressive. In 1995, the direct cost of management of osteoporotic fractures in the United States was estimated to be $13.8 billion dollars. In addition to the direct health care costs of hospitalization for fractures, physician office visits, and treatment, osteoporosis also creates extensive indirect costs related to lost productivity and institutionalized care. The incidence and effects of the disease are expected to increase with the progressive aging of the world's population.

The prevalence of low bone density and osteoporosis is striking. The condition affects 34 percent of women in their fifties, 51 percent of women in their sixties, 72 percent of women in their seventies, and 86 percent of women in their eighties. Primary care physicians, on average, see 54 women 50 years of age or older per week and encounter 16 patients with osteoporosis per week. Clinicians identifying substantially fewer cases of osteoporosis are probably failing to diagnose the condition in many patients.

The risk of development of osteoporosis varies by race and ethnicity. White and Asian women are affected more often than African American women, probably because of differences in bone mass and density. One in every five African American women is at risk of the disease, and 25 percent of African American women sustain hip fracture. Thirty-three percent of white women sustain hip fractures. Asian women have lower hip fracture rates than white women, although the prevalence of vertebral fractures is similar at 25 percent. Mexican American women are affected as well; approximately 40 to 45 percent of those older than 50 years have low bone density and 15 percent have osteoporosis.

Principal Diagnoses

Primary Osteoporosis

DEFINITION OF OSTEOPOROSIS

The World Health Organization defines osteoporosis as "a systemic skeletal disease characterized by low bone mass and micro-architectural deterioration of bone tissue, leading to enhanced bone fragility and a consequent increase in fracture risk." There are two types of bone, cortical and trabecular. Cortical bone is the compact layer that makes up the outer shell of bone. It accounts for 80 percent of the adult skeleton. The remaining 20 percent of bone is trabecular bone, the spongy, trabecular meshwork that forms the interior bone. The long bones, such as the radius and femur, consist of 90 percent cortical bone, whereas the vertebrae are mostly trabecular bone. Trabecular bone is more affected by conditions that produce rapid bone loss, but both types of bone are susceptible to fracture.

PATHOPHYSIOLOGY

Although the clinical manifestations of osteoporosis do not usually appear until late in life, the process of bone remodeling within the skeleton is lifelong. Bones, like other body tissues, are continuously undergoing change. Old bone is removed by osteoclasts in a process called *resorption,* and new bone is laid down by osteoblasts, resulting in bone formation. Bone resorption and formation are tightly coupled.

Net bone formation in childhood results in bone growth in both size and density. In the late teens, peak height is reached, but bones continue to become more dense until peak bone mass is achieved between the third and fourth decades of life. Men achieve a 10 to 15 percent greater bone mass than women. Bone mass depends on a balance between bone formation and bone resorption. Osteoporosis develops because of alterations in the balance between bone resorption and bone formation with increased turnover and loss of bone. Normal bone mass is maintained through midlife because the remodeling processes of bone resorption and formation are in equilibrium.

After peak bone mass is achieved in early adulthood, either skeletal mass is maintained, or a very gradual loss occurs until menopause. Bone loss occurs because there is an imbalance between bone removal and formation, more bone being removed than replaced. The result is a decrease in bone mass and an increase in fracture risk. The early years of menopause are associated with a rapid rate of bone loss, sometimes 5 percent per year or greater. Five to seven years after menopause, bone loss continues to occur, but at a slower rate of about 0.5 to 1 percent per year. This age-related loss of bone occurs among both men and women.

TYPES OF PRIMARY OSTEOPOROSIS

Osteoporosis may be classified as either primary or secondary. Primary osteoporosis is the most common form and occurs mainly among postmenopausal women and the elderly. Primary osteoporosis may be subdivided into two classes. Postmenopausal (type I) osteoporosis occurs among women during the decade after menopause. Declines in estrogen levels and lower estrogen-mediated osteoblastic activity are the main etiologic factors associated with primary type I osteoporosis. Bone loss is accelerated, and the most rapid rate of bone loss occurs in the trabecular bone of the vertebral bodies. Thus vertebral body compression fractures are common in the first 10 years after menopause. Cortical bone loss occurs at a slower rate, so fractures of the long bones usually occur in the seventh and eighth decades of life.

Type II, or age-related, primary osteoporosis occurs among both men and women. Both bone formation and resorption are decreased, and parathyroid hormone levels are often elevated. Bone resorption exceeds formation, resulting in bone loss. Because they do not have rapid loss of bone associated with menopause, men usually do not sustain osteoporotic fractures until 85 years of age or older.

RISK FACTORS

The major risk factors of osteoporosis are listed in Table 8-1. In general, the more risk factors present, the greater is the risk of fracture. Women should be counseled about the risk factors of osteoporosis to modify and potentially decrease the likelihood of development of the disease. Assessing risk factors may help identify those who need further evaluation with bone mineral density (BMD) testing and determine whether additional treatment is indicated.

The risk of osteoporotic fracture is associated with risks of falling, and conditions that increase the propensity for falling also increase the risk of fracture. Falls among the elderly are common, and although not all falls result in fracture, 90 percent of hip fractures are fall related. Most falls among the elderly have a multifactorial causation—a combination of intrinsic and extrinsic factors involved (Table 8-2). A fall risk assessment is an important element of the evaluation of a patient

Table 8-1

Risk Factors of Osteoporosis

Advancing age	Low calcium intake
Female sex	Cigarette smoking
White or Asian race	Alcohol abuse
Family history, heredity	Menopause
Previous fragility, fracture	Premenopausal
Low body weight	amenorrhea
Small, frail bone	Long-term use of
structure	glucocorticoids
Immobility,	
sedentary lifestyle	

Table 8-2

Intrinsic and Extrinsic Risk Factors for Falls Among the Elderly

INTRINSIC RISK FACTORS	
Demographic characteristics	**Medical conditions**
Older age	Postural hypotension
Female sex	Foot problems
White race	**Medications, alcohol**
Functional level	Number of medications used
Activities of daily living	Hypnotics
Cane or walker use	Sedatives
History of falls	Antipsychotics
Gait, balance, strength	Antidepressants
Walking speed	Antiparkinson drugs
Postural sway	Cardiac
Lower extremity strength	Diuretics
Upper extremity strength	Antihypertensives
Impaired reflexes	Alcohol
Chronic illnesses	**Sensory**
Heart disease	Vision
Parkinson's disease	Lower extremity sensory
Other neuromuscular disease	perception
Stroke	**Mental status**
Urinary incontinence	Cognitive impairment
Arthritis	Depression
Acute illness	Attitudes of invulnerability

with osteoporosis, and intervention is made if possible. Identifying and changing medications known to increase instability; referral for exercise to improve muscle strength, balance, and gait; and reduction in the use of sedative-hypnotics and total number of prescription drugs have been shown to reduce the risk of falls.

Secondary Causes of Osteoporosis

Secondary osteoporosis occurs when an underlying medical condition contributes to bone loss and may be potentially reversible if the underlying condition is identified and controlled. Although most patients with osteoporotic fractures have primary osteoporosis, it is important to consider and rule out secondary causes of osteoporosis (Table 8-3).

Among patients with vertebral compression fractures, 30 to 60 percent of men and 10 to 35 percent of women may have a secondary cause of bone loss. Secondary osteoporosis most often occurs among patients who are being treated with glucocorticoids, typically for rheumatoid arthritis, collagen vascular disease, or inflammatory bowel disease. Other causes of secondary osteoporosis that should be considered in the care of patients with vertebral compression fractures are metastatic cancer (breast, lung, prostate) and multiple myeloma.

Table 8-2

Intrinsic and Extrinsic Risk Factors for Falls Among the Elderly (continued)

EXTRINSIC (ENVIRONMENTAL) RISK FACTORS	
Home environmental hazards	Oil
Ground surfaces	Home access
Throw rugs	Stairs in ill repair
Loose carpets	Raised thresholds
Slippery floors	Absent or poorly anchored
Cords and wires on the floor	railings
Low-lying objects, e.g., toys	Lighting
Stairs with rugs or in poor	Glare from unshielded
repair	windows or lamps or
Furniture	highly polished floors
Clutter, especially causing	Low or dim light compounded
obstructed mobility	by dark-colored walls
Unstable furniture	Absence of night lights
Low-lying furniture, e.g.,	Bathroom
coffee table	Low toilet seats and no
Low chairs without armrest	secure grab bars
support or seat backs	Absence of slip-resistant,
Beds that are too high or too	strongly secured grab bars
low	Absence of nonslip surfaces
Cabinets that are too high or	or assistive devices (e.g.,
too low	tub chair)
Other	Door jambs
Poorly maintained walking aids	Community
and equipment	Traffic lights that do not allow
Improper shoes (not slip resis-	sufficient time to cross the
tant, high-heeled; too large)	street
Outdoor environment hazards	Activity related
Ground surfaces	Rising from a chair
Irregular sidewalks	Walking to bathroom
Ice or snow	Navigating unfamiliar
Uneven, variable surfaces,	environments
(e.g., holes covered by	Physical restraint use in long-
grass, rocks)	term care facilities

SOURCE: Adapted with permission from JA Grisso, E Capezuti, A Schwartz: *Falls as Risk Factors for Fractures.* New York, NY, Academic Press, 1996.

Thyroid disease is common among women and may be accompanied by osteoporosis. Hyperthyroidism is a secondary cause of osteoporosis, and thyroid function testing is indicated for patients with newly diagnosed osteoporosis. Women with hypothyroidism who receive excess thyroid hormone also may have bone loss. The availability of the sensitive thyroid-stimulating hormone assay has made the clinical management of hypothyroidism more precise. Excessive thyroid replacement will likely be a less common cause of secondary osteoporosis in the future.

Table 8-3

Secondary Causes of Osteoporosis

Endocrine diseases	Medications
Hyperthyroidism	Glucocorticoids
Hypercortisolism	Excess thyroid
Hyperparathyroidism	hormone
Hyperprolactinemia	Anticonvulsants
Hypogonadism	Chronic heparin
Acromegaly	therapy
Nutritional conditions	Other diseases
Anorexia nervosa	Systemic
Malabsorption	mastocytosis
Chronic liver disease	Multiple myeloma
Alcoholism	Bone metastasis
Calcium deficiency	Chronic renal
Hypovitaminosis D	disease
	Rheumatoid arthritis

Typical Presentation

Osteoporosis is an asymptomatic process; however, all patients with osteoporosis are susceptible to fractures. As a result, the only symptom of osteoporosis is pain from a fracture. The site of the fracture determines the location of pain.

The clinical hallmark of the disease is a fragility fracture, defined as an osteoporosis-related fracture. Approximately 1.5 million fragility fractures occur each year. The most common sites of fracture are the vertebrae, the proximal femur or hip, and the distal forearm or wrist. Almost one-half of the annual fractures are vertebral compression fractures. Wrist fractures account for one-fourth of fractures, and the others are hip fractures. Fifty percent of white women experience an osteoporotic fracture at some point in their lifetimes.

The risk is also present, but lower, among non-white women. One in five men older than 65 years sustain fractures due to osteoporosis.

Vertebral compression fractures are a common cause of acute and chronic back pain, disability, and disfigurement. Vertebral fractures may result in loss of height, kyphosis, or curvature of the upper thoracic spine. Pain from an acute fracture can be severe, and generally lasts for 6 to 8 weeks. Women who have had one compression fracture are at the highest risk of fracturing again within the next year. Multiple vertebral fractures may result in loss of strength, balance, endurance, and compromised lung function.

Hip fractures are the most clinically significant consequence of osteoporosis, resulting in the greatest morbidity, mortality, and expense. The lifetime risk of death associated with an osteoporotic hip fracture is comparable to that of breast cancer. There is up to 24 percent increased mortality within 1 year of hip fracture and approximately 50 percent of survivors are incapacitated, many permanently. Almost 20 percent of women who survive hip fracture need institutionalized nursing care.

Physical Examination

A thorough medical history should include questions about menstrual history, nutrition, exercise patterns, and family history of osteoporosis. Risk factors, such as smoking, alcohol and caffeine intake, and medication use should be assessed.

There are few physical findings of osteoporosis. Signs of osteoporosis include height loss, kyphosis, and scoliosis. The presence of goiter or the cushingoid features of hypercortisolism might signal a secondary cause of osteoporosis. When an osteoporotic fracture occurs, back pain is the prominent symptom, and the physical findings are related to the location of fracture.

Postmenopausal women should have their height measured once a year to assess for loss of height. If a loss of height of 2 in. (5 cm) from premenopausal height has occurred, then the patient should undergo evaluation osteoporosis.

Ancillary Tests

Plain Radiographs

Osteoporosis often progresses without warning signs until a fracture occurs. Plain radiographs are useful for diagnosing acute fractures. Although they may show reduced bone density (osteopenia) among patients with osteoporosis, plain radiographs are an insensitive indicator of bone loss. By the time abnormalities are seen on plain radiographs, as much as 30 percent of bone density may be lost, so plain radiographs should not be used to screen for osteoporosis. They may, however, show osteoporotic fractures of which patients may not be aware. For example, vertebral fractures appear as characteristic wedge-shaped anterior compressions of the vertebral body, known as *codfish vertebrae* (Fig. 8-1).

Bone Mineral Density Measurement

The early diagnosis and management of osteoporosis are critical in preventing fractures. Early detection of osteoporosis is possible with one of several technologies to assess bone mineral density (BMD). BMD measurement can establish or confirm a diagnosis of osteoporosis, help determine the severity of the disease, provide a baseline to monitor changes in the condition over time or in response to therapy, and possibly predict future risk of fracture.

BMD tests measure bone absorption of radiation (usually x-rays) or high-frequency sound waves. Although each test uses a different method of measuring the energy absorbed, BMD is expressed as grams of calcium hydroxyapatite per square centimeter of bone cross section. Several methods are available for assessing BMD, and all are accurate in predicting future fracture risk. The tests differ in the body site tested, radiation dose delivered, cost, and test characteristics of accuracy and precision. Dual-energy x-ray absorptiometry (DEXA) of the hip and vertebral column is considered the standard test. It often is performed to confirm abnormal BMD measurements obtained with other techniques and to provide a baseline value to follow during therapy.

Z SCORES AND T SCORES

To standardize readings from different techniques, results are reported as standard deviation (SD) above or below the mean peak bone mass for the patient's age- and sex-matched reference (Z score) or sex-matched normal young adult reference (T score). A difference of 1 SD represents a 10 to 12 percent difference in bone density. BMD correlates with fracture risk: the relative risk of fracture increases 1.5- to 3-fold for every 1 SD decline in bone density.

The T score is the most clinically relevant value obtained from the BMD report. The World Health Organization has established criteria for defining osteoporosis on the basis of the T score from BMD measurement. Normal bone mass is defined as a BMD within 1 SD of normal young adult (T score greater than −1). A BMD between 1 and 2.5 SD less than that of a normal young adult (T score between −1 and −2.5) is categorized as low bone mass (osteopenia). Osteoporosis is defined as a BMD of 2.5 SD less than that of a normal young adult (T score of or less than −2.5). Patients with bone densities less than −2.5 and a fracture are considered to have severe osteoporosis.

MEASUREMENT TECHNIQUES

Technologies available for assessing BMD include single-energy (SXA) and dual-energy x-ray absorptiometry (DEXA), quantitative

Figure 8-1

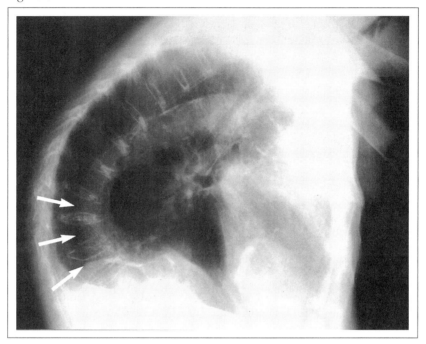

Lateral radiograph of the spine shows diffuse demineralization of the bones, anterior compression deformities of the lower spinal column (*arrows*), and kyphosis.

computed tomography (QCT), and quantitative ultrasonography (QUX). DEXA can be used to measure BMD at either central (DEXA) or peripheral body sites (pDXA). Table 8-4 summarizes the tests used to measure bone density.

DEXA scanning is accurate (90 to 99 percent), precise (98 to 99 percent), and fast and has a low radiation exposure. Central body sites commonly tested are the hip and vertebral column; pDXA scanning can be performed on the forearm, finger, or heel. SXA is an older technique used to measure heel bone density. It is accurate and precise (98 to 99 percent) and has low radiation exposure. The equipment is small and portable. In QCT a conventional CT scanner is used to provide three-dimensional, volumetric measurements (bone mineral content) reported in mg/cm³. QTC measures both trabecular and cortical bone density of the vertebrae. The radiation dose is comparable to that of a standard chest radiography

(100 rems [1 Sv]). Although precise (96 to 98 percent), QTC is not as accurate as other modalities (85 to 97 percent). A portable scanner has been developed to measure forearm BMD (pQCT). Like QCT, pQCT can differentiate cortical and trabecular bone. It is precise (98 to 99 percent) and accurate (92 to 98 percent).

INSURANCE COVERAGE

Health Care Financing Administration (HCFA) regulations provide for uniform insurance coverage of bone mass measurements for "qualified individuals." Table 8-5 lists qualifying indications for BMD BMD techniques approved by the U.S. Food and Drug Administration are included, and the frequency of allowable testing is once every 2 years. Persons being treated with long-term glucocorticoid therapy, and those with conditions that make BMD medically necessary as determined by a

Table 8-4

Techniques for Bone Mineral Density Testing

TEST	FEATURES
Dual-energy x-ray absorptiometry (DEXA)	Measures central or peripheral BMD
	Low radiation dose (10% that of chest radiograph)
	Precise and accurate measurements
	Standard for diagnosis and monitoring
Single-energy x-ray absorptiometry (SXA)	Measures peripheral BMD: wrist, finger, heel
Peripheral dual-energy x-ray absorptiometry (pDXA or pDEXA)	Low radiation dose
	Low cost; small, portable machine
Quantitative computed tomography (QCT)	Differentiates trabecular and cortical bone in the spine
	Highest radiation dose of available options
	High cost
Ultrasonography	Measures peripheral sites, mainly heel
	No radiation dose
	Low cost; portable machine
	Generally not as precise as other options but appears to predict fracture risk

ABBREVIATION: BMD, bone mineral density.

physician may be tested more frequently. A confirmatory baseline BMD measurement is allowed (for example, with DEXA) if BMD monitoring in the future will be performed with a different method than the one used initially.

For persons not enrolled in Medicare, BMD testing should be performed on the basis of the individual risk profile and when the results could influence a treatment decision. The National Osteoporosis Foundation currently recommends BMD testing for the following persons:

1. Postmenopausal women younger than 65 years with one or more risk factors (see Table 8-1) of osteoporosis besides menopause
2. All women 65 years and older regardless of additional risk factors
3. Postmenopausal women with fragility fractures
4. Women considering therapy for osteoporosis when BMD results could influence a treatment decision
5. Women who have been taking hormone therapy for prolonged periods

Laboratory Evaluation

No laboratory test can confirm the diagnosis of osteoporosis. Laboratory evaluation is used

Table 8-5

Patients with Medicare-Reimbursable Indications for Bone Mineral Density Tests

Women with estrogen deficiency at clinical risk of osteoporosis

Persons with vertebral abnormalities on radiographs indicative of osteoporosis, osteopenia, or vertebral fracture

Persons receiving or planning to receive long-term glucocorticoid therapy (equivalent to 7.5 mg or more of prednisone per day for more than 3 months)

Persons with primary hyperparathyroidism

Persons being monitored to assess the response or efficacy of an FDA-approved osteoporosis drug therapy

Table 8-6

Laboratory Evaluation to Exclude Secondary Causes of Osteoporosis

TEST	SECONDARY CAUSE OF OSTEOPOROSIS TO BE EXCLUDED
Complete blood cell count	Malnutrition
Serum urea, electrolytes	Renal osteodystrophy
Liver function tests	Alcohol abuse
Serum calcium, phosphorus, alkaline phosphatase	Osteomalacia, hyperparathyroidism, vitamin D deficiency
Thyroid-stimulating hormone	Hyperthyroidism
Serum albumin, total protein	Malnutrition, multiple myeloma
24-h urine calcium	Malnutrition, malabsorption, hyperparathyroidism
Testosterone level (men)	Hypogonadism

mainly to exclude other causes of bone loss (Table 8-6). In general, laboratory testing should include a complete blood cell count (CBC), blood chemistry tests (including electrolytes and renal and hepatic function), calcium and phosphorous levels, and thyroid-stimulating hormone level. A 24-h urine calcium level often is measured.

The CBC and blood chemistry tests help to assess for renal or hepatic disease, malabsorption or malnutrition, asymptomatic hyperparathyroidism, and multiple myeloma. Thyroid-stimulating hormone level is a screen for subclinical hyperthyroidism. Serum calcium, phosphorous, and alkaline phosphatase levels can help differentiate osteoporosis from osteomalacia and hyperparathyroidism. Low serum phosphorous and calcium levels, with high serum levels of alkaline phosphatase may suggest vitamin D deficiency. Measuring serum levels of 25-hydroxyvitamin D level may help determine the diagnosis, but levels can be variable and should not be used routinely. A low 24-h urine calcium level (less than 100 mg/24h) can suggest nutritional deficiency, malabsorption, or hyperparathyroidism. A high value (more than 300 mg/24h) may help identify those with excess skeletal loss of calcium and those in whom calcium supplementation may be harmful. Parathyroid hormone, calcitonin, or calcitriol

(1,25[OH]2 vitamin D) levels may be useful if hyperparathyroidism is suspected. For men, measurement of serum testosterone level may be indicated if hypogonadism is suspected.

The presence of multiple fragility fractures should raise a question of pathologic fracture. Serum protein electrophoresis for multiple myeloma should be considered, as should further evaluation to exclude metastatic carcinoma or a hematologic malignant disease such as leukemia or lymphoma.

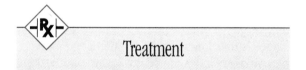

Treatment

Once osteoporosis is diagnosed, the goals of management are to decrease the clinical manifestations of the disease and to minimize future fracture risk. Management of an acute fracture also may be necessary. Optimal therapy includes a combination of pharmacologic and nonpharmacologic modalities. The nonpharmacologic interventions listed in Table 8-7 are useful guidelines for the general population for preventing osteoporosis and its consequences.

Table 8-7

Nonpharmacologic Management of Osteoporosis

> Assure adequate daily intake of calcium
> (see Table 8-8)
> Assure adequate daily intake of vitamin D:
> 400–800 IU per day
> Complete avoidance of tobacco
> Alcohol use only in moderation
> Regular weight-bearing and muscle-
> strengthening exercise
> Assessment of risk factors for fall
> Avoidance of hypnotic drugs
> Evaluation for impaired vision or hearing
> Management of gait disturbance, if present
> Proper lighting and home safety measures

Nonpharmacologic Therapy

Adequate calcium intake is essential for achieving peak bone mass and maintaining bone health. The combination of calcium and vitamin D supplementation is effective in reducing but not halting bone loss among postmenopausal women. There is evidence that the risk of fracture may be reduced with calcium therapy. National Institutes of Health NIH Consensus Conference recommendations for daily elemental calcium intakes are shown in Table 8-8. Calcium supplementation often is necessary to meet these requirements, particularly for those older than 65 years. It is important to remember that all of the pharmacologic therapies also require adequate calcium intake to ensure maximal benefit.

The typical U.S. diet provides less than 600 mg/d of calcium. Patients need to be encouraged to increase their dietary intake of calcium-rich foods. Table 8-9 contains a list of common foods with their calcium content. About 75 to 80 percent of the calcium in the U.S. diet comes from dairy products. Calcium-fortified foods, such as cereals and juices, are particularly useful for persons who do not care for milk and dairy products or who are lactose intolerant.

Calcium supplements are needed when dietary intake does not achieve the recommended level. Calcium supplements are available as calcium carbonate, phosphate, and citrate. Calcium carbonate requires gastric acid for absorption and should be taken with food. Absorption may be decreased in persons with a low level of gastric acid, such as elderly persons with acquired achlorhydria, or patients taking histamine 2 receptor blockers or proton pump inhibitors. Calcium citrate should be taken between meals. Brands vary in the amount of elemental calcium supplied.

The amount of the supplement recommended should supply the needed amount of elemental calcium on the basis of an estimate of the patient's daily calcium intake. Calcium is absorbed most efficiently if taken in small amounts throughout

Table 8-8

National Institutes of Health Consensus Conference Calcium Guidelines

AGE GROUP	DAILY CALCIUM REQUIREMENTS (mg)
11–24 y	1200
25–65 y	1000
Pregnant and lactating women	1200
Postmenopausal women not using hormone replacement therapy	1500
Postmenopausal women using hormone replacement therapy	1000
65 y and older	1500

SOURCE: Adapted with permission from NIH Consensus Development Panel on Optimal Calcium Intake:
NIH Consensus conference: optimal calcium intake. *JAMA* 272:1942–1948, 1994.

Table 8-9

Calcium Content of Common High-Calcium Foods

Food	Serving Size	Approximate Calcium Content Per Serving (mg)
Dairy		
Milk	1 cup	300
Yogurt, plain	1 cup	300
Hard cheese (swiss, cheddar, provolone, American)	1 ounce	200
Cottage cheese	1 cup	150
Vegetables		
Spinach, kale, collard greens	1/2 cup cooked	100
Broccoli	1/2 cup	50
Fish		
Sardines	3 ounces	270
Salmon with bone	3 ounces	200
Pike	3 ounces	70
Bass	3 ounces	70
Cereals		
Cheerios	1 ounce	48
Total	1 ounce	48
Wheaties	1 ounce	43
Other		
Tofu	1 cup	250
Raisins	1 cup	81
Orange juice, calcium fortified	8 ounces	300
Macaroni and cheese	1 cup	200
Pizza with cheese	1 slice	220
Almonds	1 ounce (approx. 20)	70
Orange	Medium	60
Baked beans	1 cup	150
Soybeans	1 cup	200

the day. Patients taking supplements should be encouraged to divide doses unless this would cause them to miss doses. Calcium supplements should not be taken with high-fiber meals or fiber supplements because these decrease absorption of calcium.

Adequate intake of vitamin D is important for calcium and phosphorous absorption and bone preservation. The recommended daily allowance is 400 IU daily. This can be obtained by spending 5 to 10 min in the sun each day. The elderly often are deficient in vitamin D because of decreased synthesis of vitamin D by aging skin, reduced sun exposure, decreased vitamin D intake, and impaired renal synthesis of the active metabolite. The dosage recommended for replacement is 400 to 800 IU per day. Some calcium supplements contain small amounts of vitamin D (usually 200 IU), and most multiple vitamins contain 400 IU per tablet.

Pharmacologic Therapy

Drugs to manage osteoporosis act by reducing bone resorption, stimulating bone formation, or both. Currently only antiresorptive agents are FDA-approved pharmacologic treatments for prevention or management of osteoporosis. These include treatment with hormone replacement therapy (HRT; estrogen), selective estrogen receptor modulators (raloxifene), bisphosphonates (alendronate), and calcitonin. All pharmacologic therapies require adequate intake of calcium and vitamin D to maximize effectiveness of therapy.

HORMONE REPLACEMENT THERAPY

Estrogen and estrogen-progesterone combinations are considered to be the first-line agents for preventing and managing postmenopausal osteoporosis. Estrogen reduces bone resorption, decreases postmenopausal bone loss, and increases bone density. It has been shown to decrease the risk of vertebral fracture by approximately 50 percent and of hip fracture by 25 percent. The effect of estrogen is greatest when therapy is begun at menopause, although even when started later it prevents further loss of bone for as long as the treatment is continued. Protective effects of estrogen therapy on bone have been demonstrated even among women older than 65 years. When estrogen therapy is discontinued, bone mass declines at a rate commensurate with age-associated bone loss. Table 8-10 lists the commonly prescribed estrogen and estrogen-progesterone combinations and the dosage.

NONSKELETAL BENEFITS Estrogen replacement therapy has several nonskeletal benefits. Estrogen is the agent of choice to manage menopausal vasomotor symptoms. Oral postmenopausal estrogen replacement with or without a progestin has a beneficial effect on the lipid profile by lowering low-density lipoprotein (LDL) cholesterol and raising high-density lipoprotein cholesterol. It also raises triglyceride concentrations (Table 8-11). In observational studies, use of estrogen is associated with a statistically significant reduction in total mortality and in mortality from coronary and other cardiovascular diseases. Estrogen has a neuroprotective effect and may be of benefit in the prevention and management of Alzheimer's disease (see Chap. 12).

SIDE EFFECTS HRT may cause side effects, including breast tenderness, migraine headache, and abdominal bloating. Some of these symptoms can be improved with a decrease in the dose of estrogen. Women using the transdermal method of estrogen therapy seem to have less severe side effects of breast tenderness and fluid retention. Elderly women may need a lower dose than the usual 0.625 mg conjugated equine estrogen or its equivalent to avoid side effects.

Use of unopposed estrogen increases the risk of endometrial cancer fivefold to sevenfold. The risk increases with longer duration of use, although the cancers produced are generally of low grade and stage with an excellent prognosis. When appropriate doses of progestin are given to women with an intact uterus (either continuously or cyclically), the risk of endometrial cancer is comparable with that of women not taking HRT.

A common side effect, and the most common reason women discontinue therapy, is irregular vaginal bleeding among women who have not undergone hysterectomy. Almost 50 percent of postmenopausal women taking a combined estrogen–progesterone regimen experience irregular, unpredictable bleeding during the first year of therapy. The bleeding often diminishes with time, and approximately 80 percent of women become amenorrheic within 1 year of starting

Table 8-10

Common Hormonal Formulations for Prevention of Osteoporosis

GENERIC NAME	BRAND NAME	DOSAGE
ORAL ESTROGENS		
Conjugated estrogens	Premarin	0.3–1.25 mg daily
Micronized estradiol	Estrace	0.5–2.0 mg daily
Estropiptate	Ogen	0.625–2.0 mg daily
TRANSDERMAL ESTROGENS		
Estradiol transdermal	Estraderm Alora	0.05–0.1 mg/d twice weekly
Estradiol transdermal	Vivelle	0.0375–0.1 mg/d twice weekly
Estradiol transdermal	Climara	0.05–0.1 mg/d weekly
PROGESTERONE PREPARATIONS		
Medroxyprogesterone acetate	Provera Cycrin Amen	2.5–10 mg daily
Norethindrone	Aygestin Micronor	2.5–10 mg daily
COMBINATION PREPARATIONS		
Conjugated estrogens plus medroxyprogesterone acetate	Prempro* Premphase†	1 tablet daily
Esterified estrogen plus methyltestosterone	Estratest Estratest HS	1.25 mg Estratab plus 2.5 mg methyltestosterone 0.625 mg esterified estrogen plus 1.25 mg methyltestosterone
SELECTIVE ESTROGEN-RECEPTOR MODULATOR		
Raloxifene hydrochloride	Evista	60 mg daily

*0.625 mg conjugated estrogens and 2.5 mg medroxyprogesterone acetate.
†0.625 mg conjugated estrogens and 5.0 mg medroxyprogesterone acetate (last 40 days of 28-day cycle).

treatment. Women who have this irregular bleeding during the first year may benefit from changing to a cyclical regimen to provide regularity to the vaginal bleeding. If desired, a return to the combined regimen can be attempted in 1 to 2 years with less risk of irregular bleeding.

The relation of estrogen and breast cancer is controversial, although some studies have shown a slightly increased risk of breast cancer with prolonged use (more than 5 to 10 years). Other studies have found no increased risk of breast cancer among women who have ever used hormone therapy. Although many researchers suggest that short-term use of estrogen (less than 5 years) does not increase the risk of breast cancer, there is less agreement about long-term use. A definitive conclusion is not possible with the current evidence. Patients should be counseled about the uncertainties and involved in the final decision regarding therapy.

Table 8-11

Lipid Effect of Estrogen and Raloxifene

LIPID	ESTROGEN	RALOXIFENE
Total cholesterol	↓	↓
Low-density lipoprotein cholesterol	↓	↓
High-density lipoprotein cholesterol	↑	↔
Triglycerides	↑	↔

↓, decreased; ↑, increased; ↔, no change.

The risk of gallbladder disease is increased twofold to fourfold among postmenopausal women taking estrogen. Studies have suggested that the risk of deep venous thrombosis also is increased slightly among long-term users of estrogen. Contraindications to HRT are listed in Table 8-12.

COUNSELING All menopausal women should be counseled about HRT. Risks and benefits have to be weighed and a decision made on the basis of the patient's risk profile and personal preferences. BMD testing may be useful at this time to help in making a decision. Women taking HRT must be monitored for unusual or prolonged bleeding, which necessitates further evaluation.

RALOXIFENE

Raloxifene (Evista) is a selective estrogen receptor modulator that binds to the estrogen receptor and produces tissue-specific effects. Raloxifene produces estrogen-like effects in bone and liver and antiestrogen effects in breast and uterus. Raloxifene has been shown to prevent postmenopausal bone loss and to increase BMD 1 to 2 percent over 2 years. The dose of raloxifene is 60 mg once daily.

The absolute gain in BMD is lower than that with estrogen or alendronate. Preliminary data on multiple outcomes of raloxifene use by women with osteoporosis suggest a reduction in the frequency of vertebral fractures. Other effects of raloxifene include a lowering of total cholesterol and LDL cholesterol levels but no effect on HDL or triglyceride levels (see Table 8-11). Whether treatment with raloxifene will reduce cardiovascular events among postmenopausal women is unknown.

Raloxifene may have some preventive activity on the development of breast cancer. Preliminary data from two large trials appear to suggest a reduction in the risk of breast cancer after 2 years of therapy. Thus raloxifene may provide an alternative for preserving bone density among postmenopausal women who have a personal history or strong family history of breast cancer or women who are unwilling to take estrogen because of side effects or fear of breast cancer.

Table 8-12

Contraindications to Estrogen Replacement Therapy

Known or suspected pregnancy
Undiagnosed, abnormal genital bleeding
Known or suspected cancer of the breast
Known or suspected estrogen-dependent neoplasia
Active thrombophlebitis or thromboembolic disorder

SIDE EFFECTS   Raloxifene does not cause endometrial hyperplasia or vaginal bleeding, therefore no progestin treatment is needed. Raloxifene is associated with a threefold increased risk of thromboembolic events, an increase similar to that with estrogen therapy. Unlike estrogen, however, raloxifene can increase hot flashes and should not be used by women who want to avoid this effect of menopause. Leg cramps, fatigue, and nausea are other side effects of therapy.

In summary, raloxifene acts as both an estrogen agonist and estrogen antagonist, depending on the body tissue. It is currently approved only for prevention of postmenopausal osteoporosis and has been shown to preserve bone density among postmenopausal women. Data on long-term efficacy and safety are limited, but a preliminary report suggests a beneficial effect on fracture incidence. There also may be beneficial effects on the breast and endometrium, but menopausal symptoms may worsen with treatment. Raloxifene is an option for osteoporosis prevention for women who cannot or will not take estrogen.

ALENDRONATE

Bisphosphonates, such as alendronate, etidronate, and pamidronate, are nonhormonal inhibitors of osteoclast activity and bone resorption. Bisphosphonates act only on bones and do not appear to have any effect on lipid profiles. Alendronate (Fosamax) is the only bisphosphonate indicated for both preventing and managing osteoporosis. It halts bone loss within months of starting therapy and significantly increases bone density among both older and younger postmenopausal women. Studies have documented a 40 to 50 percent reduction in the risk of osteoporotic fractures of the hip, wrist, or vertebrae. More important, women who are at the highest risk of complications from osteoporosis, such as older postmenopausal women and women with previous vertebral fractures, appear to benefit from treatment with alendronate.

Alendronate is well tolerated by many patients. Side effects are mainly gastrointestinal irritation: nausea, abdominal pain, and dyspepsia. Musculo-skeletal pain also has been reported and may respond to a short-term reduction in dosage. Alendronate can act as a direct irritant to the gastrointestinal mucosa, and esophageal or gastric erosions have been reported. The drug is contraindicated for use by patients with abnormalities of esophageal emptying, and caution should be used by patients with active peptic ulcer disease, esophagitis, or gastroesophageal reflux disease.

Alendronate is poorly absorbed and must be taken on an empty stomach with a full glass of water upon awakening. Patients must remain in an upright position for at least 30 min after taking alendronate. Because food markedly reduces absorption of the drug, patients should wait 30 to 45 min after taking alendronate before eating. Patients who cannot comply with these restrictions are not good candidates for therapy with this drug.

The optimal dose of alendronate for treatment of postmenopausal osteoporosis is 10 mg orally, once a day. Alendronate is a powerful option for women who are unwilling or not able to take HRT. Patients who have a history of thromboembolism, breast cancer, or who are refractory to treatment of osteoporosis with estrogen are candidates for alendronate therapy. Recent data also show benefit for patients who take long-term glucocorticoids and either have or are at risk of osteoporosis.

CALCITONIN

Salmon calcitonin is a polypeptide hormone that directly inhibits osteoclastic bone resorption and preserves bone mass among postmenopausal women with established osteoporosis. It is approved for managing but not for preventing osteoporosis more than 5 years after menopause. It is available although rarely used as a subcutaneous or intramuscular injection but most commonly is taken as a nasal spray formulation. One daily intranasal spray delivers 200 units of calcitonin.

Calcitonin appears to improve the BMD of the lumbar vertebrae of postmenopausal women. Studies have shown a 2 to 3 percent increase in BMD of the vertebrae with calcitonin therapy relative to calcium-supplement placebo. Calcitonin is not, however, as effective as the other agents in preventing bone loss at the hip. One study also showed a 40 percent decrease in frequency of osteoporotic vertebral fractures. No data are available on the effectiveness of calcitonin on preventing hip fractures. Thus calcitonin is considered a second-line alternative for patients who are unable to take the other treatments.

Calcitonin may be useful to patients with recent osteoporotic fractures because it appears to have an analgesic effect. Side effects are minimal; they include rhinitis and nasal irritation. Older women with symptomatic upper gastrointestinal disease and back pain due to osteoporotic fractures are excellent candidates for therapy with nasal calcitonin.

OTHER AGENTS

Sodium fluoride stimulates osteoblastic activity and new bone formation. Early studies, however, indicated that the quality of bone developed was abnormal and more prone to fracture. New data suggest that a slow-release form of fluoride will increase BMD and decrease fracture risk. At present, however, the FDA has not approved sodium fluoride as therapy for osteoporosis.

Etidronate is a bisphosphonate used in the management of Paget's disease, hypercalcemia of malignant disease, and myositis ossificans. It has been shown to increase BMD to 2 to 3 percent and to decrease the rate of new vertebral fractures but is not FDA-approved for the treatment of patients with osteoporosis. The standard dosing regimen consists of 400 mg daily for 14 days every 3 months. Side effects are gastrointestinal upset and bone pain.

Thiazide diuretics lower urinary calcium excretion, suppress parathyroid gland function, and reduce intestinal calcium absorption. Excess parathyroid hormone is known to cause bone loss. Thiazides may be useful to selected patients with hypercalciuria and secondary hyperparathyroidism.

Management of Acute Fractures

Patients with a recent fracture deserve special mention. The process of bone loss and osteo-

porosis progresses silently, and older women may have "silent" vertebral fractures. Severe pain may accompany acute vertebral fractures, as may paravertebral muscle spasm and radiation of pain due to nerve root compression. Adequate pain control is important in the care of patients recovering from vertebral compression fractures. Patients may need hospitalization for management of the acute fracture and pain control. Although vertebral fractures do not usually necessitate surgical intervention, surgery for internal fixation of the spine is a consideration in cases of nerve root or spinal cord damage.

Pain from acute fracture usually disappears gradually over a 6- to 8-week period, but it can be debilitating in the short term. Immobilization leads to rapid loss of muscle strength and bone density, and pain control is important to allow resumption of some activity during the acute period. Salmon calcitonin nasal spray may be a helpful adjunct to analgesics. It appears to decrease pain after an acute fracture. Once the fracture heals, calcitonin has no effect on musculoskeletal pain.

Physical therapy and rehabilitation are critical for improving function and reducing disability during the recovery period. The use of assistive devices such as walkers or canes often is necessary for early walking and resumption of activities of daily living. Patients at highest risk of fracture are those with recent or previous fractures. Follow-up assessment to determine medical status, understanding and compliance with treatment, and functional activity level are necessary for these patients at high risk.

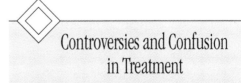

Controversies and Confusion in Treatment

One of the controversial issues in BMD testing is central versus peripheral testing. Some experts argue that the site of greatest fracture risk should be measured, such as the hip, because hip fractures are associated with higher morbidity and mortality than fractures at other sites. A reasonable alternative might be the spine, because vertebral compression fractures are the most frequent site of osteoporotic fracture. Current data suggest that peripheral measurements of the BMD of the calcaneus, distal radius, and proximal radius are as accurate as DEXA measurements at the hip, vertebrae, and calcaneus in predicting fracture risk and presence of hip fractures. The choice of BMD method should take into account the accessibility of the technology to the patient, body site, and cost. Follow-up testing after a low BMD is found with any of the testing methods is generally performed with DEXA. The same machine, site, and position are used for measurement to compare sequential test results.

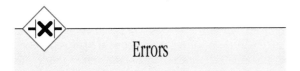

Errors

Despite the large number of women with osteoporosis, most cases are still undiagnosed and the patients untreated. The reasons are not clear, because accurate and precise diagnostic techniques are now available, as are multiple therapeutic options. Media and medical attention are increasing public awareness of osteoporosis and its potential effect on a woman's future. New guidelines that provide coverage for BMD testing of all Medicare eligible patients will allow increased screening and identification of those at risk.

Clinicians also make the error of failing to search for a secondary cause of osteoporosis. Although most patients have primary osteoporosis, it is important to consider and rule out secondary causes of osteoporosis.

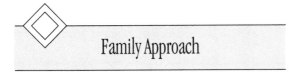

Family Approach

The prevention and management of osteoporosis can best be accomplished by the involvement of an interdisciplinary team that often includes family members at its core. Clinicians need to work with patients on the multiple factors that affect individual health status and response to disease. Exercise, diet, and other health habits, such as smoking, and the psychological response to the disease and its consequences all influence patient outcomes. The coordinated effort of physicians, nurse educators, nutritionists, physical therapists, and social workers is needed. The physician has specific technical knowledge and skills in the diagnosis and management of osteoporosis, but the involvement of other health professionals at various points in the patient's overall care will enhance patient care and patient outcomes.

Economic and family resources play a critical role, particularly for elderly persons living alone. The family support system can be a major factor for an elderly person making a decision to maintain an independent living status or move into institutionalized care. Family members may be integral to the clinician's efforts to optimize care, particularly in the areas of encouraging medication compliance, providing transportation for appointments, and diet and exercise interventions. The effort to modify the living environment to minimize the risk of falls is another area where family support may be critical. After an acute fracture, pain and disability often necessitate involvement of family members in supportive care and rehabilitation. The presence or absence of integral family involvement often is the determining factor in a decision regarding nursing home placement.

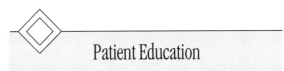

Patient Education

Osteoporosis is a growing health priority in the United States. Increased attention to the problem has resulted in legislative changes at the federal level to cover BMD testing, development of clinical standards and guidelines by national quality assurance organizations and specialty organizations, and the development and dissemination of a multitude of educational resources for both health professionals and patients.

Many information sources are available for clinicians and patients that can provide education on prevention and management of osteoporosis. The National Osteoporosis Foundation, in collaboration with a number of medical specialty societies, has developed a physician's guide to prevention and management of osteoporosis. Several versions of this guide are available for use by specialists, primary care practitioners, other health care professionals, and patients.

A wide variety of other materials are available for patient counseling and education. These include written materials, videos, and sites on the World Wide Web. Patients should be advised that caution is appropriate when reading information that appears on the Web, because scientific review of the information is not required. Web sites and additional sources of information are listed in Table 8-13.

Table 8-13

Web Sites and Additional Sources of Information About Osteoporosis

National Dairy Council
O'Hare International Center
10255 West Higgins Road, Suite 900
Rosemount, IL 60018
(800) 426-8271

National Osteoporosis Foundation
1150 17th Street NW, Suite 500
Washington, DC 20036-4603
(202) 223-2226 or (800) 223-9994
nofmail@nof.org or http://www.nof.org

Office of Medical Application Research, NIH
PO Box 2577
Kensington, MD 20891
(800) NIH-OMAR
http://text.nlm.nih.gov

Older Women's League
666 11th Street NW, Suite 700
Washington, DC 20001
(202) 783-6686 or (800) 825-3695

Osteoporosis & Related Bone Diseases National Resource Center
    (ORBD-NRC)
1150 17th Street NW, Suite 500
Washington, DC 20036-4603
(202) 223-0344
http://www.osteo.org

Emerging Concepts

Biochemical Markers of Bone Activity

Although several biochemical markers of bone activity are available, their use in clinical practice is still unclear. Biochemical markers provide information about the bone remodeling process through measurement of the enzymatic activity of osteoclasts or osteoblasts or of the bone matrix components released into the circulation during formation or resorption. A variety of markers have been used mainly for research application (Table 8-14).

The use of biochemical markers in clinical practice is evolving. They may be useful in identifying women with rapid bone turnover who might benefit from preventive treatments. Monitoring the early therapeutic response of patients with established osteoporosis is another possibility. Finally, markers may be useful in identifying women who are losing bone mass despite treatment, for example, with HRT. Insurance coverage of these tests is also evolving, and HCFA coverage of selected biochemical bone markers is expected.

Combination Bisphosphonate and Hormone Therapy

The effectiveness and safety of the combined use of hormone and bisphosphonate therapy for osteo-

porosis is being investigated. Combined therapy has been shown to increase BMD compared with either the single-treatment regimens or placebo, and the effect appears to be additive. Whether combined therapy will reduce fracture rates more than single agents is not yet known, and data on long-term safety and effect on bone quality are not available. At present, routine use of combined therapy is not recommended.

Economic Impact

Osteoporosis affects millions of postmenopausal women. The disease affects more women than heart attack, stroke, and breast cancer combined. More than 1.5 million women sustain osteoporotic fractures each year, compared with more than 500,000 women who have heart attacks, 228,000 with stroke, and 184,000 with breast cancer. The cost to society is almost 14 billion dollars per year, greater than the cost for either congestive heart failure or asthma. In 1995, osteoporosis was the presumed cause of more than 400,000 hospital admissions, almost 2.5 million physician visits, and 180,000 nursing home admissions.

Given the demographics of an aging population, the magnitude of the problem is expected to increase. Without the implementation of comprehensive prevention and treatment programs, the cost of the disease is estimated to triple by the

Table 8-14

Biochemical Markers of Bone Activity

MARKERS OF BONE FORMATION	MARKERS OF BONE RESORPTION
Alkaline phosphatase (bone specific)	Hydroxyproline
Osteocalcin	Pyridinium cross-links
Procollagen type 1 (PICP)	Collagen type I cross-linked carboxyterminal propeptide
Procollagen type 1 *N*-terminal propeptide (PINP)	*N*-telopeptide
	Collagen type I cross-linked *C*-telopeptide (cross-laps)

year 2040. Primary care, which emphasizes health promotion and disease prevention, is critical in the effort to reduce the impact of this disease. The cost-effectiveness of current modalities in preventing and managing this disease in the primary care setting (as opposed to acute in-patient management of fractures and their complications) is clear. The increased public emphasis on the disease, early identification and treatment of those at risk, and the development and dissemination of recommendations and guidelines for diagnosis and management of the disease reflect this awareness.

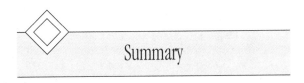

Summary

Osteoporosis is the most common skeletal bone disorder worldwide and has a high morbidity and mortality. It is a systemic skeletal disease characterized by low bone density and increased risk of fracture. It is defined by a BMD T score of −2.5 or more below the young adult reference mean. Risk factors of the disease are multiple, but female sex and postmenopausal status are most important. Sixty percent of women 70 to 79 years of age and 80 percent of women 80 years and older are affected.

Osteoporosis is asymptomatic and goes unrecognized and often undiagnosed until clinical consequences occur. The clinical hallmark of the disease is fragility fracture. The most common sites of fracture are the vertebrae, wrist, and hip. Vertebral fractures lead to loss of height, kyphosis, and chronic back pain. Hip fractures cause the greatest morbidity, mortality, and expense to the health care system.

Early diagnosis and treatment are essential to reduce the morbidity and mortality associated with this disease. BMD measurement can help predict the risk of future fracture, and effective treatment is available to reduce the risk of fracture. Optimal calcium and vitamin D intake are important throughout life for prevention, for treat-

ment, and as an adjunct to the pharmacologic agents used to manage established osteoporosis.

Pharmacologic therapy should be individualized to maximize efficacy and minimize associated risks. Estrogen replacement therapy is the current first-line therapy for preventing and managing postmenopausal osteoporosis. Raloxifene, a selective estrogen receptor modulator, is a promising new drug currently approved by the FDA only for the prevention of osteoporosis. Alendronate is a potent nonhormonal bisphosphonate that increases bone density and decreases risk of future fractures of the hip and vertebrae. Nasal calcitonin is a safe, reasonably effective agent with potential analgesic activity in the setting of acute fracture.

Preventive measures include optimal calcium intake, smoking cessation, moderation of alcohol use, weight-bearing exercise, and prevention of falls. Physical therapy and rehabilitation are important components of tertiary prevention among patients with fractures due to osteoporosis.

Bibliography

American Association of Clinical Endocrinologists: *Clinical Practice Guidelines for the Prevention and Treatment of Postmenopausal Osteoporosis.* Jacksonville, FL; AACE; 1996.

Boning Up on Osteoporosis: A Guide to Prevention and Treatment. Washington, DC: National Osteoporosis Foundation; 1997.

Castellsague J, Perez Gutthann S, Garcia Rodriguez LA: Recent epidemiological studies of the association between hormone replacement therapy and venous thromboembolism: a review. *Drug Saf* 18:117, 1998.

Cauley JA, Seeley DG, Enstraud K, et al: Estrogen replacement therapy and fractures in older women. *Ann Intern Med* 122:9, 1995.

Colditz GA, Hankinson SE, Hunter DJ, et al: The use of estrogens and progestins and the risk of breast cancer in postmenopausal women. *N Engl J Med* 332: 1589, 1995.

Consensus Development Conference: Prophylaxis and treatment of osteoporosis. *Am J Med* 90:107, 1991.

Cummings SR, Nevitt MC, Browner WS, et al: Risk factors for hip fractures in white women: study of Osteoporotic Fractures Research Group. *N Engl J Med* 332:767, 1995.

De Groen PC, Lubbe DF, Hirsch, LJ, et al: Esophagitis associated with the use of alendronate. *N Engl J Med* 335:1016, 1996.

Ettinger B, Black S, Cummings H, et al: Raloxifene reduces the risk of incident vertebral fractures: 24-month interim analysis [abstr.]. *Osteoporis Int* 8(suppl 3):11, 1998.

Gennari C, Agnusdei D, Camporeale A: Use of calcitonin in the treatment of bone pain associated with osteoporosis. *Calcif Tissue Int* 49(suppl 2):S9, 1991.

Grimes DA: Weighing the benefits and risks of hormone replacement therapy after menopause. *Contracept Rep* 6:4, 1995.

Grisso JA, Capezuti E, Schwartz A: *Falls as Risk Factors for Fractures.* New York: Academic Press; 1996.

Health Oasis, Mayo Clinic: "Bone up: your lifestyle with diet and exercise. http://www.mayohealth.org/mayo/9605/htm/osteo_1 sb.htm. Accessed May 3, 1999.

Hulley S, Grady D, Bush T, et al: Randomized trial of estrogen plus progestin for secondary prevention of coronary heart disease in postmenopausal women. *JAMA* 280:605, 1998.

Khovidhunkit W, Shoback D: Clinical effects of raloxifene hydrochloride in women. *Ann Intern Med* 130:431, 1999.

Liberman UA, Weiss SR, Broll J, et al: Effect of oral alendronate on bone mineral density and the incidence of fractures in postmenopausal osteoporosis: the Alendronate Phase III Osteoporosis Treatment Study Group. *N Engl J Med* 333:1437, 1995.

Lyritis GP, Tsakalakos N, Magiasis B, et al: Analgesic effect of salmon calcitonin in osteoporotic vertebral fractures: a double blind placebo-controlled clinical study. *Calcif Tissue Int* 49:369, 1991.

Maricic MJ, Silverman SL, Chestnut C, et al: Salmon-calcitonin nasal spray prevents vertebral fractures in established osteoporosis: further interim results of the PROOF study (abstr.) *Arthritis Rheum* 41(suppl): S129, 1998.

National Osteoporosis Foundation: *Physician's Guide to Prevention and Treatment of Osteoporosis.* Belle Mead, NJ; Excerpta Medica; 1998.

NIH Consensus Development Panel on Optimal Calcium Intake: NIH Consensus conference: optimal calcium intake *JAMA* 272:1942, 1994.

Osteoporosis and Related Bone Diseases, National Resource Center: *Fast Facts on Osteoporosis.* Washington, DC: ORBD-NRC; 1996.

Osteoporosis and Related Bone Diseases, National Resource Center: *Latino Women and Osteoporosis.* Washington, DC: ORBD-NRC; 1996.

Overgaard K, Hansen MA, Jensen SB, et al: Effect of salcatonin given intranasally on bone mass and fracture rates in established osteoporosis: a dose-response study. *BMJ* 305:556, 1992.

Ray NF, Chan JK, Thamer M, et al: Medical expenditures for the treatment of osteoporotic fractures in the United States in 1995: report from the National Osteoporosis Foundation. *J Bone Miner Res* 12:24, 1997.

Saag KG, Emkaj R, Schnitzer TJ, et al: Alendronate for the prevention and treatment of glucocorticoid-induced osteoporosis. *N Engl J Med* 339:292, 1998.

Stampfer MJ, Colditz GA: Estrogen replacement therapy and coronary heart disease: a qualitative assessment of the epidemiological evidence. *Prev Med* 21:47, 1991.

The Calcium Information Resource: Calcium calculator. http://www.calciuminfo.com/calculator/calc.htm. Accessed May 3, 1999.

The Writing Group for the PEPI Trial: Effects of estrogen or estrogen/progestin regimens on heart disease risk factors in postmenopausal women. *JAMA* 273: 199, 1995.

Tresolini CP, GOld DT, Lee LS (eds): *Working with Patients to Prevent, Treat, and Manage Osteoporosis: A Curriculum Guide for the Health Professions,* 2nd ed. San Francisco: National Fund for Medical Education; 1998.

Wimalawansa SJ: A four-year randomized controlled trial of hormone replacement and bisphosphonate, alone or in combination, in women with postmenopausal osteoporosis. *Am J Med* 104:219, 1998.

World Health Organization: Assessment of fracture risk and its application to screening for postmenopausal osteoporosis: report of a WHO Study Group. *World Health Organ Tech Rep Ser* 843:1, 1994.

Ursula McClymont
Niharika N. Suchak

Chapter 9

Joint Pains

Errors
  Failure to Differentiate Periarticular Disease
    from Other Causes of Joint Pain
  Overuse of NSAIDs in the Treatment of
    Osteoarthritis
  Failure to Consider the Diagnosis of Septic
    Arthritis in a Patient with Chronic Arthritis

Patient Education
Emerging Concepts
  New Oral Treatments for Osteoarthritis
  New Treatments for Osteoarthritis of the Knee
    Autogenous Cartilage Implantation
    Autogenous Osteochondral Grafting
    Hyaluronic Acid Injection
  New Treatments for Rheumatoid Arthritis

The diagnosis and management of joint pain in elderly patients can be a difficult process, and one that is often complicated by diagnostic uncertainty because of atypical manifestations, the presence of comorbid conditions, and an increased frequency of adverse drug events. In this chapter, we review the common disorders that cause non-traumatic joint pain in the elderly and an approach to the diagnosis and management of these conditions.

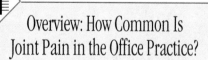

Overview: How Common Is Joint Pain in the Office Practice?

Joint pain is a very common symptom in the elderly. Arthritis ranked first among the ten most prevalent chronic health problems in a survey conducted in 1989 by the National Center for Health Statistics. The estimated prevalence rate of arthritis in 1990 was 49.4 percent for people aged 65 years and over, as compared with 5.1 percent for people aged 44 years and under. Activity limitation associated with arthritis in the 65 years and older age group was estimated at 11.6 percent versus 2.8 percent in the general U.S. population. Not only is joint pain common, but it can also affect mobility, quality of life, and independence.

Principal Diagnoses

Table 9-1 lists the common causes of joint pains in the elderly under two broad categories, articular and periarticular. The most frequently encountered of these causes are discussed below.

Osteoarthritis

Osteoarthritis (OA) is a degenerative process of articular surfaces that result in pain and diminished function. The etiology is believed to be multifactorial. The prevalence of OA increases with age. OA can be classified as primary or idiopathic (no obvious antecedent insult), or secondary (obvious antecedent insult). Women are more commonly affected than men. Approximately 33 percent of the population aged 25 to 74 years have radiographic evidence of OA involving the hand, foot, knee, or hip. It is estimated that more than 60 percent of all persons over age 70 suffer from OA.

The pathogenesis of osteoarthritis involves a complex series of interactions culminating with destabilization of the normal balance of synthesis and degradation of articular cartilage. Although several risk factors have been identified, there is no single factor that initiates the destruction of

Table 9-1

Common Causes of Joint Pains

ARTICULAR	PERIARTICULAR
Osteoarthritis	Polymyalgia rheumatica
Rheumatoid arthritis*	Bursitis
Crystal-associated arthritis: gout, pseudogout	Tendinitis
Septic arthritis	
Systemic lupus erythematosus*	
Spondyloarthropathies	
Osteoporosis (vertebral compression fractures)	
Malignancy related arthritis*	

*May have extraarticular manifestations.

cartilage in OA. Risk factors for OA include older age, female gender, previous trauma, mechanical stress (especially in OA of the knee), and previous inflammatory arthritis (i.e., gout, rheumatoid arthritis). Several cross-sectional studies have shown an association between obesity and OA, although the mechanism is unclear.

Periarticular Disease

A common source of joint pain complaints in the elderly results from soft tissue damage, usually secondary to trauma. Repetitive motion or acute trauma may damage the tendons and bursae associated with joints that endure daily stresses (i.e., shoulder, knee, and hip). In the elderly, biceps tendinitis, rotator cuff tendinitis (RCT), subacromial bursitis, lateral epicondylitis, olecranon bursitis, trochanteric bursitis, and anserine bursitis are the most common soft-tissue syndromes (Table 9-2).

Table 9-2

Common Causes of Periarticular Pain

NAME	LOCATION OF PAIN COMPLAINT	POINT TENDERNESS	COMMENTS
Biceps tendinitis	Anterior shoulder	Bicipital groove	
Rotator cuff tendinitis	Shoulder and radiates down the lateral arm	Greater tuberosity of the humerus	Pain is reproducible with shoulder abduction or flexion
Subacromial bursitis	Pain frequently radiates down the arm	Lateral shoulder, especially over the subacromial space	Pain with abduction and flexion of the shoulder
Lateral epicondylitis	Elbow	Lateral epicondyle	Resisting wrist dorsiflexion
Olecranon bursitis	Elbow	Olecranon process	Usually present with a mass over the olecranon process
Trochanteric bursitis	Lateral hip, which sometimes radiates to the knee	Greater trochanter	Pain is worse with walking and lying on the affected side
Anserine bursitis	Experienced with knee flexion	Medial aspect of the proximal tibia	Especially walking upstairs

Bursae are fluid-filled sacs between muscles, tendons, and bone which serve to reduce friction between these structures. Inflammation of these structures results in significant pain or dysfunction of the involved joint (stiffness secondary to decreased mobility).

SHOULDER

The locations of the structures involved make shoulders vulnerable to damage. The long head of the biceps travels in the bicipital groove to insert above the glenoid process. The rotator cuff is composed of four muscles (supraspinatus, infraspinatus, teres minor, and subscapularis). The rotator cuff mediates the major functions of the shoulder (abduction, adduction, external rotation, and internal rotation) and is often damaged by repetitive shoulder activities; the supraspinatus muscle is most frequently affected. The most frequent type of shoulder bursitis is subacromial bursitis; the bursa is located between the deltoid muscle and the shoulder capsule and the acromion.

ELBOW

The elbow's primary function is to allow pronation and supination of the forearm. The most frequent causes of elbow pain are epicondylitis and olecranon bursitis. Lateral epicondylitis (tennis elbow) results from overuse or damage to the extensor carpi radialis brevis tendon. Olecranon bursitis is most commonly caused by trauma; the olecranon bursa lies between the skin and olecranon process. It is this superficial location that makes it prone to trauma (traumatic bursitis) and infection (septic bursitis). Septic olecranon bursitis is usually caused by common skin pathogens introduced by trauma to the skin and occasionally by seeding from other sites of infection.

HIP

Bursitis-induced hip pain is almost always due to trochanteric bursitis. The trochanteric bursae are located between the tendon of the gluteus maximus and the greater trochanter.

KNEE

The anserine bursae are located adjacent to the knee at the junction of the sartorius, gracilis, and semitendinosus tendons. It is the most common bursitis causing knee pain and is seen typically in elderly, overweight women.

Polymyalgia Rheumatica

Polymyalgia rheumatica (PMR) is a clinical syndrome of unknown etiology characterized by pain and stiffness in the neck, shoulder girdle, and pelvic girdle. The incidence of PMR increases with age, and the disease is rarely diagnosed in those below the age of 50 years. The mean annual incidence of PMR has been reported to be 54 per 100,000 members of the population 50 years of age and older. The prevalence of PMR is estimated at 550 per 100,000 aged 50 years and older. PMR is roughly twice as common in women as in men. It is much more common among people of northern European descent. It is rare among people of African and Asian descent.

PMR is often associated with temporal arteritis, frequently occurring in the same patient. The nature and cause of the association, however, is not known. PMR, which is predominantly a synovitis/bursitis, and temporal arteritis, which is predominantly a vasculitis, are nosologic terms used to define typical clinical syndromes. Some consider the two to be syndromes at either end of the spectrum of one disease, with temporal arteritis the more severe and PMR the less severe expression of the syndrome.

It is thought that the specific musculoskeletal symptoms in PMR are due to underlying synovitis as well as proximal bursitis. Despite the absence of vascular symptoms, however, PMR has been shown to involve blood vessels, as evidenced by abnormalities in temporal artery biopsy specimens from patients with PMR. Muscle also can be affected by vasculitis as has been observed in muscle biopsy specimens.

The cause of PMR is not known. It is also not clear why there is such a high prevalence in older persons. An increased prevalence of antibodies to adenovirus and respiratory syncytial virus in patients with PMR has been interpreted as evidence of a possible infectious cause of the disease. Cell-mediated immune responses appear to play a greater role as compared to humoral immune mechanisms. The predominance in the white population, familial aggregation, and the association with HLA-DR4 antigen favor a genetic predisposition. The association of PMR with HLA-DR4 may explain the lower incidence of PMR in blacks. Caucasians are four times more likely to have HLA-DR4 than African-Americans.

Calcium Pyrophosphate Deposition Disease

Calcium pyrophosphate deposition (CPPD) disease is an arthropathy caused by the deposition of calcium pyrophosphate crystals in joints, and most commonly affects the knee. The incidence of CPPD increases with age. Because symptoms resemble those seen in gout, the disease is often called "pseudogout." Although CPPD resembles gout clinically, the mechanism of cartilage calcification in CPPD is unclear, and there are familial forms of the disease. CPPD is more common than gout.

Gout

Gout is a mono- or polyarticular arthritis resulting from the deposition of monosodium urate monohydrate crystals in joint or soft tissue. Years of systemic hyperuricemia (generally serum uric acid levels > 7.0 mg/dL) usually precede crystal formation in joints. The prevalence of gout in men is twice that in women. Men most commonly develop the disease after the age of 40 years, with a peak incidence in the decade of the 50s. Women usually develop the disease after menopause.

The hyperuricemia of gout involves increased uric acid production, decreased uric acid excretion, or a combination of both. It is estimated that approximately 10 percent of gout patients overproduce uric acid (urinary uric acid secretion of > 800 mg/day). Several conditions are associated with hyperuricemia and gout (Table 9-3). Most patients are underexcretors of uric acid. The main route of uric acid elimination is renal, primarily via the proximal tubules. Medications or diseases that affect the proximal tubules can alter uric acid excretion. The condition most commonly associated with overproduction and under-secretion of uric acid is excessive alcohol intake.

Rheumatoid Arthritis

Rheumatoid arthritis (RA) is a chronic, inflammatory, systemic disease that produces its most prominent manifestations in the diarthrodial (hinged) joints. RA is a relatively common medical problem in the elderly. Its estimated prevalence in the U.S. adult population is somewhere between 1 to 2 percent. The highest incidence is found in the fourth and fifth decades of life, but new cases continue to arise into the ninth decade. The mean annual incidence of RA has been reported to be 77 per 100,000 population 50 years of age and older. Several surveys have

Table 9-3

Medications and Diseases Associated with Gout

MEDICATIONS	DISEASES
Salicylates	Myeloproliferative disease
Diuretics	Lymphoproliferative disease
Alcohol	Psoriasis
Pyrazinamide	Obesity
Ethambutol	Hemolytic anemia
Nicotinic acid	

shown that approximately 20 to 30 percent of RA presents after age 60.

The etiology of RA is unknown. It is believed that genetic predisposition and environmental triggers play major roles. The possibility of an infectious etiology of RA has been investigated extensively, without yielding convincing evidence. Genetic and environmental factors are believed to control the progression, extent, and pattern of the inflammatory response. RA has been noted to possess several features typical of a complex genetic disease, such as incomplete penetrance, genetic variance, and involvement of multiple genes. The clinical risk for developing RA is highly associated with HLA-DR, which is a major histocompatibility complex (MHC) class II molecule and is present on all antigen-presenting cells.

RA is characterized by an intense inflammatory, proliferative synovitis that may erode adjacent bone. The rheumatoid joint produces many destructive enzymes and cytokines, which produce their effects within the synovium, the vascular endothelium of synovial vessels, the synovial fluid, and peripherally in serum. These inflammatory mediators promote granulocyte extravasation, B-cell proliferation with antibody production (including rheumatoid factor), vascular hyperplasia, thrombocytosis, anemia, cartilage degradation, and bone destruction. The end result is joint space narrowing.

RA has tremendous public health implications due to the related disability, home health requirements, health care costs, increased mortality in severe cases, and reduced life expectancy. Disability for rheumatoid-factor-positive patients develops early because a high percentage of joints ultimately affected in these patients are involved in the first years of disease. Seronegativity is associated with a more favorable prognosis. The mortality in RA patients arises from various secondary conditions such as infections, fractures, gastrointestinal bleeding, lymphoproliferative malignancy, or myocardial infarction.

Predictors for increased RA mortality include increased severity of disease at baseline, many involved joints, poor functional status, advanced age, and lower educational achievement. Other indicators of poor prognosis include elevated ESR and the presence of extraarticular manifestations. The extraarticular manifestations of RA include rheumatoid nodules, Sjögren's syndrome, episcleritis and scleritis, interstitial lung disease, pericardial disease, systemic vasculitis, and Felty's syndrome. The primary methods used for determination of prognosis during the first 2 years of disease include the history, joint examination, and functional assessment.

Septic Arthritis

An infectious process causes septic arthritis. The elderly are at an increased risk of developing septic arthritis (SA) because of comorbid medical diseases such as rheumatoid arthritis, diabetes mellitus, peripheral vascular disease, and prosthetic joints. SA in older persons is almost always due to nongonococcal organisms. The most common cause of SA in the elderly is gram-positive bacteria. *Staphylococcus aureus* is the predominant organism followed by *Streptococcus* species (groups A, B, C, and G). Gram-negative bacilli and anaerobes (especially with prosthetic joints) also cause SA. Lyme disease may also present as a septic monarthritis, 5 to 6 months following the initial infection.

Septic arthritis usually results from hematogenous spread of organisms (i.e., from skin infections), but direct invasion (i.e., introduction of bacteria when injecting a joint) and contiguous infection (i.e., bursitis) also occurs. Hours after bacteria enter the joint space, there is an intense inflammatory response that eventually leads to protease and cytokine-mediated degradation of cartilage. The inoculum size and host preexisting conditions (i.e., joint disease) determine the severity of the inflammatory reaction and subsequent structural damage. Prompt diagnosis and treatment can decrease the duration of disease and sequelae.

Typical Presentation

Osteoarthritis

Pain is usually the presenting complaint. Other complaints can include morning stiffness, joint swelling, crepitus, joint deformity, and deficits in range of motion (ROM). The pain is mild-to-moderate in intensity, worsened by the use of the involved joint, and improved with rest. Patients also commonly report stiffness after inactivity that improves with use of the joint. Stiffness can last from 5 to 30 min and can involve one or more joints.

OA is usually insidious in onset. Early in the course of the disease, the pain is usually localized. Pain at rest or during the night usually indicates severe disease.

Joint involvement varies, with the knee and hip being the most commonly affected joints. Primary OA also affects distal interphalangeal joints, proximal interphalangeal joints, base of the thumb (first metacarpal joint), first metatarsophalangeal joint, and the spine (cervical and lumbar).

Polymyalgia Rheumatica

The onset of PMR is usually insidious, but can be abrupt. Before diagnosis, vague symptoms may be present for greater than 1 month. The most common symptoms are aches and stiffness involving the proximal muscle girdles and the neck. Some patients can also have symptoms such as joint synovitis, tenosynovitis, and carpal tunnel syndrome.

Systemic signs and symptoms occur in about one third of patients, including fever, night sweats, malaise or fatigue, anorexia, weight loss, and depression. Some patients complain of headaches, jaw claudication, facial sensitivity to touch, blurred vision, or decreased visual acuity. These visual symptoms should alert the clinician to the possible presence of concomitant temporal arteritis.

The common features in the various published sets of diagnostic criteria for PMR are pain and stiffness in any of the following: neck and torso, shoulders and upper arms, hips and thighs; age greater than 50 years; and exclusion of other diagnoses except temporal arteritis. The presence of morning stiffness lasting over 1 h and persistence of symptoms for more than 2 weeks supports the diagnosis.

Calcium Pyrophosphate Deposition Disease

CPPD typically presents with the acute onset of a severe, monoarticular arthritis involving a large joint such as the knee. Smaller joints, however, such as the wrist or ankle, can also be affected. Unlike gout, the first metatarsophalangeal joint is usually not affected. CPPD can be associated with systemic symptoms such as fatigue, fever, and morning stiffness.

The affected joint is usually swollen, warm, and erythematous. The disease can also cause a polyarthritis. CPPD has been associated with several medical conditions (Table 9-4). Attacks of pseudogout are usually self-limited, lasting for 1 to 14 days. CPPD can also be chronic with episodic attacks mimicking RA or gout.

Gout

The natural progression of gout involves three stages: asymptomatic hyperuricemia, acute gout,

Table 9-4

Conditions Associated with Calcium Pyrophosphate Deposition Disease

Hypothyroidism
Hypomagnesemia
Hypophosphatemia
Hyperparathyroidism
Hemochromatosis

and chronic tophaceous gout (CTG). Asymptomatic hyperuricemia (an elevation in uric acid levels without clinical manifestations of gout) is not a disease, and most patients with hyperuricemia will not develop gout. Patients who will later develop gout usually only do so after at least 15 years of hyperuricemia.

Most acute gouty attacks (~ 90 percent) involve the first metatarsophalangeal (MTP) joint. The pain experienced by the patient usually begins in the night or early morning. The affected joint is exquisitely tender and sensitive even to light touch (i.e., touch of the bed sheet). The onset of pain is rapid and associated with local signs of inflammation (i.e., erythema, edema, and warmth) that can mimic cellulitis. Systemic symptoms (fever or chills) may also be present.

Acute gout is a self-limited disease. The pain usually reaches its peak within 12 h and lasts a few days to weeks. Classically, the pain is intense and severe; however, some patients only experience mild discomfort. There is usually a symptom-free period between acute attacks.

Although the first MTP joint is most commonly affected, gout can be polyarticular (10 percent to 13 percent), affecting ankles, knees, wrist, elbow, instep, and fingers. There are many other conditions that can cause first MTP joint pain including stress fractures, septic arthritis, and pseudogout.

The time between first and second gouty attacks can range from 6 months to greater than 20 years. The majority of recurrences occur within 2 years of the initial attack. Many individuals only experience one attack. As acute attacks increase in frequency and duration, patients eventually develop persistent symptoms with no symptom-free periods and progress to developing tophi (deposits of sodium urate crystals usually over bony prominences).

Tophaceous gout is the consequence of the chronic inability to efficiently excrete urate. It is characterized by polyarticular pain without pain-free periods. Tophi can develop in any area. Tophi cause joint destruction by the enzymes that are released and the pressure they exert. The average time between the initial attack and the development of CTG is 10 years; however, on rare occasions, patients have presented with CTG at initial presentation. The joints are constantly painful and swollen with periods of acute flares. It is during this phase of the disease that polyarticular involvement is most frequent, and the condition can mimic rheumatoid arthritis.

Rheumatoid Arthritis

"Elderly-onset" rheumatoid arthritis (EORA) can present with features similar to those seen in younger patients. Constitutional symptoms such as fatigue, weight loss, and generalized stiffness can precede or accompany the insidious onset of arthritis in the small joints of hands and feet, wrists, and knees. A characteristic feature is prolonged morning stiffness of the inflamed joints.

Based on the few studies that have addressed EORA specifically, a subset of patients with EORA can exhibit a clinical picture that is quite different than that seen in younger patients. This subgroup is characterized by abrupt onset, involvement of larger joints (i.e., shoulders and knees), prominent constitutional symptoms, less propensity to progress to extraarticular manifestations, and a near equal sex distribution. In younger RA patients, the usual female to male ratio is 3:1. A comparison between traditional or younger-onset RA (YORA) and elderly-onset RA (EORA) is shown in Table 9-5.

The joints of the hand are commonly affected in RA. In the absence of involvement of the hands, a definite diagnosis of RA can be made with a positive rheumatoid factor or presence of a rheumatoid nodule. By definition, the diagnosis of RA cannot be considered until the disease has been present for at least several weeks. Therefore, the diagnosis of RA is usually presumptive, early in its course.

Septic Arthritis

Septic arthritis typically presents with local signs of inflammation (pain, swelling, and erythema) and

Table 9-5

Clinical Features of Younger-Onset Rheumatoid Arthritis (YORA) versus Elderly-Onset
Rheumatoid Arthritis (EORA)

CLINICAL FEATURE	YORA	EORA
Age of onset	30–50 years	> 60 years
Onset	Gradual	Abrupt
Number of joints	Multiple	Few
Type of joints	Small, distal	Large, proximal
Morning stiffness	Moderate	Severe and prolonged
Sedimentation rate	Normal to high	Significantly high
Rheumatoid factor	Seropositive	Seronegative
Vasculitis	Common	Uncommon
Secondary Sjögren's syndrome	Rare	Common

systemic signs of infection (malaise, anorexia, and fever). Although the disease can be polyarticular, it most commonly affects a single joint (usually the knee). Pain is usually acute, severe, and present with rest and activity. Although the onset of pain is usually acute, it can be insidious. When a patient presents with an acutely inflamed joint, it should be presumed to be SA until proven otherwise.

Septic arthritis is a true medical emergency because of the propensity for rapid joint destruction and the development of osteomyelitis. To decrease the high morbidity and mortality (case fatality rate of 5 to 15 percent) associated with this disease, quick diagnosis and treatment is needed. SA can mimic or coexist with RA, gout, or pseudogout.

Physical Examination

General Examination

Table 9-6 shows the important elements of the joint examination. In general, the focus of the examination should be on the affected joint(s).

The examiner should look for swelling of the joint. Swelling can represent either soft-tissue swelling or joint space effusion.

Bony enlargement and nodules are often found in OA. Heberden's nodes are bony nodules of the

Table 9-6

Elements of the Joint Examination

Inspection for
Swelling
Deformity
Erythema
Alignment
Active range of motion
Palpation for
Warmth
Swelling
Deformity
Passive range of motion
Crepitus
Pattern of joint involvement
Symmetric versus nonsymmetric
Large versus small joint involvement
Monarthritis versus polyarthritis

distal interphalangeal joints. Bouchard's nodes are of the proximal interphalangeal joints. Malalignment of the joint can be found in OA and RA. The deformity of RA typically involves the proximal interphalangeal joints of the hands and wrists.

Erythema and warmth are indicators of inflammatory or infectious changes associated with acute inflammatory arthritis or septic arthritis. A doughy consistency to the joint is a nonspecific finding, but it also suggests an inflammatory process (synovitis).

The examiner should actively and passively range the affected joint. Pain that occurs with active ranging, but not with passive ranging, usually suggests a periarticular problem. An inflamed joint will usually be painful with both actively and passively ranging the joint. While ranging the joint, crepitus may be detected that can be either audible, palpable, or both. This finding is a characteristic but a nonspecific finding in patients with OA.

The distribution and location of affected joints can also provide clues to the diagnosis of underlying disorders. Multiple, symmetric joint involvement (polyarthritis) is characteristic of RA or SLE. Septic arthritis and gout typically involve a single joint (monoarthritis). Symmetric swelling of the second and third MCP joints, and fusiform swelling of the fingers, is suggestive of RA. Many extra-articular features of RA and the characteristic symmetric joint findings may not be obvious in the first several weeks of the disease.

Periarticular Disease

Table 9-2 shows the characteristic location of common periarticular diseases. Biceps tendinitis pain is often localized to the anterior shoulder and is reproducible with palpation over the bicipital groove. A simple test for biceps tendinitis is where the patient flexes the elbow and then supinates the forearm/hand against the examiner's resistance (Yergason's sign). This maneuver will reproduce pain of biceps tendinitis.

Rotator cuff pain most often originates in the shoulder and radiates down the lateral arm. Pain is reproducible with shoulder abduction or flexion. On physical examination, there is pain over the greater tuberosity of the humerus. RCT can often be diagnosed by having the patient abduct the arm to 90° and hold it. Pain and weakness will make the task impossible, and the arm will drop to the patient's side. Pain can also inhibit activities of daily living that require upper extremity abduction (i.e., combing hair, getting food from cabinet).

Subacromial bursitis often accompanies RCT and is characterized by shoulder pain with abduction and flexion of the shoulder; the pain frequently radiates down the arm. Physical examination can reveal pain with palpation over the lateral shoulder, especially over the subacromial space. Patients with subacromial bursitis will often demonstrate the "painful arc," where the patient is able to abduct to approximately 50° with minimal discomfort but experiences intolerable pain between 50 and 120°. Once passive abduction movement is taken past 120°, the pain decreases.

The pain of lateral epicondylitis is often reproducible with palpation distal to the lateral epicondyle or by actively resisting wrist dorsiflexion. Traumatic bursitis can occur from the simple act of resting the elbow on a hard surface for prolonged periods. Patients usually present with a mass over the olecranon process that is painful to palpation. Septic bursitis presents as a local cellulitis with pain, warmth, redness, erythema, and edema.

The pain of trochanteric bursitis is present at the lateral hip. Often, the pain is described as a dull ache, which sometimes radiates to the knee. Walking or lying on the affected side often exacerbates the pain. Patients with trochanteric bursitis most often complain of pain when he or she, during sleep, rolls onto the affected side. On physical examination, the hip joint often has good range of motion and has minimal pain; however, palpating over the greater trochanter causes severe pain. Anserine bursitis pain is experienced with knee flexion (especially walking upstairs). Patients with anserine bursitis can complain of stiffness suggesting arthritis, but typically, the pain is localized to the medial aspect of the proximal tibia.

Ancillary Tests

Ancillary tests for the evaluation of joint pain fall into four categories: laboratory testing, synovial fluid analysis, imaging studies, and other.

Laboratory Tests

Laboratory tests for joint pain problems lack the sensitivity and specificity required for diagnostic studies recommended for the general population. Laboratory tests are most valuable when used selectively. Laboratory blood testing is nonspecific and insensitive for diagnosing most elderly patients with joint pain. Frequently ordered tests include erythrocyte sedimentation rate, rheumatoid factor, antinuclear antibody, and uric acid levels. With the exception of diagnostic joint aspiration, other laboratory tests, such as standard serologic tests for rheumatic disease, should be used mainly for determination of prognosis or planning treatment.

ACUTE PHASE REACTANTS

The most commonly ordered acute phase reactant is the erythrocyte sedimentation rate (ESR). An elevated ESR can be associated with an inflammatory process, but it is not specific for inflammatory arthritides and can be elevated in many other conditions, such as malignancies, infections, and others. An elevated ESR is most helpful in patients with PMR or temporal arteritis (TA), where it is usually higher than 50 mm/h. Unfortunately, a normal ESR does not rule out PMR or TA. Some patients with RA can also have a very high ESR. The ESR is also useful in following the course of PMR. A fall in ESR is correlated with clinical improvement.

RHEUMATOID FACTOR

Rheumatoid factors (RF), first identified in the 1940s, are autoantibodies reactive with the Fc portion of immunoglobulin G (IgG) molecules. There are two widely used assays for RF. In the sensitized sheep cell agglutination (SSCA) test, the presence of RF is noted by the agglutination of sheep RBCs coated with nonagglutinating concentrations of rabbit IgG. Latex beads coated with human IgG are used in place of sheep RBCs and rabbit IgG in the latex fixation test (LFT). Titers tend to be higher with the LFT than with the SSCA. The SSCA is slightly more specific than the LFT for RA. RF is found in the serum of approximately 75 percent of adult patients with RA.

In elderly patients, a cautious approach to the interpretation of standard serologic tests for rheumatic disease is needed for two reasons. First, the reference range of normal results generated in healthy young adults may not be appropriate for the elderly. Second, the RF has many false-positive and false-negative results. Some patients with RA can be seronegative, especially early in the course of the disease. The false-positive rate of RF also increases with age.

The sensitivity and specificity of RF can also depend on the method of assay. In the general population, the RF by LFT has sensitivity of 75 percent and a specificity of 95 percent. RF (by LFT), however, has a false-positive rate between 10 to 15 percent in healthy elderly (> 65 years) persons as compared to 2 to 5 percent of healthy younger (30 to 50 years) subjects. The false-positive rate of RF using the SSCA test is 2 to 7 percent in the elderly as compared to 2 percent in the younger population. Thus, the specificity of RF testing in a geriatric population is lower than in a younger population.

ANTINUCLEAR ANTIBODIES

Although not common in the elderly, late-onset systemic lupus erythematosus (SLE) can occur. Antinuclear antibodies (ANA) are commonly present in patients with SLE; however, the increased prevalence of ANA and other autoantibodies with aging can complicate the interpretation of serologic findings in late-onset SLE. The positive predictive value of the ANA tends to increase with progressively higher antibody titers. Some studies have demonstrated an increased frequency of autoantibodies directed against SSA/Ro and SSB/La autoantigens in late-onset SLE. Antibodies to double-stranded DNA (dsDNA), which are highly specific and sensitive for SLE, can be used to substantiate the diagnosis and monitor disease activity in late-onset SLE.

URIC ACID

An elevated serum uric acid level in the presence of a monarticular, inflammatory arthritis supports a diagnosis of gout, but does not exclude the diagnosis if normal. The presence of crystals in synovial fluid is the definitive test for gout.

Synovial Fluid Examination

Aspiration and examination of synovial fluid is indicated in a patient with an inflamed joint with or without fever. The diagnosis of CPPD and gout can be made through analysis of joint fluid with phase contrast polarized-light microscopy. Whereas gout has negatively birefringent crystals, in CPPD, they appear as positively birefringent rhomboid structures within white blood cells. If septic arthritis is suspected, joint aspiration and fluid analysis is imperative to limit the amount of joint destruction.

A definitive diagnosis of septic arthritis can only be made by identifying organisms by Gram stain and culture. The distinguishing characteristics of synovial fluid analysis are shown in Table 9-7.

Imaging Studies

PLAIN RADIOGRAPHS

Table 9-8 lists the indications for obtaining plain radiographs. In the absence of these indications, plain x-rays are usually not helpful. Patients with inflammatory arthritis frequently have no radiographic changes in the first year of symptoms.

Radiography can be used to identify and quantify disease progression in OA. Over 70 percent of patients over 65 years of age have radiographic features of OA. Early in the course of the disease, findings on plain radiograph include asymmetric joint space narrowing and subchondral bony sclerosis and bone cysts (Fig. 9-1). As the disease progresses, marginal osteophytes and subchondral bone cysts develop.

A typical x-ray finding of CPPD is chondrocalcinosis (calcification of hyaline and fibrous cartilage). Many people with chondrocalcinosis, however, do not have CPPD. Other radiographic findings include subchondral cysts, joint space narrowing, and osteophyte formation.

Table 9-7

Synovial Fluid Analysis in Common Arthritides

FLUID SAMPLE	LEUKOCYTE COUNT (PER mL)	POLYMORPHONUCLEAR LEUKOCYTES (PERCENT)	CULTURE	CRYSTALS
Normal fluid	< 200	< 25	Negative	Negative
Osteoarthritis	100–2000	< 25	Negative	Negative
Gout	2000–60,000	40–75	Negative	Negatively birefringent crystals
Calcium pyrophosphate deposition disease	2000–60,000	40–75	Negative	Positively birefringent crystals
Rheumatoid arthritis	2000–60,000	45–75	Negative	Negative
Septic arthritis	80,000–100,000	75–100	Positive	Negative

SOURCE: Modified with permission from Swedberg JA: Osteoarthritis. In: Weiss BD (ed): *20 Common Problems in Primary Care.* New York: McGraw-Hill; 1999;300.

Table 9-8

Indications for Plain Radiographs in Patients with Joint Pain

> History of trauma
> Loss of joint function (e.g., inability to bear weight or decreased range of motion)
> Persistent joint pain despite conservative treatment
> Suspicion of a fracture or infection

SPECIAL IMAGING STUDIES

More expensive imaging studies, such as MRI, should be reserved for specific problems. MRI is excellent for assessing soft tissue such as rotator cuff tears or spinal cord or root compression. CT is particularly useful in assessing bony abnormalities.

Other Testing

When temporal arteritis is suspected, temporal artery biopsy should be performed. Tenderness over the temporal artery does not necessarily correlate with involvement of the artery. If the diagnosis is suspected, biopsy should be performed regardless of the absence of temporal artery tenderness.

Algorithm

A diagnostic algorithm for joint pain is shown in Figure 9-2. The first step in diagnosing the cause of the joint pain is to determine if the patient truly has a joint problem or a periarticular problem

Figure 9-1

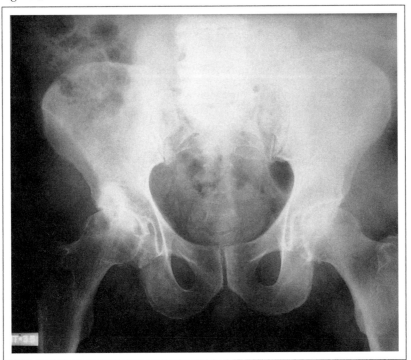

This radiograph of the hips shows the typical findings of osteoarthritis in the right hip including joint space narrowing, subchondral sclerosis, and cyst formation.

Figure 9-2

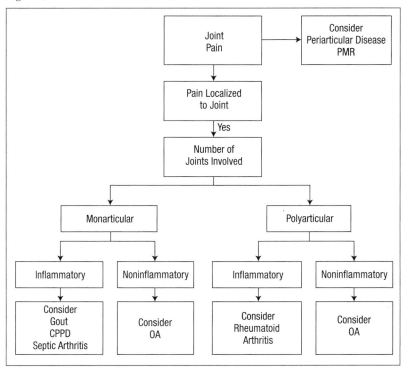

A diagnostic algorithm for joint pain.

such as bursitis, tendinitis, or PMR. The next key differentiating factors are the number of joints involved and the presence of inflammation. Predominately single joint involvement is a monarticular process, whereas multiple joint involvement is termed polyarticular. The presence of warmth, swelling, effusion, or erythema is indicative of inflammation or infection.

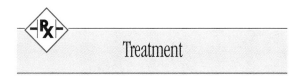

Treatment

Osteoarthritis

A multidisciplinary approach is required that uses both nonpharmacologic and pharmacologic treat-

ments. Surgical therapy also has a role in the treatment of osteoarthritis.

NONPHARMACOLOGIC TREATMENTS

Table 9-9 lists the nonpharmacologic treatments for osteoarthritis. Education is extremely valuable for the patient with osteoarthritis as well as other types of chronic arthritis. Several studies show the efficacy of educational and self-management programs. The benefits of these programs include improved ability to cope with illness, a general feeling of well-being, and decreased pain and disability.

Physical therapy is effective in maintaining good joint motion and muscle strength. Strengthening muscles decreases the amount of load across diseased joints as the weight is dispersed to the periarticular musculature. Physical modalities such as heat can be useful in pain management. Occupa-

Table 9-9

Nonpharmacologic Management of Osteoarthritis

EDUCATION
Education of patient and counseling to improve coping skills, management of stress, and understanding of the disease process Self-help information and resources
SOCIAL AND PSYCHOLOGICAL
Encouragement of social interaction (involvement in activities with family, friends, and community) Support groups Coordination of support services
EXERCISE
General conditioning with low-impact aerobic exercises, such as walking or aquatics Stretching and strengthening exercise for muscles around affected joints (isometric and/or isotonic exercises) Maintain range of motion and balance Treatment of coexisting diseases that might interfere with exercise ability
PHYSICAL MODALITIES
Application of heat: hydrotherapy, paraffin baths, short-wave or microwave diathermy, ultrasound Applications of ice (cold) for spasm or to limit swelling Use of transcutaneous electrical nerve stimulation, especially for lumbar spine, hip, or knee involvement
JOINT PROTECTION
Reduction of body weight to ideal weight Modified use of affected joint and development of strategies for daily activities Tailoring of level and length of activity to degree of symptoms with rest periods at regular intervals Use of walking aids, such as canes and walkers Splints, orthotics, and appropriate shoes: wedges or shoe inserts stress on the joint, cushioning of the soles to protect joints, nonslip soles to provide traction Use of assistive devices: grab bars, bath seats, mobile shower heads, dressing sticks, large tool grips, and utensil handles

SOURCE: Reprinted with permission from Swedberg JA: Osteoarthritis. In: Weiss BD (ed): *20 Common Problems in Primary Care*. New York: McGraw-Hill; 1999;302.

tional therapy can increase function by teaching the patient how to better perform activities of daily living (ADLs) and instrumental activities of daily living (IADLs).

The use of assistive devices also decreases pain by decreasing loading forces on affected joints by as much as 30 to 40 percent. Another load-reducing intervention is weight reduction. Excess weight places an additional stress on weight-bearing joints. Appropriate footwear and orthotic devices such as wedges can also decrease the stress on joints.

PHARMACOLOGIC TREATMENTS

A stepped approach to management of pain should be taken. Acetaminophen is the drug of first choice in the treatment of pain in patients with osteoarthritis. It is as effective as nonsteroidal anti-inflammatory drugs (NSAIDs) but has fewer gastrointestinal (GI) side effects. Doses up to 4000 mg/day can be used.

Topical analgesics (i.e., capsaicin or methylsalicylate cream) can be a useful adjuvant therapy for patients who receive minimal relief with analgesics or NSAIDs.

If there is no response to acetaminophen, then an NSAID can be added or used alone. NSAIDs act by inhibiting the production of prostaglandins. There are two forms of cyclooxygenase enzymes (COX-1 and COX-2) that are involved in prostaglandin production. COX-1 is primarily involved in the production of prostaglandins that protect the lining of the gastrointestinal tract, particularly the stomach, whereas COX-2 is primarily involved with joint inflammation. The older NSAIDs inhibit both COX-1 and COX-2. The new COX-2 inhibitors are more selective. COX-2 inhibitors can cause GI side effects, including dyspepsia and gastroduodenal ulcers, but at a lower rate than nonselective COX inhibitors.

NSAIDs, as a class of analgesic drugs, are of equal effectiveness. They do vary by their potential GI side effects. They have a minimal effect on platelets. NSAIDs inhibit prostaglandin-mediated dilation of renal blood vessels. Elderly patients with already compromised renal function are more susceptible to develop worsening renal function when taking NSAIDs. This potential adverse effect on renal function should be monitored. Although rare, they can also cause liver toxicity.

In patients with severe osteoarthritis who are not candidates for joint replacement, tramadol (ultram) 50 mg four times daily or an opioid analgesic can also be effective.

Patients with a joint effusion can benefit from arthrocentesis with removal of fluid and intra-articular steroid injection. This treatment is usually effective in relieving acute joint pain for up to 6 weeks. Intraarticular steroid injection can be repeated several times per year.

AVOIDING TOXIC EFFECTS OF NSAIDs Gastrointestinal hemorrhage and perforated ulcer resulting from an NSAID-induced ulcer can be a costly and potentially life-threatening event. There are three ways in which these side effects can be avoided. The clinician can avoid the use of NSAIDs. Acetaminophen with or without a topical analgesic agent is very effective in the treatment of the pain associated with osteoarthritis. A second strategy would be to use one of the new COX-2 inhibitors [celebrex], rofecoxib [vioxx] in patients who are at high risk for NSAID-induced ulcers (Table 9-10).

A third strategy is to prescribe a prophylactic agent in addition to the NSAID for patients who are at high risk for NSAID-induced ulcers. Misoprostol (200 μg four times daily) has been shown to be effective and is FDA approved for this indication. Although proton pump inhibitors (omeprazole, 20 mg daily) appear to also be effective, they are not FDA approved for this purpose. Misoprostol has been shown to be beneficial in the prevention of both gastric and duodenal ulcers. It may, however, induce adverse side effects such as diarrhea. H_2-receptor antagonists are not recommended.

Table 9-10

Risk Factors for NSAID-Induced Ulcers

Age > 60 years
Prior history of
Peptic ulcer disease
Gastrointestinal bleeding
High NSAID dose
Concurrent use of
Corticosteroids
Anticoagulants

SOURCE: Reproduced with permission from Lanza FL, Members of the Ad Hoc Committee on Practice Parameters of the American College of Gastroenterology: A guideline for the treatment and prevention of NSAID-induced ulcers. *Am J Gastroenterol* 93:2037, 1998.

SURGICAL TREATMENT

When medical management of osteoarthritis fails as evidenced by uncontrolled pain or increasing disability, the patient should be referred to an orthopedic surgeon for evaluation for joint replacement. Hip and knee replacements have been shown to decrease pain and improve patient function and quality of life. For osteoarthritis of the knee, arthroscopy with debridement of cartilage and washout of the joint space is an alternative to total knee replacement.

Periarticular Disease

The treatment of bursitis and tendinitis is similar. It includes rest, warm compresses, range-of-motion exercises, muscle-strengthening exercises, weight reduction on weight-bearing joints, and NSAIDs. Steroid injection into the affected area provides effective pain relief but should be done only by an experienced practitioner to avoid tendon rupture or other damage. If pain or difficulties with range of motion persists after 4 to 6 months of conservative therapy for RTC, then a rotator cuff tear should be ruled out by MRI. Patients with tears should be referred for surgical repair.

Polymyalgia Rheumatica

The aim of treating patients with PMR is to relieve troublesome symptoms and prevent vascular complications from an underlying vasculitis. The approach to treatment differs based on whether temporal arteritis is present.

PMR WITHOUT TEMPORAL ARTERITIS

Corticosteroids are the drugs of choice. Patients with PMR usually promptly improve symptomatically once treatment with low doses of prednisone is begun. Dramatic symptomatic relief is often noted within the first few days of therapy.

A prompt response to corticosteroids can be regarded as confirmation of the diagnosis. Failure of patients to improve clinically within days of beginning corticosteroids should strongly suggest alternative diagnoses. An initial dose of prednisone 10 to 15 mg may be sufficient to relieve the symptoms, although doses of 15 to 30 mg may be needed. The lowest dose necessary to control symptoms should be prescribed, and treatment should be continued only as long as absolutely necessary, due to the numerous adverse effects of corticosteroid therapy. Corticosteroids relieve the symptoms of PMR, but there is no evidence to suggest that they alter the course or duration of the disease.

The prednisone dose should be tapered using the patient's symptoms and the ESR as the guide. The majority of patients usually have to be treated for at least 1 year with either a daily or every other day dose of prednisone. In some patients, after 4 to 8 weeks, the prednisone can be switched to an NSAID if their symptoms completely resolve and the ESR normalizes.

Patients with PMR, but without temporal arteritis, should always be instructed to report symptoms associated with temporal arteritis such as headache or visual disturbance.

PMR WITH TEMPORAL ARTERITIS

Higher dosages of corticosteroids are necessary to treat patients with temporal arteritis (40 to 60 mg prednisone). Dose reduction requires careful monitoring of the patient's symptoms as well as ESR level, which should be assessed every 2 to 3 weeks. Once symptoms have resolved and the ESR has returned to normal, dose reductions below the level of 15 mg can be achieved. This is done in steps of 1 to 2.5 mg every 2 to 4 weeks, with close monitoring for recurrence of symptoms or a rising ESR. Once the dose has been reduced to 5 mg/day, a more gradual taper (decreasing doses by 1 mg/month) often is necessary to prevent symptom relapse. A maintenance dose of prednisone of 2.5 mg to 7.5 mg is usually reached within 6 to 12 months. The duration of treatment varies according to the patient. No laboratory test can predict when therapy should be discontinued. After a symptom-free period of 6 to 12 months with a normal ESR on a maintenance dose of 2.5 mg of prednisone, therapy can usually be discontinued.

RELAPSES

Relapses associated with new elevation of ESR are usually due to reducing the corticosteroid dose too quickly. Spontaneous disease exacerbations, however, also occur more frequently in the first 2 years, independent of the corticosteroid regimen. The prednisone dose should be temporarily increased, followed by reductions in smaller decrements at longer intervals, in these situations.

ADJUNCTIVE THERAPY

There is conflicting opinion regarding the use of methotrexate as a corticosteroid-sparing drug in the treatment of PMR. Also, methotrexate has its own adverse side effects and does not obviate the need for corticosteroids altogether. The use of methotrexate or other drugs is generally reserved for special circumstances such as the presence of severe comorbid conditions that are exacerbated by corticosteroid therapy.

Most patients achieve complete remission that is often maintained after withdrawal of treatment. Overall life expectancy among patients with PMR is essentially similar to the general population. It is important to note that corticosteroid-related side effects are a potentially dangerous complication of treatment of PMR.

Calcium Pyrophosphate Deposition Disease

The first line of therapy in treating CPDD is NSAIDs. Indomethacin is effective in controlling acute attacks. Oral colchicine, although not as effective as in acute gout, can be beneficial in acute attacks. Intraarticular steroids can also be beneficial in the acute phase or in recurrent attacks that do not respond to NSAID. As with other rheumatic diseases, if the disease is unresponsive to conservative therapy, and there is significant joint destruction, joint replacement should be considered.

Gout

The treatment of gout can be divided into treatment of the acute gouty attack and long-term treatment.

TREATMENT OF ACUTE GOUTY ARTHRITIS

The aim of therapy for an acute gouty arthritis is to alleviate pain. There are several therapies available for treating pain in gout including NSAIDs, colchicine, corticosteroids, and ACTH. Whichever medication is chosen, it should be started early and continued for at least 24 h after resolution of symptoms. NSAIDs are used most frequently to treat acute gout. As a class, they are equally effective.

Colchicine is also effective. The initial oral dose is 1.2 mg, followed by 0.6 mg every hour until the pain resolves (usually within 48 h) or unacceptable side effects (nausea, diarrhea) develop. The maximum daily dose is 6 mg/day dose. Colchicine's main effect is inhibition of phagocytosis of urate crystals by neutrophils. The drug can also be given intravenously, not to exceed a total dose of 4 mg/day and no more than 3 mg intravenously per dose. Although the drug is effective, its hematologic and CNS side effects have limited its use, especially in patients with renal insufficiency.

Glucocorticoids are effective in patients who do not respond to NSAIDs or colchicine. Prednisone is usually given at a dosage of 20 to 40 mg/day for 1 week and then tapered. Intraarticular steroid injections can also be beneficial but should be given only if a joint aspirate is sterile.

ACTH can also be used to treat gout, especially in polyarticular gout. It is administered as 40 to

80 IU intramuscularly and can be repeated every 6 to 12 h for several days. This method of administration is associated with fewer side effects.

Nonpharmacologic treatment includes short-term bed rest for 24 to 48 h, especially in patients who have lower extremity acute attacks. The use of warm compresses should be avoided in acute gouty arthritis as it appears to worsen the crystal-induced inflammation.

LONG-TERM TREATMENT

The long-term treatment of gout involves the normalization of hyperuricemia, thus preventing further gouty attacks. The treatment of hyperuricemia may also resolve tophi. There are two treatment options: inhibiting the synthesis of or increasing the excretion of urate. The goal of therapy is to achieve serum uric acid concentrations below 6.4 mg/dL, the level at which the extracellular fluid becomes saturated and deposition of urate crystals occurs.

Allopurinol is the drug of choice because of its effectiveness and ease of use. It should be used in patients with a history of nephrolithiasis or who are hyperexcretors of uric acid (> 800 mg/24 h). Allopurinol in doses of 100 to 200 mg per day is usually adequate to decrease uric acid levels to normal range. Allopurinol should be used in patients who excrete large amounts of uric acid in the urine daily because of a greater risk of urolithiasis.

Uricosuric medications (probenecid, sulfinpyrazone) can be used in patients who excrete low levels of uric acid in their urine and who have good renal function and no history of renal disease. These agents act by inhibiting uric acid resorption by the distal tubule, thus increasing the uric acid load in the urine. This action can cause probenecid-induced nephrolithiasis. These medications have minimal benefits in patients with creatinine clearance less than 50 mL/min. In patients whose hyperuricemia is difficult to control, combinations of allopurinol and probenecid can be used.

Rheumatoid Arthritis

There is no known cure for RA or any methods for its prevention. The treatment of RA arising de novo in the elderly is similar to that in younger patients. Optimal management includes early diagnosis and timely introduction of agents that reduce the probability of irreversible joint damage. Although the ultimate goal of treating RA is to induce a complete remission, this occurs only in rare cases. Complete remission is defined as the absence of (1) symptoms of active inflammatory joint pain (in contrast to mechanical joint pain); (2) morning stiffness; (3) fatigue; (4) synovitis on joint examination; (5) progression of radiographic damage on sequential radiographs; and (6) elevated erythrocyte sedimentation rate (ESR) or C-reactive protein (CRP) levels.

NONPHARMACOLOGIC TREATMENTS

Managed or coordinated multidisciplinary care through a team effort can be effective in the maintenance of function and productivity of patients with RA. The initial cornerstones of nonpharmacologic treatment are education and physical therapy. Patients with RA should be advised to perform regular stretching and strengthening exercises. Resistance training is known to improve strength, gait, and balance; help in the control of pain; and alleviate fatigue.

PHARMACOLOGIC TREATMENTS

INITIAL THERAPY   The initial drug treatment of RA commonly involves the use of nonsteroidal anti-inflammatory drugs (NSAIDs) with an aim to reduce joint pain and swelling and improve function. NSAIDs provide analgesic and anti-inflammatory effects, but do not alter the course of the disease. There are no significant differences in efficacy among the NSAIDs, although there are some differences in the incidence of side effects. Nonacetylated salicylates and ibuprofen have the lowest gastrointestinal (GI) complication risk and, therefore, should be preferred for initial use in elderly patients. The American College of Rheumatology NSAID monitoring guidelines recommends baseline tests (CBC, AST/ALT, creatinine) followed by an annual CBC (with additional AST/ ALT for diclofenac, and creatinine for concomitant ACE inhibitor or diuretic therapy).

GLUCOCORTICOIDS   Low-dose oral glucocorticoids (< 10 mg prednisone daily) and local injections of glucocorticoids are often highly effective in providing relief of symptoms in patients with active RA. They appear to slow the rate of joint damage. The adverse effects of long-term use of systemic glucocorticoids limit their use. Injecting one or few of the most involved joints early in the course of the disease can provide local and even systemic benefit. The same joint should not be injected more than once within a 3-month period.

Appropriate candidates for glucocorticoid therapy are patients with major functional disability due to active RA. Glucocorticoid therapy should not be used in patients with minimal disability or disease activity or in those with chronic disability due to destructive bone changes without active inflammation. Short-term use of low-dose oral glucocorticoids can also suppress disease activity and improve functional status during the initiation period of a disease-modifying antirheumatic drug.

DISEASE-MODIFYING ANTIRHEUMATIC DRUGS   All patients whose RA remains active despite adequate treatment with NSAIDs and those with erosive disease are candidates for more aggressive therapy. Disease-modifying antirheumatic drugs (DMARDs) are as effective in elderly patients as in younger patients, but the elderly are at increased risk of developing adverse effects. These drugs have the potential to reduce or prevent joint damage and preserve joint integrity and function. The most commonly used DMARDs are hydroxychloroquine (HCQ), sulfasalazine (SSZ), methotrexate (MTX), gold salts, D-penicillamine (DP), and azathioprine (AZA). The initiation of DMARD therapy should not be delayed for any patient with an established diagnosis who, in spite of adequate treatment with NSAIDs, has ongoing signs and symptoms of active RA.

There has been a recent trend toward the use of DMARDs early in the course of disease. This trend reflects the recognition of the acceleration of erosive changes in the first few years of disease. The main aim of DMARD use early in the course of the disease is to intervene before joints are destroyed. The DMARDs have a slow onset of action, and clinical benefit accrues over several months. These drugs appear to affect different inflammatory and immune pathways, thus making it possible to use drug combinations for an additive effect. Treatment must be sustained to maintain clinical efficacy.

SURGICAL TREATMENT

The surgical management of RA remains a critical option in the overall care of a disabled patient. Joint deformities that are permanent rather than temporary during regional inflammatory synovitis, and impair important functional goals, should be considered for surgical correction.

Septic Arthritis

Treatment of septic arthritis includes intravenous antibiotics and orthopedic referral for drainage of the involved joint. Antibiotic choice should be tailored to cover the common organisms (gram-positive cocci and gram-negative bacilli). Nafcillin or vancomycin, if methicillin-resistant *Staphylococcus aureus* is suspected, and an aminoglycoside (renal dose adjusted) may be started initially until a specific organism is identified.

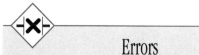

Errors

Failure to Differentiate Periarticular Disease from Other Causes of Joint Pain

Although many elderly patients attribute their musculoskeletal symptoms to arthritis, quite often these symptoms are related to diseases of the soft-tissue structures within and around the joints. Soft-tissue joint disease was detected in 18 percent of referrals to an arthritis clinic over a 26-month period.

Overuse of NSAIDs in the Treatment of Osteoarthritis

NSAIDs are overused by clinicians. Acetaminophen has been shown to be just as effective in controlling the pain of osteoarthritis. NSAIDs can cause serious renal and gastrointestinal side effects. Acetaminophen has minimal risk of toxicity and is also less expensive.

Failure to Consider the Diagnosis of Septic Arthritis in a Patient with Chronic Arthritis

Because of the presence of an underlying chronic arthritis, clinicians may fail to consider septic arthritis when there is exacerbation of arthritic symptoms. Septic arthritis should always be considered in a patient who experiences an acute flare of his or her arthritis. The presence of malaise, fever, or other systemic symptoms, or erythema in a single joint, can help the clinician differentiate a simple exacerbation from suspicion of a septic joint. If the symptoms of the exacerbation are atypical for that patient, septic arthritis should also be considered.

Patient Education

The benefits of education and self-management programs for patients with osteoarthritis and rheumatoid arthritis are well documented. The non-pharmacologic treatments for osteoarthritis (see Table 9-9) can be used in other arthritides, such as rheumatoid arthritis, and should be reviewed with patients. Where available, patients should be referred to self-management educational programs.

There are many excellent resources for patients (Table 9-11). The Arthritis Foundation has local chapters in many areas. They not only provide information and educational programs for patients and families but they also are advocates for public policies favorable to patients with arthritis.

Emerging Concepts

New Oral Treatments for Osteoarthritis

Oral glucosamine and chondroitin sulfate have received attention as chondroprotective agents. They have also been touted for their ability to improve cartilage and modify the progression of osteoarthritis. Their effectiveness has been shown in in vitro and animal experiments, but their clinical effectiveness is debated. Some small studies demonstrate a modest relief in pain. Large, well-

Table 9-11

Resources for Patients and Families

National Arthritis and Musculoskeletal and Skin Diseases Information Clearinghouse
  1 AMS Circle
  Bethesda, MD 20892
  301-495-4484
  www.nih.gov/niams

The Arthritis Foundation
  1330 West Peachtree Street
  Atlanta, GA 30309
  800-283-7800
  www.arthritis.org

The Arthritis Helpbook
  By Kate Lorig, RN, PhD and James F. Fries, MD
  Perseus, 1995

The American College of Rheumatology
  www.rheumatology.org

controlled randomized clinical trials are needed to demonstrate their role in the management of osteoarthritis.

New Treatments for Osteoarthritis of the Knee

The treatment of osteoarthritis has been limited to mainly analgesia and joint replacement surgery for patients with disabling pain or loss of function. Three new treatments have been studied with good short-term results.

AUTOGENOUS CARTILAGE IMPLANTATION

Autogenous cartilage implantation uses articular cartilage obtained arthroscopically. In an open procedure, cultured chondrocytes are injected in the focal areas of cartilage damage. Candidates for this procedure have focal areas of cartilage damage, ligamentous stability, and no other anatomic abnormalities. Several studies with 2 to 10 years of follow-up show as many as 90 percent of selected patients report an improvement. More long-term, randomized trials are needed before this procedure proliferates.

AUTOGENOUS OSTEOCHONDRAL GRAFTING

In autogenous osteochondral grafting, a core of bone and autogenous cartilage from another area of the distal femur are transferred into an articular defect. Limited studies show promising results; however, more long-term studies are needed before this procedure is used widely.

HYALURONIC ACID INJECTION

One of the deficits found in patients with osteoarthritis is decreased viscosity and elasticity of their synovial fluid. Visco-supplementation, or injection of the joint with hyaluronic acid, has been shown to restore the normal viscosity of the synovial fluid. Patients improve after injection, and individuals with mild disease show the most improvement. The injections can be repeated.

After injection, patients use less NSAIDs. Once again, more studies are needed.

New Treatments for Rheumatoid Arthritis

Many biologic products are under investigation for the treatment of RA. Several proinflammatory actions of tumor necrosis factor alpha (TNF-α) may contribute to its role in the pathogenesis of RA. A tumor necrosis factor antagonist is currently awaiting FDA approval for use in the treatment of RA.

Bibliography

American College of Rheumatology Ad Hoc Committee on Clinical Guidelines: guidelines for the management of rheumatoid arthritis. *Arthritis Rheum* 39:713, 1996.

Anderson RJ: Rheumatoid arthritis: B. clinical and laboratory features. In: Klippel JH (ed): *Primer on the Rheumatic Diseases*, 11th ed. Atlanta: Arthritis Foundation;1997:161.

Arnett FC, Edworthy SM, Bloch DA, et al: The American Rheumatism Association 1987 revised criteria for the classification of rheumatoid arthritis. *Arthritis Rheum* 31:3:315, 1988.

Baum J: Joint pain. *Postgrad Med* 85:311, 1989.

Bengtsson B: Polymyalgia rheumatica. In: Klippel JH (ed): *Primer on the Rheumatic Diseases*, 11th ed. Atlanta: Arthritis Foundation; 1997:305.

Block J, Schnitzer T: Therapeutic approaches to osteoarthritis. *Hosp Prac* Feb:159, 1997.

Bradley DJ, Brandt KD, Katz BP, et al: Comparison of an anti-inflammatory dose of ibubrofen, an analgesic dose of ibuprofen, and acetominophen in the treatment of patients with osteoarthritis of the knee. *N Engl J Med* 325:87, 1991.

Creamer P, Hockberg M: Osteoarthritis. *Lancet* 350:503, 1997.

Evans JM, Hunder GG: Polymyalgia rheumatica and giant cell arteritis. *Clin Geriatr Med* 14:455, 1998.

Freundlich B, Leventhal L: Signs and symptoms of musculoskeletal disorders: C. Diffuse pain syndromes. In: Klippel JH (ed): *Primer on the Rheumatic Diseases*, 11th ed. Atlanta: Arthritis Foundation; 1997:123.

Goronzy JJ, Weyand CM: Rheumatoid arthritis: A. Epidemiology, pathology, and pathogenesis. In: Klippel JH (ed): *Primer on the Rheumatic Diseases*, 11th ed. Atlanta: Arthritis Foundation; 1997:155.

Healey LA: Polymyalgia rheumatica and seronegative rheumatoid arthritis may be the same entity. *J Rheumatol* 19:270, 1992.

Hochberg MC, Altman RD, Brandt KD, et al: Guidelines for the medical management of osteoarthritis: Part I. Osteoarthritis of the hip. *Arthritis Rheum* 38:1535, 1995.

Hochberg MC, Altman RD, Brandt KD, et al: Guidelines for the medical management of osteoarthritis: Part II. Osteoarthritis of the knee. *Arthritis Rheum* 38:1541, 1995.

Holland NW, Gonzalez EB: Soft tissue problems in older adults. *Clin Geriatr Med* 14:601, 1998.

Koch M, Dezi A, Ferrarid F, et al: Prevention of nonsteroidal anti-inflammatory drug-induced gastrointestinal mucosal injury. *Arch Intern Med* 156:2321, 1996.

Lanza FL, Members of the Ad Hoc Committee on Practice Parameters of the American College of Gastroenterology: A guideline for the treatment and prevention of NSAID-induced ulcers. *Am J Gastroenterol* 93:2037, 1998.

LaPrade RF, Swiontkowski MF: New horizons in the treatment of osteoarthritis of the knee. *JAMA* 281:876, 1999.

Michet CJ, Evans JM, Fleming KC, et al: Common rheumatologic diseases in elderly patients. *Mayo Clin Proc* 70:1205, 1995.

Mishra N, Kammer G: Clinical expression of autoimmune diseases in older adults. *Clin Geriatr Med* 14:515, 1998.

National Center for Health Statistics: Current estimates from the National Health Interview Survey, 1989. *Vital and Health Statistics*, Series 10, No. 176. October, 1990.

Salvarani C, Macchioni P, Boiardi L: Polymyalgia rheumatica. *Lancet* 350:43, 1997.

Sewell KL: Rheumatoid arthritis in older adults. *Clin Geriatr Med* 14:475, 1998.

Sorenson LB, Blair JM: Rheumatologic diseases. In: Cassel CK, Cohen HJ, Larson EB, et al (eds): *Geriatric Medicine*, 3rd ed. New York: Springer-Verlag; 1997:449.

Superio-Cabuslay E, Ward MM, Lorig KR: Patient education interventions in osteoarthritis and rheumatoid arthritis: a meta-analytic comparison with nonsteroidal anti-inflammatory drug treatment. *Arthritis Care Res* 9:292, 1996.

Towheed TE, Anastassiades TP, Houpt J, et al: Glucosamine sulfate in osteoarthritis (Protocol for a Cochrane Review). In: The Cochrane Library, Issue 2, 1999. Oxford: Update Software.

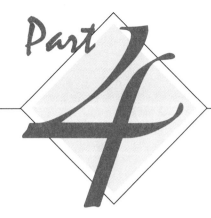

Part 4

Neuropsychiatric Problems

Patrick P. Coll

Chapter
10

Sleep Disorders

Overview: How Common Are Sleep Disorders Among Older Primary Care Patients?

From an economic perspective, unless you happen to be in the bedding business or produce and sell hypnotics, sleep is a complete waste of time. We spend almost one-third of our lives in a partly conscious state called *sleep* that is as yet a poorly understood phenomenon. Persons older than 90 years have slept for 30 years.

However wasteful sleep may appear to an economist, it is vital to our integrity as human beings, and such is the case for all complex life forms. Sleep is restorative and potentially as critical to survival as breathing and urination. Sleep deprivation increases daytime sleepiness and is implicated in many falls and accidents, which cause mortality and morbidity among elderly persons. Sleep-related respiratory disorders can have serious and potentially life-threatening pulmonary, neurologic, and cardiovascular sequelae, including hypertension, arrhythmias, and sudden death.

We sleep during most of our in utero existence and spend most of the first year of life asleep. Sometime during the first year of life most of us develop a circadian rhythm, sleeping somewhere between 6 and 8 h, usually during the night. Many patients, especially those who are older, report difficulties with sleep, usually insufficient sleep or difficulty falling or staying asleep. It is important for health care providers to understand the range of normal sleeping patterns, to appreciate changes in sleep with age, to be versed in how to obtain relevant information pertaining to sleeping difficulties, to know the common sleep and sleep-related pathologic conditions, and know how to effectively treat them.

Sleep disorders are common among all age groups but are particularly common among older patients. The Gallup Organization found in a 1995 survey that approximately 50 percent of Americans had ever had difficulty sleeping and 12 percent reported they had frequent difficulty sleeping. Older patients are more likely to report sleep disturbances, and women are more likely than men to report a sleep-related problem. In a large study of community-dwelling older men and women in Italy, investigators found a 36 percent prevalence of insomnia for men and 54 percent for women. Only 26 percent of men in the study and 21 percent of women reported no difficulty with sleeping. The same study found that persons who used hypnotic medications on a regular basis were more likely to report that they did not feel rested on wakening in the morning. Older persons are more likely to report difficulty getting to sleep, staying asleep, and finding sleep restorative. Family members are likely to report that the elder has difficulty maintaining daytime alertness. Numerous studies have shown that patients in institutional settings such as nursing homes and hospitals have a very high prevalence of sleep-related difficulties.

Sleep disorders are second only to the common cold as a reason for older persons to see a physician. As many as one-half of community-dwelling elderly persons use sleep medications, either over-the-counter or prescription. Persons older than 60 years are prescribed sedative-hypnotic agents almost twice as often as are persons between the ages of 40 and 59 years. Most patients in long-term care facilities are prescribed hypnotic medications at some stage during their stay. More than 60 percent of all persons older than 60 years snore during sleep. Evidence suggests a link between loud snoring and risk of cardiovascular disease and hypertension.

Younger persons with sleeping difficulties are more likely to miss work, receive a poor work performance evaluation, lose a job, and be involved in a motor vehicle accident. This may be as much related to associated conditions such as depression and anxiety as it is to lack of sleep. The image of an older person napping on a park bench or in a chair often is considered a phenomenon of aging and may be a cause of concern among patients, family, or nursing facility staff. It also, however, may be an indication of a sleep disorder worthy of further investigation.

Pathophysiology of Sleep

Normal Sleep

Although there is great individual variability in sleep patterns, in general the total sleep time for elderly persons is less than that of younger adults. Normal sleep architecture changes with the advance in years. The amount of sleep needed to stay alert during the day varies from person to person. On average, it is 8 h. Almost everyone tires early in the next day without the usual amount of sleep the previous night. Not only the duration but also the continuity of sleep is important. We feel more rested after 8 h of uninterrupted sleep than we do after 8 h with interruptions.

Normal sleep occurs in cycles ushered in by a short, presleep wake period. Then a number of cycles of non–rapid eye movement (NREM) sleep alternate with rapid eye movement (REM) sleep. NREM sleep is divided into four stages. The first two stages are light sleep, and the latter two stages are deep sleep. Uninterrupted, there are several cycles during the course of a night's sleep. REM sleep encompasses 20 percent of the total amount of sleep and is associated with dreaming and lability of heart rate, blood pressure, and respiration. REM sleep occurs at approximately 90-min cycles, the duration increasing throughout the night. Disruption of these cycles by periods of wakefulness leads to inadequate sleep.

Changes in Sleep with Age

Older persons frequently have slightly delayed onset sleep and frequent shifts in sleep stages. When examined in a sleep laboratory, older patients have less deep sleep, represented by less time spent in the deeper and more restorative stage 3 and stage 4 sleep. They also have less REM sleep. Older patients also tend to wake up more during the night because of age-associated physiologic processes and disease-related changes.

Recent sleep analysis suggests that, contrary to previous opinion, we do not need less sleep as we age. The amount of sleep needed may depend on how active the older person is during daytime hours. There does appear to be an increasing tendency for older persons to sleep less at night, to become somnolent late in the day or early evening, and to awaken early in the morning. This is called *advanced sleep phase syndrome*. Sleep latency testing also shows that older persons have shortened sleep latency during the day, which leads to occasional to frequent daytime napping. Other older persons have completely desynchronized sleep patterns and as a result are always asleep during the day and awake at night. Others still have irregular sleep–wake cycles and fragmented sleep and wakefulness. Daytime napping may compound the problem by reducing the urge for sleep at the conventional bedtime.

Principal Diagnoses

Although the physiologic features of normal sleep change with aging, sleep can be disrupted by many other factors. Table 10-1 lists the common causes of sleep disruption among older patients.

Medication Side Effects

Many elderly patients take multiple prescription and over-the-counter medications. Sleep disruption is a direct side effect of many medications. Commonly implicated medications include aminophylline, phenytoin, serotonin reuptake inhibitors, levodopa, and over-the-counter decongestants. Caffeine, nicotine, herbal remedies, and antihistamines can contribute to or exacerbate the sleep problems of elderly persons. Nightmares have been associated with the chronic use of quinidine, glucocorticoids, and some β-blockers. Withdrawal from sedative-hypnotic medications or alcohol can

Table 10-1

Common Sleep Disorders Among Older Persons

Medication side effects
Psychophysiologic insomnia
Advanced sleep phase syndrome
Nighttime wakening
Institutional insomnia
Dementia and depression
Nocturnal myoclonus
Sleep apnea
Sundowning
Jet lag
REM behavior disorder

dramatically alter sleep patterns. Patients taking sedating medications such as α-methyldopa, clonidine, and major tranquilizers may report daytime somnolence and difficulty sleeping at night. Medical conditions such as uremia, hypercalcemia, and hypothyroidism often are associated with a chronic state of lethargy that may manifest as a sleep-related problem.

Psychophysiologic Insomnia

As defined in International Classification of Sleep Disorders, psychophysiologic insomnia is "a disorder of somatized tension and learned sleeping prevention associations that result in a complaint of insomnia and associated decreased functioning during wakefulness." Patients report that they fall asleep easily although watching television or reading in the living room but begin to feel tension and anxiety when they go to bed. Most often the anxiety initially is related to external circumstances such as finances or family difficulties but becomes directed at the lack of sleep as wakefulness continues. Physical or mental stimulation, caffeine, or alcohol may exacerbate the problem. Psychophysiologic insomnia usually is of short duration; is situational, as after the death of a spouse or loved one; and responds well to short courses of treatment aimed at correcting the pre-

cipitating cause and eliminating exacerbating factors such as excessive alcohol or caffeine use.

Advanced Sleep Phase Syndrome

With age the circadian clock may advance so that rather than becoming sleepy at 10 or 11 P.M., older persons become sleepy earlier in the evening. As they become sleepy, these persons may retire at 8 P.M. and fall soundly asleep. Some of them may nap for an hour or more during the day. On awakening at 3:00 A.M., they wonder why they cannot stay asleep. A new diurnal pattern may thus become established.

Some older persons, especially if they live alone or have vision impairment, go to bed early, at least in part because of boredom. They also wake early in the morning and cannot get back to sleep. Alcohol consumption in the evening is initially sedating. As the alcohol is metabolized, however, a rebound state of hyperarousal occurs in the early hours of the morning and exacerbates this condition. These patients often come to the clinician looking for something to help them sleep through the night.

Nighttime Wakening

Pain, dyspnea, urinary frequency, reflux esophagitis, and other symptoms can interfere with normal sleep. The need to urinate is the most common cause of nighttime wakening among older patients. This is particularly common among older men with benign prostatic hyperplasia, but is also common among women. Patients with congestive heart failure may become dyspneic with recumbency or when sleeping. Recumbency causes mobilization of extravascular fluid and consequent dyspnea. Taking fluids, alcohol, diuretics, or caffeine late in the day exacerbates the problem. Older patients may wake spontaneously without needing to urinate because of decreased deep sleep cycles. Pain caused by arthritis and myoclonic muscle jerks or dyspnea caused by congestive heart failure or chronic obstructive pulmonary disease also can cause wakening episodes.

Institutional Insomnia

Many patients admitted to hospitals and skilled nursing homes have insomnia. This may be related to concerns regarding the illness, but is in large part related to the environment in which they are trying to sleep. Hospitals and nursing homes are noisy. Patients have to assume the schedule of the facility in terms of when they go to bed and when they arise. This may not match their usual diurnal rhythm. Residents of a facility may be left sitting in chairs without stimulation for hours on end, resulting in excessive daytime napping with resultant nighttime insomnia. They may have a roommate whose snoring, wakening, medical machinery, or watching of television keeps them awake. When they finally do get to sleep, a nurse checking their condition or an alarm may waken them. Many patients undergo surgical procedures tired and ill prepared because they had to be at the hospital at 6:00 A.M. the day of the operation and had to take an hour-long car trip to get there. Intensive care settings are among the most difficult places to get sufficient uninterrupted sleep. The effect on response to treatment and psychological well-being is almost certainly negative.

Dementia and Depression

DEMENTIA

Disturbances of sleep and sleep–wake rhythms are common among patients with dementia. Loss of sleep among caregivers because of the patient's nighttime insomnia and wandering is one of the primary reasons for the institutionalization of persons with dementia. Impaired sleep among patients with Alzheimer's disease is related at least in part to the disruption of neuronal pathways that initiate and maintain sleep. When patients with dementia are compared with those without dementia, more

disrupted sleep is found and more arousals occur. Even greater decreases in stages 3 and 4 NREM sleep are found when these patients undergo testing in sleep laboratories. For some patients with dementia, sleep may be less disturbed than for healthy age-matched controls.

The nucleus basalis of Meynert, a part of the brain particularly affected by Alzheimer's disease, has been demonstrated in animal experiments to have a sleep-regulating function. The aforementioned factors related to institutionalization may further contribute to sleep disturbances among patients with dementia.

DEPRESSION

Depression is associated with frequent arousals and early-morning awakening that may exacerbate already disrupted age-related sleep patterns. Depressive symptoms (dysthymia) are common among older persons and occur because of the greater likelihood of physical impairment, loss of loved ones, and the need to live in more restricted living arrangements because of increased frailty. Patients with depression and dysthymia have characteristic sleep encephalograms (EEGs)—delayed sleep onset, prolonged first REM period, decreases in NREM (slow-wave sleep), frequent arousals, and early-morning awakening. There is some evidence that EEG patterns of patients revert toward normal with treatment and that this may be a useful way to monitor the effectiveness of therapy.

Patients with a recent loss are at risk of insomnia. Bereavement is associated with a strong likelihood of sleep disturbance, which may become persistent.

Nocturnal Myoclonus

Nocturnal myoclonus, also called *periodic limb movement disorder,* is characterized by repetitive, stereotypical, periodic jerking movements of the limbs that occur at regular intervals during a night's sleep. These movements typically involve hip flexion, knee flexion, and foot extension. Partners may report being kicked during the night and commonly the bedclothes are in disarray by morning.

Nocturnal myoclonus is a primary disorder of sleep and is of unknown causation. It has been described in association with sleep apnea syndrome, uremia, and chronic arthritis. The incidence increases with age, and there may be a familial association. Nocturnal myoclonus occurs most commonly during light NREM sleep and is frequently associated with arousal. Symptoms are variable and can be debilitating, yet habituation is common. Studies conducted in sleep laboratories have indicated that as many as 40 percent of patients older than 65 years experience nocturnal myoclonus at least some of the time. A much smaller percentage of persons ever report insomnia resulting from jerking limb movements. This suggests that different persons have different propensities to arousal from nocturnal myoclonus.

Nocturnal myoclonus is related to the restless leg syndrome. Restless leg syndrome is characterized by intense discomfort in the legs that occurs when the person is at rest and most often in the evening. Patients feel discomfort and a desire to move around. Restless leg syndrome may impair the onset of sleep. Aggravating factors for both conditions include use of antihistamines, caffeine, anemia, diuretics, and antidepressants. Both nocturnal myoclonus and restless leg syndrome are associated with sleep apnea.

Sleep Apnea

Sleep apnea is defined as five apneic or ten hypopneic and apneic episodes per hour of sleep. Patients with sleep apnea may have hundreds of these episodes per night. An apneic episode is cessation of nasobuccal airflow for at least 10 s. A hypopneic episode is at least a 50 percent reduction in flow for the same period. This frequently causes repeated episodes of arousal to which the person is oblivious, but it can cause awakening. Episodes of apnea or hypopnea are punctuated by stuttered gasps for breath. The patient may report insomnia but is more likely to recognize excessive daytime somnolence that impairs performance

and can have serious consequences. Daytime somnolence often is associated with accident-prone behavior and, occasionally, forgetfulness.

Intermittent nighttime snoring, particularly when the patient is supine, is characteristic. The snoring often is sufficient to wake both bed partner and snorer. In the context of unexplained right-sided heart failure, arrhythmias, hypertension, or bradycardia, sleep-related respiratory disorders should be considered. Hypnotic medications, especially benzodiazepines, may worsen sleep apnea and should be avoided by patients known or believed to have sleep apnea.

Sleep apnea is divided into central apnea, caused by a central nervous system disorder (reduction in central respiratory drive), and obstructive apnea, caused by obstruction of the airflow tract (partial occlusion of the upper respiratory tract). Risk factors of sleep apnea include male sex, obesity, hypothyroidism, chronic obstructive pulmonary disease, and certain neurodegenerative disorders (Shy-Drager syndrome, seizure disorders) and cardiovascular diseases.

The number of apneic and hypopneic episodes increases with age. As many as 75 percent of elderly persons may have more than 10 apneic or hypopneic episodes per hour. Most cases of sleep apnea among older patients are caused by an obstruction of the airway.

Sundowning

A disruptive reversal of the sleep–wake cycle may occur among patients who have acute or chronic organic brain dysfunction. This is commonly called *sundowning* or *sundown syndrome*. Although used frequently, the term is not well described. *Sundowning* is the term generally ascribed to patients with dementia who are somnolent during the day and become increasingly alert and agitated in the early evening and early night. The term is used more often to describe patients who live in institutions than those who reside in their own homes. The patient may exhibit fear of being left alone or be restless and feel the need to pace. Recently institutionalized patients with dementia may become verbally demanding and abusive, refuse care, pull out intravenous lines, or sleep during the day.

Jet Lag

Many older persons travel on a regular basis. Travel across more than two or three time zones, especially going east, causes jet lag among most persons. It is a wonderful example of how our circadian sleep pattern is entrained by light. After traveling east over several time zones, the traveler begins to feel sleepy at the usual bedtime in the home time zone. This makes it difficult to sleep in the evening and difficult to wake up in the morning in the new time zone. Adjustment to a diurnal rhythm more in step with the new time zone can take several days.

REM Behavior Disorder

REM behavior disorder is a rare condition characterized by intense muscular activity during REM sleep when normally somatic muscle activity is largely paralyzed. This disorder is caused by disinhibition of the normal paralysis of muscle during REM sleep. In contrast, narcolepsy and cataplexy (usually a disorder affecting younger persons) are characterized by sudden onset of REM activity that causes sudden paralysis and loss of muscle tone. Patients with REM behavior disorder dream and at the same time experience excessive muscle activity, often thrashing about the bed.

Typical Presentation

Patients with sleep-related difficulties have various symptoms. They may report excessive tiredness during the day, frequent waking during the night, early waking, or inability getting to sleep. Excessive tiredness during the day may be associated with sleep apnea, which is a potentially dangerous and life-threatening condition. Difficulty getting to sleep may be caused by psychophysiologic insomnia or excessive use of stimulants late in the day. Nighttime wakening may be caused by pain, nocturia, or periodic leg movements. Early wakening is common in advanced phase sleep syndrome, excessive sleeping during the day, and depression.

Health care providers should inquire about insomnia or other sleeping difficulties during routine clinical evaluations. If the patient is unable to give a good history, caregivers and family should be asked to provide information. If a problem is identified, additional detail is required. Important questions to pose to the patient are listed in Table 10-2. Medications that should be discussed because of their potential effect on sleep are diuretics, decongestants, asthma medication, and those containing caffeine, which include many over-the-counter cold medications.

It may be useful to have the patient complete a 2-week sleep–wake diary to chronicle sleep and wake-time symptoms, perceptions of sleepiness, and the quality and quantity of sleep. The diary should include the time the patient goes to bed, time it takes to fall asleep, number of episodes of wakening and duration of each, estimated total time asleep, number and duration of daytime naps, and how refreshed the patient generally feels during the day. It is important to have a partner corroborate the diary perceptions, because it is common for patients to over- and underestimate the length of time asleep and the quality of sleep.

Physical Examination

Findings at physical examination usually are nonspecific. Morbid obesity, however, should alert the physician to the possibility of obstructive sleep apnea. Physical signs of congestive heart failure and chronic obstructive pulmonary disease also may suggest that a sleep-related respiratory disorder should be considered. It is important to

Table 10-2

Important Questions to Explore with Patients with Insomnia

How long has there been a problem?
Does insomnia come and go, or is it chronic?
Which of the following do you have difficulty with: getting to sleep, staying asleep, awakening early, or
    waking up several times at night?
How long does it generally take you to get to sleep, and how often and how long are you awake during
    the night?
Is the insomnia associated with pain, nocturia, or leg spasms?
Do you snore, or does your partner tell you that you snore?
Do you consume caffeinated beverages or alcohol during the evening or at night?
Which prescription or over-the-counter medications do you take?
Do you exercise late in the evening?
Is your difficulty with sleep associated with worrying or anxiety?
Do you spend a lot of time in bed reading or watching television before trying to go to sleep?
Do you nap during the day, and if so, for how long ?

look for signs and symptoms of arthritis, congestive heart failure, incontinence, and other painful conditions that may cause symptoms that interfere with sleep. An evaluation for depression and for cognitive dysfunction should be included in the evaluation of all older patients with sleep-related difficulties. Few other findings at physical examination direct the clinician in the diagnosis of insomnia.

Ancillary Tests

There is no routine set of laboratory tests to perform for patients with insomnia. All patients should undergo testing for a metabolic cause of sleepiness. At a minimum this should include thyroid function studies, liver function studies, and measurement of serum calcium, hemoglobin, urea, creatinine, and if indicated, blood levels of medications.

Referral to a sleep laboratory is indicated if the cause of a persistent sleep disorder is unclear from the history, examination, and review of the sleep diary. Other indications for referral include suspicion of a serious sleep-related respiratory disorder and evaluation for sleep-related myoclonus or persistent insomnia. The effect of interventions such as continuous positive airway pressure (CPAP) also can be tested in a sleep laboratory.

The patient usually spends 1 or 2 days at the sleep center. A complete history interview, physical examination, neuropsychological testing, and laboratory studies are conducted, and 1 or 2 nights of sleep are observed and monitored. Sleep latency, total sleep time, awakenings, and phase shifts in sleep are measured. Continuous EEG monitoring of sleep–wake uroelectric activity is performed. Other monitoring includes pulse oximetry, tibialis anterior electromyography, external oculography, penile strain-gauge monitoring, continuous electrocardiography, blood pressure, and temperature. If indicated, as often is the case among older persons, continuous measurement of esophageal pH and manometric studies of the upper airways can be performed.

Algorithm

Figure 10-1 shows an algorithm for the evaluation of the major causes of insomnia. The first decision point is consideration of the diagnosis of sleep apnea. If the diagnosis of sleep apnea is considered, the patient should be referred for a sleep study. If the diagnosis of sleep apnea is not considered or ruled out with a sleep study, the patient should be asked to keep a sleep diary. If the patient documents sufficient duration of sleep, the diagnosis of advanced sleep phase syndrome should be considered. If not, the algorithm guides the clinician through the most common causes of sleep interruption, such as pain, heartburn, nocturia, anxiety, depression, and dementia.

Treatment

General Measures

Because many factors influence the normal sleep–wake cycle among older adults, the approach to treating older persons with sleep symptoms must be highly individualized. All patients should be informed that there is no absolute ideal number of hours for normal sleep. Someone who sleeps an hour during the day and goes to sleep early in the evening only to wake in the middle of the night should not be given a prescription for a hypnotic medication to help get back to sleep. This person is probably getting a sufficient amount of sleep.

SLEEP HABITS

The patient or staff should be instructed in good sleep habits or nonpharmacologic approaches to insomnia (Table 10-3). Unless planning to have sex

Table 10-3

Nonpharmacologic Approaches to Insomnia

Create an appropriate environment for sleep (minimize noise, appropriate lighting and heat).
Avoid stimulants (alcohol, caffeine, exercise) late in the day.
Avoid spending time in bed reading or watching television.
Perform relaxation techniques.
Drink a small amount of warm milk before bedtime.
Exercise during the day.

or go to sleep, the patient should not go to bed. Patients with insomnia should be discouraged from spending a large amount of time reading or watching television in bed. This is as true for seniors in institutions as it is for those who live at home.

SLEEP ENVIRONMENT

It is important to create an environment that is conducive to sleep. Noise should be reduced to a minimum, and temperature and lighting should be appropriate for sleep. Many institutional environments are not conducive to sleep because of excessive noise, lighting, and temperatures that are too warm or cold. Daytime activity and regular exercise should be encouraged. Stimulants such as caffeine and nicotine should not be consumed before sleep. If possible, diuretics should be taken many hours before bedtime.

Time spent in bed during the night should be kept to 7 to 8 h, and daytime naps to less than 1 h. Patients with a circadian rhythm disorder or whose sleep–wake cycle is out of phase with the environment may benefit from modification of the environment to enhance external cues. This includes regular daytime scheduling of meals, exercise, and administration of medications together and a reduction of nocturnal stimulation.

Figure 10-1

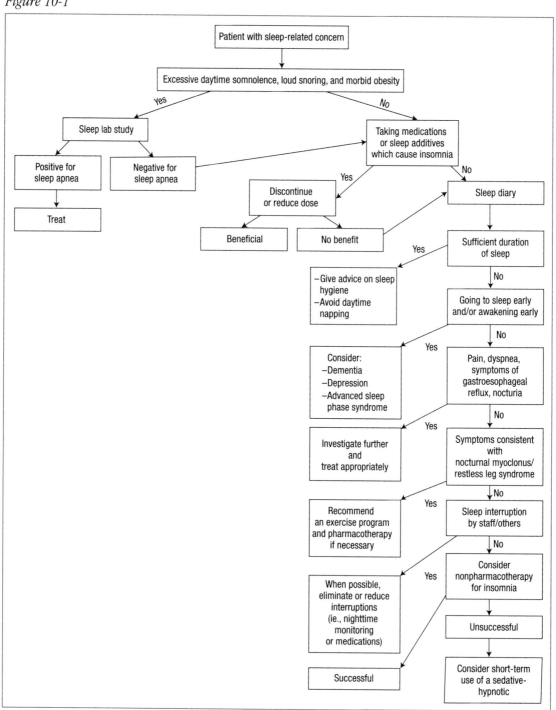

Algorithm.

RESPONSE TO INSOMNIA

Patients unable to get to sleep after 30 min should be counseled to get out of bed and go to another room. Once they feel sleepy, they should go back to bed. It is unreasonable to expect to go to sleep at 8 P.M. and sleep past 4 A.M. One can partly alleviate advanced sleep phase syndrome by making a concerted effort to go to bed later. Bright light therapy late in the day has been described as an effective therapy for advanced sleep phase syndrome among some patients.

RELAXATION TECHNIQUES

Relaxation techniques may be helpful for persons with psychophysiologic insomnia. It should be recommended that the patient not focus on thoughts that cause them worry or anxiety. Thoughts should focus on pleasant images or a simple object. Muscle relaxation may be helpful. Patients should be instructed to first tense all the muscles in the body and beginning with their feet consciously relax the main muscle groups moving toward the head and neck. A gentle massage by a bed partner or staff member may help. Soothing music may help some but distract others. A nonpharmacologic sleep protocol tested at a university teaching hospital demonstrated a 23 percent reduction in the use of sedative-hypnotic medication among older patients. The interventions used included a drink of warm milk, a gentle massage, and soothing music.

Pharmacologic Treatment

SEDATIVE-HYPNOTIC AGENTS

Elderly patients account for 12 percent of the population yet use 40 percent of all sedative-hypnotic medications prescribed despite there being little evidence that long-term or repeated dosing of hypnotics is beneficial. Sedative-hypnotics are appropriate only for the short-term management of insomnia. This is especially true in the care of older patients, who are at higher risk of drug-related complications, including drug tolerance, dependence, drug-drug and drug-disease interactions, hangover effects, and severe withdrawal effects than are younger persons. Benzodiazepines with long half-lives, such as flurazepam and diazepam, are likely to worsen undiagnosed sleep apnea syndrome and sleep problems caused by depression. There is evidence that regular use of long-acting sedative-hypnotic medications is associated with adverse daytime effects, such as impaired cognition, increased risk of injurious falls, and impaired psychomotor functioning. Chronic use of benzodiazepines may cause habituation, loss of efficacy, tolerance, and drug-induced insomnia. Short-acting agents may cause rebound insomnia, impaired psychomotor performance, and unusual behavioral effects.

Medications to be avoided in the treatment of persons with insomnia are listed in Table 10-4. In addition to the aforementioned sedative-hypnotics, several other medications should be avoided. Chloral hydrate (Noctec) has been used for many years to treat patients with insomnia. It is rapidly metabolized to its active form, trichloroethanol. The potential for gastrointestinal side effects, interaction with protein-bound medications, and morning hangover among some patients suggests that this agent be avoided by older patients. Antihistamines should be avoided in the management of insomnia, especially among older men, because of their anticholinergic effects and the potential for causing urinary retention, postural hypotension, and confusion.

Table 10-4

Medications to Avoid in the Treatment of Older Patients with Insomnia

Alprazolam (Xanax)
Chloral hydrate (Noctec)
Diazepam (Valium)
Diphenhydramine hydrochloride (Benadryl)
Flurazepam (Dalmane)

Physicians often are under considerable pressure from patients, family members, and other health care providers to prescribe hypnotic medications. It is almost always simpler and frequently tempting to reach for a prescription pad and meet the request. At least a brief sleep history should be taken and an attempt at nonpharmacologic therapy made first. It is important to avoid routine prescription of or standing orders for hypnotic agents, as was commonly the practice for all hospitalized patients and many nursing home residents a short time ago.

Hypnotic medications should be prescribed in the smallest possible dose for a short period of time (Table 10-5). Chronic use of hypnotic medications should be strongly discouraged. Zolpidem tartrate (Ambien) 5 mg should be considered as a first pharmacologic agent, increasing to a maximum dose of 10 mg if necessary. Zolpidem is a hypnotic agent with a chemical structure unrelated to that of benzodiazepines, barbiturates, or any other drugs with known hypnotic effects. It acts on a γ-aminobutyric acid–benzodiazepine complex and shares some of the pharmacologic effects of benzodiazepines. It does not, however, cause muscle relaxation or have an antiseizure effect. Zolpidem is less likely than benzodiazepines to contribute to amnesia and appears to be generally well tolerated by older patients. Tolerance and dependency may potentially occur.

Benzodiazepines can cause toxicity, tolerance, and physical and psychological dependency, especially among elderly patients. Dosing should be initiated at the lowest possible potential effective dose and slowly increased, if tolerated. It is preferable to use an agent that is short acting, such as temazepam (Restoril). Temazepam is slowly absorbed and should be taken about 30 min before bedtime. A reasonable starting dose for elderly patients is 7.5 mg, but the dose can be increased to 15 or 30 mg if tolerated. Diazepam (Valium) and flurazepam (Dalmane) should be avoided by older patients because of a long half-life (48 and 72 h, respectively). Alprazolam (Xanax) is not recommended as a hypnotic because of the likelihood of dependency, tolerance, and risk of withdrawal among older persons. Triazolam (Halcion) can be considered, but both triazolam and alprazolam have been reported to induce transient global amnesia.

Other medications that may be considered are sedating antidepressants, such as nortriptyline (Pamelor), doxepin (Adapin, Sinequan), and trazodone (Desyrel), especially if the patient has depression.

Management of Specific Conditions

MEDICATION SIDE EFFECTS

Whenever possible, the clinician should attempt to reduce or discontinue medications believed to cause or contribute to insomnia. The clinician also should consider the potential effects of over-the-counter medications, such as decongestants, and caffeine-containing foods and beverages.

Table 10-5

Hypnotics to Consider in Treating Older Patients with Insomnia

GENERIC NAME	TRADE NAME	DOSE RANGE (mg)
Doxepin	Adapin, Sinequan	10–50
Nortriptyline	Pamelor	10–50
Temazepam	Restoril	7.5–30
Trazadone	Desyrel	50–100
Triazolam	Halcion	0.125–0.25
Zolpidem tartrate	Ambien	5–10

PSYCHOPHYSIOLOGIC INSOMNIA

The patient should be instructed in relaxation techniques (see earlier). Many patients with psychophysiologic insomnia use benzodiazepines for relief of the anxiety that contributes to insomnia. It is often difficult to persuade these patients to replace the anxiolytic medication with a relaxation exercise, but the attempt should be made.

ADVANCED SLEEP PHASE SYNDROME

Advanced sleep phase syndrome is a challenging condition to manage. It may help to keep the patient stimulated late in the day with exercise or other forms of recreation, such as a card game. A small amount of caffeine may help, but may have the undesired effect of preventing sleep when it is more appropriate to do so. Bright light therapy, which has been reported to ameliorate seasonal affective disorder, also may be helpful. A variety of light sources are available with a light intensity equivalent to a bright sunny day. The lights are turned on early in the evening and left on for 1 to 2 h. A light with no ultraviolet radiation is recommended.

NIGHTTIME WAKENING

The clinician needs to address the cause of the nighttime wakening. If the cause is nocturia, the patient may try reducing fluid intake late in the day. Reducing or eliminating alcohol also may decrease nocturia. Therapy for congestive heart failure also may decrease the frequency of nighttime wakening due to nocturia. If benign prostatic hyperplasia is present, therapy for the disease may reduce the frequency of nocturia (see Chap. 7). If nighttime wakening is due to pain, an analgesic may be taken at bedtime.

INSTITUTIONAL INSOMNIA

Hospitals, nursing homes, and residential care facilities need to institute policies to help patients and residents achieve satisfactory sleep. Unless absolutely necessary, the patient should not be wakened during the night for administration of medication or recording of vital signs. Nighttime noise from staff or equipment should be minimized. The use of heavy drapes or window blinds can reduce outside light, which may impair sleep. Patients should be kept stimulated during the day, especially if they are napping frequently. Nonpharmacologic interventions, such as a warm glass of milk or a massage late in the evening, have been shown to be effective in the management of institutional insomnia.

DEMENTIA AND DEPRESSION

If insomnia is associated with depression, the clinician needs to address the underlying depression (see Chap. 11). A sedating antidepressant, such as trazodone, may relieve the insomnia. Trazodone has a small risk of inducing priapism. Many patients with dementia experience insomnia due to increased agitation at night. This may be reduced with an evening dose of an anxiolytic medication or risperidone (see Chap. 12).

NOCTURNAL MYOCLONUS (RESTLESS LEG SYNDROME)

Low-dose levodopa combined with carbidopa (Sinemet) has been used successfully to treat some patients with nocturnal myoclonus. Carbidopa-levodopa (25/100-mg formulation) may be started in a dose of one-half tablet before bedtime. The dose can be increased in increments of one-half tablet every 3 or 4 days to a maximum of two tablets per day.

Pergolide starting at doses of 0.05 mg and gradually increasing to 0.5 mg has been used successfully in the management of restless leg syndrome and periodic limb movement disorder. Other drugs that have been tried in the management of restless leg syndrome include bromocriptine, carbamazepine, and clonazepam. The Restless Leg Syndrome Foundation has a Web site that provides useful information (http://www.rls.org).

SLEEP APNEA

There are specific effective therapies for moderate to severe sleep apnea syndrome. Decisions about intervening should be made only after evaluation at a sleep referral center. Weight loss can be helpful.

Definitive therapy for sleep apnea usually involves CPAP during sleep. It is accomplished by means of having the patient wear a tight-fitting nasal mask. A variety of masks and a variety of adaptive devices are available for the tubing to make this therapy less of an inconvenience during sleep. Humidification and warming of air administered with CPAP can reduce nasal drying and irritation. Some CPAP machines have an automatic setting. These machines deliver a higher pressure only when there is a reduction in air flow. The patient can get to sleep without the irritation of high-pressure CPAP. The average monthly rental fee for the equipment needed to deliver CPAP is $200. Surgical interventions, such as widening the upper airway, often eliminate snoring. The procedure may ameliorate apnea and improve daytime alertness and functioning Medroxyprogesterone and protriptyline may benefit some persons with sleep apnea.

SUNDOWNING

Sundowning is frequently associated with delirium. If a reversible cause of delirium is suspected, it should be sought and the patient treated. Inouye et al reduced the incidence of delirium among older hospitalized patients using a variety of interventions, including interventions to promote healthy sleeping. Keeping patients active during the day and preventing daytime napping also may help reduce sundowning episodes and insomnia associated with dementia. Sedative medications given late in the day may cause paradoxical arousal and should be suspected as a contributing factor in sundowning and insomnia associated with dementia.

JET LAG

There are many suggestions to minimize the effects of and disruption caused by jet lag. Trav-elers going east over several time zones should avoid alcohol, caffeine, and a heavy meal. If traveling at night they should try to sleep but avoid taking hypnotics. On arrival, if it is early in the morning, rather than going to sleep immediately, travelers should consider taking some exercise and spending as much time as possible outside during daylight hours. Most travelers do not have access to bright light therapy, which has been shown to be of benefit in decreasing the effects of jet lag.

REM SLEEP DISORDERS

Patients with REM behavior disorders may be effectively treated with long-acting benzodiazepines, such as clonazepam.

Controversies

Melatonin

Melatonin is secreted by the pineal gland at night and may be important in the regulation of sleep. Melatonin secretion has been demonstrated to decrease with age. Many patients take melatonin (in doses up to 3 mg) to help them sleep, and there is clinical evidence to suggest that it can be an effective hypnotic for some patients. Improved induction, maintenance, and quality of sleep have been reported among older patients. One study of mice showed that regular nightly use of melatonin increased life span. Melatonin, including slow-release forms, is available in most health food stores.

Sedative-Hypnotics

All hypnotics are approved only for short-term use, yet many patients have chronic and persistent insomnia. Where and when possible, non-pharmacologic means should be used to manage insomnia. Some patients, however, respond well to the use of hypnotics. As long as nonpharmacologic means of treatment have been exhausted, it is not unreasonable to continue use of these agents. The effectiveness of continued use of hypnotic medications should be reevaluated on a regular basis. It is important, however, to continue to monitor the patient for adverse effects of the use of the medication and to suggest that use be kept to an absolute minimum.

Sleep Studies

Most patients with insomnia do not need a sleep study. Sleep studies are time consuming and expensive and should be reserved for patients who may have sleep apnea, narcolepsy, or insomnia resistant to standard forms of therapy. Other potential indications for ordering sleep studies are monitoring the effectiveness of pharmacologic interventions or CPAP and progression of sleep apnea syndrome.

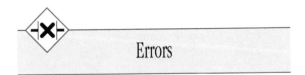

Errors

The most common error in the management of insomnia is excessive use of sedative-hypnotics. This includes the use of routine as needed (prn) orders for administration of hypnotics to hospitalized patients and nursing home residents. Federal regulations require that ongoing use of sedative-hypnotics in nursing homes be monitored. In the outpatient setting, clinicians should be vigilant about prescribing sedative-hypnotics on an as needed basis or continually refilling these medications without monitoring effectiveness.

Another common error is inappropriate use of long-acting hypnotics to treat older patients. These medications have a long half-life because of age-related changes in pharmacokinetic properties. This can cause morning drowsiness and may be a factor in a large number of falls and accidents.

Antihistamines often are prescribed as hypnotics for older patients when these agents should be avoided because of their propensity to cause confusion and urinary retention.

Not Taking a Sleep History

A common error is not to ask an older patient about sleep-related problems. Clinicians and patients may believe that what they are experiencing is a normal part of aging. Patients may believe that the clinician has little to offer in terms of treatment, especially if they want to avoid the use of hypnotics. It is therefore important for clinicians to ask older patients routinely whether they are having difficulty sleeping.

Failure to Diagnose Sleep Apnea

A common error is failure to consider or miss the diagnosis of sleep apnea. The potential consequences of failing to diagnose sleep apnea syndrome may be devastating. A patient does not have to be obese to have sleep apnea. Snoring is so prevalent that this symptom may be ignored if a patient has insomnia or excessive daytime somnolence. If the clinician has any suspicion that sleep apnea is present, the patient should be referred for a sleep study.

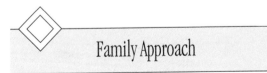

Family Approach

Involving family members early in the management of insomnia is important. It may be a family member who raises the problem to begin with. Some family members have an impression that there is a problem with insomnia when the patient has no perceived difficulty in this regard. Other family members need to be convinced that there is not a problem and that the issue being raised is within the realm of normality. A spouse may be of great assistance in helping a patient comply with suggested relaxation treatments and may be able to provide a relaxing massage at night to help the patient get to sleep.

Insomnia can be a family problem, particularly for patients with dementia. Loss of sleep for a primary caregiver compromises the ability to cope with a loved one during the day. This may be a predisposing factor for premature institutionalization. A family member's input and assistance are essential if a hypnotic medication is prescribed for a community-living patient with marked memory impairment. Patients who take a hypnotic agent before going to bed may wake in the middle of the night, forget they have already taken a pill, and take another. This problem is more likely to occur among patients with memory impairment. A spouse or family member can secure the medication so that it is not used inappropriately.

Patient Education

Patients should be educated about good sleep hygiene. Tables 10-6 and 10-7 list things to do and avoid to help someone get a good night's sleep. These tables may be used as patient handouts. Table 10-8 lists several resources for patients with sleep difficulties.

Emerging Concepts

The standard test for the diagnosis of sleep apnea is an overnight study. This can be costly in terms of both money and time. Many patients find the experience difficult. Other methods are being examined, including partial night or daytime studies, use of portable sleep-monitoring devices that could be used in the home, focused questionnaires, mea-

surements of neck circumference, endoscopic measurements of the nasopharynx, and imaging studies (plain radiography, magnetic resonance imaging, computed tomography) of the head and neck, the result of which could be predictive of sleep apnea. These methods could lead to less expensive, faster, and more accurate diagnosis of sleep apnea.

Table 10-6

Things to Do to Get a Better Night's Sleep

Go to bed at the same time each day.
Get up at the same time each day.
Get regular exercise each day.
Keep the temperature in your bedroom
    comfortable.
Keep the bedroom quiet when sleeping.
Keep the bedroom dark when sleeping.
Use your bed only for sleep and sex.
Take medicines only as directed.
When you go to bed, relax your muscles,
    beginning with your feet and working your
    way up to your head.

Table 10-7

Ways to Avoid Worsening Insomnia

Don't exercise before going to bed.
Don't engage in stimulating activity before bed.
Avoid caffeine, especially late in the day.
Don't read or watch television in bed.
Don't use alcohol to help you sleep.
Don't take another person's sleeping pills.
Don't lie in bed awake for more than half an
    hour. Get up and perform quiet activity, and
    return to bed when you are sleepy. Do this as
    many times a night as you need to.

Table 10-8
Sources of Information on Sleep Disorders

American Sleep Disorders Association 6301 Bandel Rd, Suite 101 Rochester, MN 55901 *http//www.asda.org* National Center on Sleep Disorders Research Two Rockledge Center, Suite 7024 6701 Rockledge Dr, MSC 7920 Bethesda, MD 20892-7920 (301) 435-0199 Fax (301) 480-3451 National Heart, Lung and Blood Institute NHLBI Information Center PO Box 30105 Bethesda, MD 20824-0105 (301) 251-1222 Fax (301) 251-1223 The Sleep Foundation *http//www.sleepfoundation.org* Sleep Net *http//www.sleepnet.com*

Bibliography

Ancoli-Israel S: Sleep problems in older adults: putting myths to bed. *Geriatrics* 52:20, 1997.

Bachman DL: Sleep disorder with aging: evaluation and treatment. *Geriatrics* 47:53, 1992.

Bonn D: Melatonin's multifarious marvels: miracle or myth? *Lancet* 347:184, 1996.

Cadieux RJ, Adams DG: Sleep disorders in older patients: conservative treatment is usually enough. *Postgrad Med* 91:403, 1992.

Gallup Organization: *Sleep in America: 1995.* Princeton, NJ: The Gallup Organization; 1995.

Garfinkel D, Laudon M, Nof D, Zisapel N: Improvement of sleep quality in elderly people by controlled-release melatonin. *Lancet* 346:541, 1995.

Haimov I, Laudon M, Zisapel N, et al: Sleep disorders and melatonin rhythms in elderly people. *BMJ* 309:167, 1994.

Haimov I, Lavie P, Laudon M, et al: Melatonin replacement therapy of elderly insomniacs. *Sleep* 18:598, 1995.

Inouye S, Bogardus S, Charpentier P, et al: A multicomponent intervention to prevent delirium in hospitalized patients. *N Engl J Med* 340:669, 1999.

International Classification of Sleep Disorders Diagnostic and Coding Manual. Rochester, MN: American Sleep Disorders Association; 1990.

Maggi S, Langlois JA, Minicuci N, et al: Sleep complaints in community-dwelling older persons: prevalence, associated factors, and reported causes. *J Am Geriatr Soc* 46:161, 1998.

McCall WV: Management of primary sleep disorders among elderly persons. *Psychiatr Serv* 46:49, 1995.

McDowell JA, Mion LC, Lydon TJ, Inouye SK: A nonpharmacologic sleep protocol for hospitalized older patients. *J Am Geriatr Soc* 46:700, 1998.

Middelkoop HA, Kerkhof GA, Smilde-van den Doel DA, et al: Sleep and aging: the effect of institutionalization on subjective and objective characteristics of sleep. *Age Aging* 23:411, 1994.

Prinz PN, Vitiello MV, Raskind MA, Thorpy MJ: Geriatrics: sleep disorders and aging. *N Engl J Med* 323:520, 1990.

Swift CG, Shapiro CM: ABC of sleep disorders: sleep and sleep problems in elderly people. *BMJ* 306:1468, 1993.

Systemic Review of the Literature Regarding the Diagnosis of Sleep Apnea: Summary. Evidence Report/Technology Assessment: no. 1. Rockville, MD, , US Department of Health and Human Services, Public Health Service, Agency for Health Care Policy and Research, 1998. Available at http://ahcpr.gov/clinic/apnea.htm. Accessed April 29, 1999.

Vitiello MV, Bliwise DL, Prinz PN: Sleep in Alzheimer's disease and the sundown syndrome. *Neurology* 42(7 suppl 6):83, 1992.

Walsh JK, Hartman PG, Kowall JP: Sleep disorders medicine: basic science, technical considerations and clinical aspects. In: Chokroverty S (ed): *Insomnia.* Boston: Butterworth-Heinemann; 1994; 219.

Wooten V: Sleep disorders in geriatric patients. *Clin Geriatr Med* 8:427, 1992.

Joseph J. Gallo
Junius Gonzales

Chapter

11

Depression and Other Mood Disorders

Overview: How Common Is Depression Among Older Primary Care Patients?

Depression among older primary care patients is a common problem. Patients may have a variety of symptoms, including memory problems, unexplained somatic disorders such as dizziness, or sleep disturbance. Depressed patients sometimes do not adhere to prescribed medical or diet therapy. Attempts to control multiple somatic symptoms and anxiety may lead to polypharmacy. Depression is associated with additional disability associated from chronic diseases such as arthritis and diabetes. Evaluation for depression is essential in planning for terminal care and in executing advance directives. Yet depression remains among the most difficult geriatric syndromes to recognize, assess, and manage in primary care.

About 6 percent of all patients who visit a primary care physician meet criteria for having major depression, but most studies of primary care patients do not include persons older than 65 years. Community surveys around the world have reported rates of major depression from 3 percent to about 15 percent of older persons. If "minor" depression (depression that does not meet full standard criteria for major depression but which

may impair everyday functioning) is included, the rates are higher, ranging from 6 percent in Sweden to more than 20 percent in studies of older primary care patients in Finland and the United Kingdom. Rates of depression among older persons with serious medical illness are higher still, around 40 percent among patients with stroke, 35 percent with cancer, 25 percent with Parkinson's disease, 20 percent with cardiovascular disease, and 10 percent with diabetes.

Although methodologic differences probably account for the variations in reported rates, there is little doubt that depression is a common cause of disability. Major depression, which was the fourth leading cause of disability in 1990 worldwide, will be second only to heart disease in 2020, according to the World Health Organization. Older adults with depression, even if symptoms do not meet the full criteria for major depression, are at increased risk of functional and cognitive decline. In addition, suicide rates increase with advancing age and appear to be increasing among the elderly throughout the world.

Older adults with mental disorders frequently consult a primary care physician, not a specialist in mental health, so that the primary health care setting is pivotal in the early assessment and management of the mental disturbances of late life. Although depression is an important issue for older patients, there is evidence that despite effective therapies for depression, undertreatment may be common. The reasons are complex and related to clinician, patient, and practice characteristics. A major reason that older adults with depression often do not receive adequate treatment of depression relates to a tendency of older adults to seek medical attention with somatic symptoms and to deny feeling depressed. William Styron, describing his experience with depression in his later years in the book *Darkness Visible* (Vintage Books, New York, 1990, page 36) wrote, "When I was first laid low by the disease, I felt a strong need, among other things, to register a strong protest against the word, 'depression'."

Principal Diagnoses

Major Depression

Standard criteria for major depression include depressed mood or loss of interest in activities that usually please the patient (inability to experience pleasure), and at least four of the following symptoms: appetite disturbance; sleep disturbance; fatigue; psychomotor agitation or retardation; feelings of worthlessness, sinfulness, or guilt; trouble concentrating; and thoughts of death or suicidal ideation. Symptoms are not transient and should be present nearly every day for 2 weeks or more.

Depression may be present among persons with fewer symptoms or with less intense symptoms. Nonverbal clues, such as stooped posture, slow movement, and slowed speech (psychomotor retardation) may signal depression. In the context of a severe life event or chronic medical illness, it is easy to ascribe symptoms to something other than depression.

Dysthymia

Dysthymia is a form of chronic depression that may occur with major depression (Table 11-1).

Dysthymia is characterized by a depressed mood for most of the day, more days than not, for at least 2 years, and without more than a 2-month symptom-free period. It is also accompanied by two or more of the following symptoms: poor appetite or overeating, insomnia or hypersomnia, low energy or fatigue, low self-esteem, poor concentration or difficulty making decisions, feelings of hopelessness. Dysthymia should be differentiated from major depression that is in remission or partially treated. Patients who experience dysthymia and who have met criteria for major depression in the past are said to have *double depression*. Dysthymia is important to recognize because the patient may take longer to respond to antidepressant therapy or may be less likely to respond to therapy at all.

Bereavement

Bereavement is a life event that is strongly associated with depression in late life, but is not a mental disorder. Older persons commonly experience loss of a spouse, a child, a grandchild, or other close relatives and friends. It is normal to feel sadness, to lose interest in activities, to have trouble sleeping and eating, and to think a great deal about death after the loss of a loved one. Some older persons who have lost a loved one report hearing or seeing the deceased person, which is normal after a death. The loss of a familiar pet may precipitate grief for some persons.

Persons who have experienced a loss usually do not have feelings of worthlessness or suicidal ideation as part of the depression syndrome. Refusing to see or to talk to others may be important signals of pathologic grief. Older adults with these symptoms should be considered for further assessment and treatment rather than being told the depression is ascribed to the loss.

In any case, bereaved older persons need careful follow-up care because they may be at risk of a number of adverse outcomes, such as heart problems, in addition to major depression. Older adults with a depression syndrome persisting more than

Table 11-1

Diagnostic Criteria for a Major Depressive Episode

A. Five (or more) of the following symptoms have been present during the same 2-week period and represent a change from previous functioning; at least one of the symptoms is either (1) depressed mood or (2) loss of interest or pleasure. NOTE: Do not include symptoms that are clearly due to a general medical condition or mood-incongruent delusion or hallucinations.

  1. Depressed mood most of the day, nearly every day, as indicated by either subjective report (e.g., feels sad or empty) or observation made by others (e.g., appears tearful). NOTE: Among children and adolescents, can be irritable mood.

  2. Markedly diminished interest or pleasure in all, or almost all, activities most of the day, nearly every day, as indicated by either subjective account or observation made by others.

  3. Substantial weight loss when not dieting or weight gain (e.g., a change of more than 5 percent of body weight in a month) or a decrease or increase in appetite nearly every day. NOTE: Among children, consider failure to make expected weight gains.

  4. Insomnia or hypersomnia nearly every day.

  5. Psychomotor agitation or retardation nearly every day, observable by others, not merely subjective feelings of restlessness or being slowed down.

  6. Fatigue or loss of energy nearly every day.

  7. Feelings of worthlessness or excessive or inappropriate guilt, which may be delusional, nearly every day, not merely self-reproach or guilt about being sick.

  8. Diminished ability to think or concentrate or indecisiveness, nearly every day, either by subjective account or as observed by others.

  9. Recurrent thoughts of death, not just fear of dying, recurrent suicidal ideation without a specific plan, or a suicide attempt or a specific plan for committing suicide.

B. The symptoms do not meet criteria for a mixed episode (mania).

C. The symptoms cause clinically significant distress or impairment in social, occupational, or other important areas of functioning.

D. The symptoms are not due to the direct physiologic effects of a substance (e.g., a drug of abuse, a medication) or a general medical condition (e.g., hypothyroidism).

E. The symptoms are not better accounted for by bereavement, that is, after the loss of a loved one, the symptoms persist for longer than 2 months or are characterized by marked functional impairment, morbid preoccupation with worthlessness, suicidal ideation, psychotic symptoms, or psychomotor retardation.

SOURCE: Adapted with permission from American Psychiatric Association: *Diagnostic and Statistical Manual of Mental Disorders, DSM-IV,* 4th ed. Washington, DC: American Psychiatric Association; 1994.

2 months after a loss are candidates for therapy for depression.

Dementia of Depression

Dementia is a syndrome characterized by loss of intellectual capacity involving not only memory but also cognition, language, visuospatial skills, and personality. All five components need not be impaired, but they frequently are impaired to varying degrees. Depression can mimic dementia, and a number of studies have found that depressive symptoms among older persons can be a harbinger of cognitive impairment. Clues that cognitive impairment may be caused by depression include recent onset and rapid progression, a family or personal history of affective disorders, and vigorous reports of poor memory.

Depression can coexist with dementia. As many as 20 percent of persons with Alzheimer's disease have a major depressive syndrome. Treatment with antidepressants may be the only way to prove that concomitant depression exists.

Depression Associated with Medical Conditions and Medications

A number of medical conditions may cause symptoms of depression, including endocrine disorders, cerebrovascular disease, and cancer. Hyperthyroidism typically manifests with fatigue, palpitations, proximal muscle weakness, diaphoresis, and weight loss. Among older persons, hyperthyroidism may manifest primarily as apathy and weight loss. Hypothyroidism also may cause symptoms of depression, although cognitive changes such as memory impairment are thought to be more common. Depression may occur early in the course of Cushing's syndrome.

Hyperparathyroidism resulting in elevated serum calcium levels can manifest as depression, even at mild elevations of serum calcium. Patients with diabetes mellitus may have depression, which has been related to poor control of blood sugar. Strokes near the left frontoparietal lobes are more likely than strokes in other regions to cause depression. The depression is not necessarily associated with the extent of functional impairment. The development of depression also may be associated with a diagnosis of cancer.

Many medications have been associated with depression, although this association sometimes is difficult to evaluate because depression is so common among persons with medical illnesses. Reserpine, β-blockers, clonidine, and methyldopa are antihypertensive agents that have been implicated in the development of depression. Exogenous steroid ingestion may be associated with psychosis and depression. Withdrawal from stimulants, ben-

zodiazepines, and barbiturates has been associated with the development of depression.

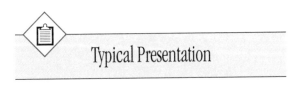

Typical Presentation

Primary Symptoms of Depression

MOOD CHANGE

It seems obvious that depression should imply that the person experiences "depression" or sadness. However, older adults are less likely to report sadness than are younger adults. Lehmann and Rabins reported that "up to one-third of older people who suffer from major depression do not describe their mood as depressed." Guidelines from the American Psychiatric Association on treating patients with depression state that the elderly appear to be less likely to report subjective dysphoria but are more likely to have vegetative signs and cognitive disturbance. Patients may express mood disturbance as vague reports of feeling "bad," "lousy," "crummy," or "blah" rather than feeling sad, blue, or depressed.

A question such as "How are your spirits today?" may open a discussion related to depression. It is important to ask about depression specifically. If a patient does not report a change in mood, the clinician should still consider the diagnosis of depression when other symptoms or signs of depression syndrome are present.

ANHEDONIA

An inability to derive pleasure from life is at the core of symptoms related to depression. Depressed patients may lose their zest for life and may not derive the usual satisfaction from everyday objects or events. This has been described as a loss of *vital sense*. When assessing older patients it is useful to ask whether there are activities that they once enjoyed but no longer do. Although it is tempting to ascribe restriction of activity to physical illness, there is increasing evidence that depression adds disability to medical problems such as diabetes, arthritis, and heart disease. A feeling of a loss of feeling may be expressed as no longer enjoying being with grandchildren or losing a sense of closeness to God.

Patients who deny having suicidal thoughts may report feeling that it would be just as well to fall asleep and not wake up. Lack of interest in self-care, such as adherence to medical therapy or diet, can also reflect loss of initiative and anhedonia. Mentally healthy older adults maintain a zest for living, even in the face of hardship.

Because of age-related changes in work and social roles, there may be less opportunity for older patients with depression to reveal diminished functioning. For this reason, anhedonia may be difficult to assess among older persons. In assessments for anhedonia, the focus should be on self-care activities, such as dressing, shopping, and cooking, and whether the loss of activities is out of proportion to that of other persons with a similar level of severity of medical illness.

PSYCHOMOTOR AGITATION OR RETARDATION

Psychomotor agitation or retardation can be defined as motor and cognitive underactivity or overactivity. Psychomotor agitation expresses itself as restlessness, constant pacing, and fidgeting. Psychomotor retardation manifests as slowed movement and speech. Some investigations have shown that older adults with depression are more likely to have psychomotor retardation than are younger persons with depression. Psychomotor changes may best be identified through careful observation of the patient by others rather than by self-report of the patient. The *psycho* or cognitive component of psychomotor change may be difficult to differentiate from trouble concentrating. Psychomotor slowing may increase time to respond to questions or lead to frequent answers of "I don't know." The cognitive equivalent of psychomotor agitation consists of ruminations or worries that

are not productive and seem to be internally driven.

FEELINGS OF WORTHLESSNESS, SINFULNESS, OR GUILT

Depressed patients often have poor self-esteem and may experience feelings of worthlessness or guilt. Older depressed patients may feel that they are not as good as other persons or that they are a burden on family and other caregivers. Sometimes depressed older patients do not adhere to medical therapy or will resist referral to medical specialists because they do not feel they are worthy of the expense and attention. Other patients may view their illness as a punishment for past deeds. Because of a sense of worthlessness or fear of being a burden on others, help for physical or functional problems may not be sought by older patients. These patients' feelings may engender an attitude of hopelessness on the part of the clinician. Clinicians need to avoid adopting this attitude. To ascertain whether a patient has such thoughts, it is useful to ask, "Do you feel that you are good as other people?" "Why do you think you are ill now?" and "Do you feel that you are a burden?"

APPETITE DISTURBANCE

Several investigators have found that older adults with depression were more likely to report weight loss or appetite disturbance than depressed younger adults. Among younger persons, depression can sometimes manifest as increased, rather than decreased, appetite. Weight loss and diminished appetite are nonspecific symptoms of illness that may signal thyroid disease, cancer, or other disorders. They must be considered in relation to other indications that depression might be present.

SLEEP DISTURBANCE

Disturbed sleep is a cardinal symptom of depression, especially among older persons. Abnormalities in the sleep–wake cycle suggest that a fundamental biologic mechanism accounts for the association between depression and sleep disturbance (Chap. 10). Sometimes older persons who report sleep problems harbor attitudes about what normal sleep in old age should be like, so education about normal sleep may be helpful. When a patient reports sleep problems, the clinician should review the other symptoms of depression. Early morning awakening, not feeling rested when waking, or trouble staying asleep are characteristic of depression.

FATIGUE

Older persons with depression often report feeling tired all the time. Lack of energy can be a sign of a medical condition such as anemia, congestive heart failure, or chronic pulmonary disease. Unlike fatigue from medical conditions that may be most evident with exertion, fatigue caused by depression may be described as feeling that one just cannot get going.

TROUBLE CONCENTRATING

Trouble concentrating and thinking frequently accompanies depression. This may be expressed as inability to make decisions or to complete complex tasks. Among depressed older adults, reports of memory impairment can be prominent. Older adults with depression sometimes describe memory loss without objective evidence of impairment on simple tests of memory. These patients should be evaluated for symptoms of depression, and careful follow-up care should be provided to detect signs of dementia.

THOUGHTS OF DEATH OR SUICIDAL IDEATION

Thoughts of death are not by themselves abnormal among older persons; suicidal ideation, however, is not normal. For a sample of older primary care patients, Callahan and colleagues estimated the prevalence of suicidal ideation at 0.7 to 1.2 percent. The severity of depressive symptoms and functional impairment varied widely among patients report-

ing suicidal ideation. No demographic or clinical variables differentiated depressed suicidal patients from depressed nonsuicidal patients. Only one-half of the patients with suicidal ideation reported a history of depression, and none reported a history of alcohol abuse.

Skoog interviewed 494 adults 85 years and older and found a 1-month prevalence of any suicidal thoughts of 9.6 percent among men and 18.7 percent among women. In this sample, suicidal ideation was strongly associated with depression. Only 6.2 percent of the participants who did not meet criteria for depression or anxiety endorsed any suicidal thoughts, whereas almost 50 percent of the persons meeting criteria for having depression harbored suicidal ideation. Suicidal feelings were associated with treatment with anxiolytics but not antidepressants, suggesting that clinicians were not adequately assessing or managing symptoms of depression.

Severe physical illness does not figure prominently in suicide committed by older persons. Few older persons who have committed suicide have had a terminal or serious illness. However, some patients believe that they have a serious illness, perhaps because they have misinterpreted the meaning of symptoms or test results. Most older adults with physical illness, even cancer, are not suicidal. To address this issue, it is important to emphasize that professionals who deal with the elderly should ask patients about the meaning of their illness and how they are coping. Older persons who commit suicide are more likely than younger persons to have depression that is unaccompanied by other psychiatric conditions, such as substance abuse. Most older patients who attempt suicide are having their first episode of depression. Purported risk factors of suicide among older persons are presented in Table 11-2.

Patients are less likely to commit suicide if they are asked about such intentions by the health care team. Asking about suicidal thoughts can defuse a suicide attempt because asking shows concern for the patient, helps rally social and other support, and begins the process of healing. In evaluating patients who may be depressed it is critical to ask

Table 11-2

Risk Factors of Suicide Among Older Persons

> History of previous suicide attempts or suicidal
> ideation
> Male sex
> White race
> Living alone or socially isolated
> Recent loss or bereavement
> Feelings of hopelessness, helplessness, or that
> life is a burden
> Physical illness
> Alcohol abuse
> Sleeplessness
> Firearms in home

whether they have had thoughts of self-harm. In asking about suicidal thoughts, an examiner can say "Sometimes persons in your situation think about harming themselves. Have you had such feelings?"

Patients thinking about suicide should be asked if they have a plan for hurting themselves. For example, does the patient have a gun at home? Patients who are actively suicidal have a plan and often the means to carry it out. Intentionality can be assessed by asking "How close do you feel to doing something?" or "What might make you act on your feelings?" Patients with passive suicidal ideation may wish to fall asleep and not wake up, without active planning; this form of ideation should be addressed and taken seriously.

Other Symptoms of Depression Among Older Adults

ANXIETY AND WORRIES

Worry and nervous tension are common presentations of depression among older persons. Symptoms of anxiety are important because many clinicians focus on those symptoms and do not consider depression among patients with such

symptoms. Patients may feel jittery, nervous, fearful, or afraid. Studies show that patients with symptoms of both anxiety and depression are more likely to receive a benzodiazepine than more appropriate therapy for depression. Patients with anxiety should be carefully assessed for depression and treated initially with an antidepressant if clinical clues of depression exist.

HOPELESSNESS AND HELPLESSNESS

Hopelessness is an important symptom to ask about when examining older patients with physical illness and functional impairment. Hopelessness, not sadness, has been associated with suicidal ideation and suicide. Statements such as "What's the use?" or "I might as well be dead" should prompt an assessment rather than assurances that all is well. It is important to ask older patients how they are coping with the illness, whether they feel helpless or hopeless about their life, and what concerns they have about the future.

UNEXPLAINED SOMATIC PROBLEMS

Older patients with depression may have somatic symptoms for which a medical cause cannot be found or that appear to be out of proportion to the extent of medical illness. Persons who express somatic symptoms as a manifestation of depression may be less likely than persons with psychological symptoms to have positive attitudes about mental illness and are less willing to mention psychological symptoms to the doctor.

Somatic presentations of depression are among the most challenging situations faced by primary care physicians. Patients may be worried that a serious illness such as cancer accounts for the symptoms. Clinicians may be concerned about missing hidden disease that mimics depression. Therefore it is important to address psychological distress while considering the medical possibilities. The medical evaluation should include a careful review of all associated or causative medical conditions and medications.

IRRITABILITY

Grouchiness is taken as a stereotypical characteristic of old age, but as among children and adolescents, irritability can be a symptom of depression. Older adults with a reputation for having a "short fuse" or for snapping at others may be experiencing depression they have difficulty expressing in other ways. If other key symptoms such as sleep and appetite disturbance exist, depression should be suspected.

POOR ADHERENCE TO MEDICAL OR DIET THERAPY

Patients who are frustrating to deal with may be depressed. Older persons who do not make expected progress in rehabilitation should be assessed for depression.

PSYCHOSIS

Less common manifestations of depression among the elderly include psychotic symptoms, including hallucinations and delusions. Psychotic symptoms are critical to consider because they have implications for treatment and prognosis.

Hallucinations are false sensory perceptions. Visual hallucinations may occur among older patients with severe depression but also may indicate an organic pathologic condition such as a tumor, metabolic disorder, or dementia. Auditory hallucinations, such as hearing voices, are characteristic of schizophrenia but also can occur with depression. Because the patient may deny the presence of hallucinations, family or friends should be asked about them.

Delusions are false beliefs held with conviction (not a misinterpretation based on false reasoning). The content of the delusion may concern persecution, guilt, poverty, or the body (somatic delusions). Patients with a somatic delusion may believe they have cancer despite evidence to the contrary. A patient may not volunteer hallucinations and delusions because to the patient these are normal perceptions and ideas.

Additional Clinical Clues to Depression Among Older Adults

Women are at higher risk of depression than are men, even in later life. Whether this is due to biologic or social factors is not clear. Women with less than a high school education appear to be at especially high risk.

The amount and quality of social support available to an older patient can help identify patients who may have difficulty coping with stressful life events. Older persons who take comfort from religious practices may be less prone to depression. A family history of depression is thought to be less relevant for older than for younger depressed persons.

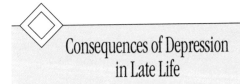

Consequences of Depression in Late Life

Whether symptoms meet full standard criteria for depression, depressive symptoms among older adults have important consequences. Depression among older adults appears to be associated with poor prognosis, especially when accompanied by physical illness. Among older adult ambulatory patients with depression in one study, after 1 to 2 years about one-third continued to have symptoms, one-third had improved, and one-third had died. Among older primary care patients with clinically significant depression, almost one-half continued to meet criteria for depression at short-term (6 month) and long-term (2 year) follow-up evaluations.

Schulberg reported that adults 60 years and older who had major depression and were assessed in primary care settings had markedly impaired social and physical function despite intact cognitive function and mild depressive symptoms. At 6-month follow-up assessment, these patients were unlikely to be free of symptoms and had persistent disability.

Increasing levels of depression were independently associated with functional impairment after 4 years of follow-up study among persons 71 years and older.

In another investigation based on a 13-year follow-up study of adults 50 years and older, subsyndromal depression was associated with a number of adverse functional, cognitive, and emotional outcomes. Older persons with depressive symptoms without sadness (hopelessness, worthlessness, thoughts of death, wanting to die, or suicide) were at increased risk of functional impairment in activities of daily living, instrumental activities of daily living, psychological distress, and death. These follow-up results strongly suggest that it is critical to consider depression in the care of older patients and that depression is associated with poor functional outcomes.

Physical Examination

Physical examination provides an opportunity to find evidence of occult conditions associated with depressive illness and that affect therapeutic decisions. Blood pressure and pulse should be obtained with the patient supine and standing, because medications used to manage depression sometimes cause or exacerbate orthostatic hypotension. Sensory deficits, such as hearing or vision loss, have been associated with psychotic symptoms among older patients and should be considered. Cerebrovascular disease, especially left hemisphere frontal lobe disorders, is commonly associated with depressive symptoms. Right-sided motor or sensory symptoms and signs suggest these disorders.

Hyperthyroidism may cause tremor, psychomotor agitation, tachycardia or atrial fibrillation, bounding pulses, warm moist skin, thinning hair, and hyperreflexia. Among older persons, however, hyperthyroidism may manifest primarily as apathy and weight loss. Hypothyroidism may cause constipation, slowed reflexes, and cognitive impairment.

Cushing's syndrome may cause central obesity, hypertension, hirsutism, proximal muscle weakness, and easy bruisability. Parkinson's disease may cause tremor and difficulty walking. Vitamin B_{12} and folate deficiency may manifest as difficulty walking, paresthesia, and loss of position or vibratory sense, especially in the feet. A thorough physical examination to look for evidence of cancer, including rectal and gynecologic examinations, should be performed when appropriate. Urinary retention may be caused by the anticholinergic activities of some medications used to manage depression and may be detected as an enlarged bladder at physical examination.

Ancillary Tests

A basic laboratory evaluation for depression in the care of older adults includes a complete blood cell count, chemistry profile, serum calcium level, and thyroid function tests. An electrocardiogram should be obtained for a baseline determination of QT interval and rhythm before antidepressant medication is instituted. Electrolyte abnormalities may reflect an underlying adrenal disorder, whereas anemia or macrocytosis may suggest vitamin B_{12} or folate deficiency. Other studies can be considered depending on the situation. For example, history or physical examination findings that suggest stroke or dementia might warrant an imaging study of the brain and additional evaluation. Specific symptoms, such as weight loss or constipation, may necessitate further evaluation, such as imaging of the colon.

Assessment Scales

The use of standardized questionnaires sometimes can be useful to screen patients for depression, to help educate patients and caregivers about depression, and to follow the course of depressive symptoms over time. A number of instruments to measure depressive symptoms may be useful in the primary care setting. For the most part, these questionnaires are sensitive but not specific. Most persons with clinically significant depression score above the recommended threshold, but many persons who score above the recommended threshold do not have depression. If the cutoff score is set at a lower level, more older patients are identified as being potentially depressed, but evaluation is needed to determine whether clinically significant depression is present.

Two questionnaires used to evaluate elderly persons for depression are the 30-item Geriatric Depression Scale (GDS) and the 20-item Center for Epidemiologic Studies Depression Scale, Revised (CES-D-R).

GERIATRIC DEPRESSION SCALE

The GDS (Table 11-3) was constructed to eliminate somatic items, such as sleep disturbance,

Table 11-3

Geriatric Depression Scale (GDS)

	YES	NO
1s. Are you basically satisfied with your life?		*
2s. Have you dropped many of your activities and interests?	*	
3s. Do you feel that your life is empty?	*	
4s. Do you often feel bored?	*	
5. Are you hopeful about the future?		*
6. Are you bothered by thoughts you can't get out of your head?	*	
7s. Are you in good spirits most of the time?		*
8s. Are you afraid that something bad is going to happen to you?	*	
9s. Do you feel happy most of the time?		*
10s. Do you often feel helpless?	*	
11. Do you often get restless or fidgety?	*	
12s. Do you prefer to stay at home rather than going out and doing new things?	*	
13. Do you frequently worry about the future?	*	
14s. Do you feel you have more problems with memory than most?	*	
15s. Do you feel it is wonderful to be alive now?		*
16. Do you often feel downhearted and blue?		*
17s. Do you feel pretty worthless the way you are now?	*	
18. Do you worry a lot about the past?	*	
19. Do you find life very exciting?		*
20. Is it hard for you to get started on new projects?	*	
21s. Do you feel full of energy?		*
22s. Do you feel that your situation is hopeless?	*	
23s. Do you think that most people are better off than you are?	*	
24. Do you frequently get upset over little things?	*	
25. Do you frequently feel like crying?	*	
26. Do you have trouble concentrating?	*	
27. Do you enjoy getting up in the morning?		*
28. Do you prefer to avoid social gatherings?	*	
29. Is it easy for you to make decisions?		*
30. Is your mind as clear as it used to be?		*

NOTE: Score one point for each response corresponding to an asterisk. Items forming the 15-item short form are indicated with an *s.*

that might not be specific to depression among older persons. The GDS is commonly used to assess depression among older persons but may not be valid when moderate cognitive impairment is present. The GDS is scored by counting 1 for each answer corresponding to depressive symptoms (asterisks in Table 11-3). A score of 11 or greater indicates clinically significant depression. A short version of the GDS consists of the 15 items designated in Table 11-3. For the short version, a score of 5 or greater may indicate clinically significant depression.

CENTER FOR EPIDEMIOLOGIC STUDIES DEPRESSION SCALE

The Center for Epidemiologic Studies Depression Scale (CES-D) was developed at the National Institute of Mental Health for use in studies of depression in community samples. A revision of the CES-D scale (Table 11-4) may be more useful than the original CES-D in screening for major depression because the content of the items is closer to the *Diagnostic and Statistical Manual of Mental Disorders* (DSM-IV) criteria than that of the original CES-D.

Table 11-4

Center for Epidemiologic Studies Depression Scale, Revised (CES-D-R)

What follows is a list of the ways you might have felt or behaved. Please check the boxes to tell me how often you have felt this way in the past week or so.	LAST WEEK				
	NOT AT ALL *OR* LESS THAN 1 DAY	1–2 DAYS	3–4 DAYS	5–7 DAYS	NEARLY EVERY DAY FOR 2 WEEKS
My appetite is poor.	☐	☐	☐	☐	☐
I could not shake off the blues.	☐	☐	☐	☐	☐
I had trouble keeping my mind on what I was doing.	☐	☐	☐	☐	☐
I felt depressed.	☐	☐	☐	☐	☐
My sleep was restless.	☐	☐	☐	☐	☐
I felt sad.	☐	☐	☐	☐	☐
I could not get going.	☐	☐	☐	☐	☐
Nothing made me happy.	☐	☐	☐	☐	☐
I felt like a bad person.	☐	☐	☐	☐	☐
I lost interest in my usual activities.	☐	☐	☐	☐	☐
I slept much more than usual.	☐	☐	☐	☐	☐
I felt like I was moving too slowly.	☐	☐	☐	☐	☐
I felt fidgety.	☐	☐	☐	☐	☐
I wished I was dead.	☐	☐	☐	☐	☐
I wanted to hurt myself.	☐	☐	☐	☐	☐
I was tired all the time.	☐	☐	☐	☐	☐
I did not like myself.	☐	☐	☐	☐	☐
I lost a lot of weight without trying to.	☐	☐	☐	☐	☐
I had a lot of trouble getting to sleep.	☐	☐	☐	☐	☐
I could not focus on the important things.	☐	☐	☐	☐	☐

NOTE: The items map onto the diagnostic criteria for major depression in Table 11-1 (namely, depressed mood in items 2, 4, and 6; anhedonia in items 8 and 10; appetite disturbance in items 1 and 18; sleep disturbance in items 5, 11, and 19; psychomotor agitation or retardation in items 12 and 13; fatigue in items 7 and 16; feelings of worthlessness or guilt in items 9 and 17; concentration difficulty in items 3 and 20; and recurrent thoughts of death in items 14 and 15). When using the CES-D-R as a scale, code each item from 0 (not at all or less than 1 day) to 3 (5 to 7 days or nearly every day for 2 weeks).

The revised instrument allows mapping of responses to the items that form the diagnostic criteria for major depression shown in Table 11-1, so that one can get an idea of whether criteria for major depression are met. Specifically, a response in the most intense category (nearly every day for 2 weeks) in five of the nine symptom groups with the additional requirement of either dysphoria or anhedonia would be consistent with a diagnosis of major depression.

The CES-D-R also may be used as a scale of depressive symptoms, much as the original CES-D has been used. Each item is coded from 0 (not at all or less than 1 day) to 3 (5 to 7 days or nearly every day for 2 weeks) so that the range of the questionnaire is 0 to 60. Scoring the CES-D-R in this way is highly correlated with the score on the original CES-D. On the basis of prior work with the CES-D, a threshold of 17 and greater may be considered a signal of significant depression. These instruments can be administered by appropriately trained nursing assistants or other personnel to monitor response to depression treatment.

MNEMONIC

Some clinicians find it useful to use a simple mnemonic to record responses to the diagnostic interview for depression. The mnemonic is SIG EM CAPS: S, sleep; I, interest; G, guilt; E, energy; M, mood; C, concentration; A, appetite; P, psychomotor retardation or agitation; and S, suicide.

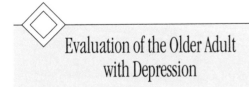

Evaluation of the Older Adult with Depression

Three questions should guide clinicians who are considering diagnosis and treatment of depression in the care of older patients: (1) Are the symptoms attributable to a medical condition or to the effects of medications? (2) Are other psychiatric conditions present? (3) What conditions are present that will modify therapy for depression? The first question should lead to a search for potentially correctable conditions. Optimizing the management of medical illnesses and withdrawal of unnecessary medications, especially psychoactive drugs, is important in the care of older patients with depression.

The answer to the second question influences treatment decisions. Concurrent psychiatric conditions such as alcohol abuse, mania, cognitive impairment, and anxiety disorders may change the approach to therapy or may prompt consultation with a specialist in mental health. For example, one should address alcohol abuse before focusing on depression. The presence of mania calls for treatment that may not be available in primary health care.

The third question highlights consideration of concurrent conditions, such as heart disease, that affect the treatment of older adults with depression. The history, physical examination, and laboratory evaluation should be focused on answering these three questions.

Evaluation of Psychiatric Comorbidity

An important question to be addressed in the evaluation of an older patient with depression is, Are other psychiatric conditions present? Other psychiatric conditions that may be associated with depressive symptoms include anxiety disorders, alcohol and other substance abuse and dependence, manic depression (bipolar disorder), schizophrenia and paraphrenia, and dementia. Each comorbidity has implications for treatment decisions and may require consultation with a specialist in mental health.

ANXIETY DISORDERS

Anxiety disorders include phobias, panic disorder, generalized anxiety disorder, and obsessive-compulsive disorder. Worry or nervous tension rather than specific anxiety syndromes such as panic disorder may be more important for older persons. Anxiety symptoms are important to understanding the process of treatment of depression. In clinical studies, older adults with anxiety and depression were more likely to discontinue antidepressant treatment, were less likely to respond to antidepressants, and had shorter time to relapse than did depressed older adults without symptoms of anxiety.

ALCOHOL USE

Alcohol consumption is common among older adults: 10 to 20 percent report daily use of alcohol. In a survey of residents of a retirement community, almost one-half reported some alcohol consumption, 15 percent reporting consumption of 1 to 6 drinks each week. Among adults 60 years and older screened in primary care practices in Wisconsin, 10.5 percent of the men and 3.9 percent of the women had responses that suggested problem alcohol use. However, the proportion of older persons who meet criteria for alcohol abuse or dependence appears to be much smaller. In the Epidemiologic Catchment Area study, for example, the 1-month prevalence of alcohol abuse or dependence was 1.93 percent for men and 0.40 percent for women 65 years and older. The incidence of alcohol abuse or dependence appears to show an upturn in rates with age among men. Alcohol abuse or dependence should be the initial focus of therapy when present and may necessitate referral to specialty mental health services. Detection of problem alcohol consumption may be facilitated by the use of brief questionnaires such as the CAGE or the AUDIT.

BIPOLAR DISORDER

Mania is elevated mood, flight of ideas, and overactivity that may be associated with grandiose or paranoid delusions, irritability, or hypersexuality. Manic depression, or bipolar disorder, is present if the patient has had even one episode of mania that occurs with episodes of depression. Among older persons, mania may be associated with an organic cause such as cerebrovascular dis-

ease or medication. Antidepressant medications used in the management of major depression can precipitate a manic episode among susceptible patients with bipolar disorder. The mainstay of therapy for bipolar disorder is a mood stabilizer (e.g., lithium, valproic acid, or carbamazepine). Patients with bipolar disorder should be referred to a specialist in mental health.

SCHIZOPHRENIA AND PARAPHRENIA

Schizophrenia is a psychotic condition resulting in thought disorder, hallucinations, and delusions. The onset usually is in young adulthood, but many patients with schizophrenia are now surviving into old age. Paraphrenia is a disorder that resembles schizophrenia but is characterized by onset in late life, paranoid delusions, and hallucinations occurring in the absence of dementia or a depressive disorder.

DEMENTIA

Cognitive impairment, present in Alzheimer's disease and other forms of dementia, affects the presentation and management of depression from several perspectives. Cognitive impairment may coexist with depression and obfuscate the diagnosis of depression. Cognitive impairment of a patient with a personal or family history of affective disorder should raise suspicion that depression may be contributing to cognitive changes. Cognitive impairment may dominate the clinical signs and symptoms and interfere with the reporting of depressive symptoms. Depression may be an early indication of developing dementia; a common pathophysiologic mechanism may underlie both depression and dementia. Devanand and coworkers found that depressed mood at baseline was associated with an almost threefold risk of Alzheimer's disease over the course of a follow-up period, even after adjustment for age, sex, and educational status. Among older adults, it appears that these disorders (dementia and depression) sometimes evolve into a common presentation. Although cognitive impairment should not deter therapy for depression when indicated, careful follow-up care allows more appropriate therapeutic decisions over time.

Evaluation of Conditions That May Modify Treatment

The presence of medical conditions may affect therapeutic decisions. For example, antidepressants that are less likely to cause cardiac conduction abnormalities (e.g., selective serotonin re-uptake inhibitors) should be prescribed for patients with heart disease. Patients with seizure disorders may be at increased seizure risk if given some antidepressant medications (e.g., bupropion). Hepatic or renal disease may affect the clearance of antidepressant medicines.

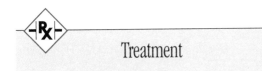

Treatment

Despite the availability of safe and effective treatment, most older adults with depression do not receive any treatment. The key to treating older persons with depression is initial recognition of depression. Older patients often have concurrent physical illnesses that may obscure the diagnosis of depression and that must be considered in treatment decisions. Two important considerations in the management of depression are that (1) depression is often a chronic illness and (2) long-term follow-up care of the patient is essential. For these reasons, the primary care setting is well suited for continuing, coordinated care of older persons with depression.

The Agency for Health Care Policy and Research clinical practice guidelines for primary care of patients with depression summarize phases of therapy for depression. After days, weeks, or months of symptoms, the depression syndrome develops. Appropriate treatment may result in a response as evidenced by decreasing symptoms and improved functioning within 6 to 12 weeks. Relapse can occur at any time if sustained treatment for 4 to 9 months is not provided. In some cases, maintenance therapy for longer periods may be warranted. An overview of the management strategy is shown in Fig. 11-1. The essential feature illustrated in the algorithm is monitoring for effectiveness of treatment.

Counseling

Counseling should be an integral component of all treatment regimens for depression among older persons. Although formal psychotherapy sessions may be recommended for some patients, the techniques used by psychotherapists can be implemented by primary care practitioners to supplement routine pharmacologic management of depression. The basic components of counseling can be summarized in the concepts of empathize, encourage, and educate. These concepts involve supportive listening, encouraging the patient to engage in pleasurable activities, and educating the patient about depression and its management. The need to incorporate these three basic elements in the encounter is especially critical in the care of older patients and their families because the diagnosis of depression may not be readily accepted.

Although drug therapy is effective therapy for depression in late life, there are a number of compelling reasons to offer psychosocial therapy for depression to older primary care patients. First, older patients and families may prefer nondrug therapy. Older adults rate their willingness to try counseling higher than use of medication to manage depression. Once in therapy, older adults may be more likely to adhere to psychotherapy than are younger persons. Second, older adults have more adverse reactions to medications. Because many patients are already taking multiple medications for medical conditions, alternatives to pharmacotherapy may be useful. Third, many problems of old age involve psychosocial stressors, such as death of loved ones, family conflict,

Figure 11-1

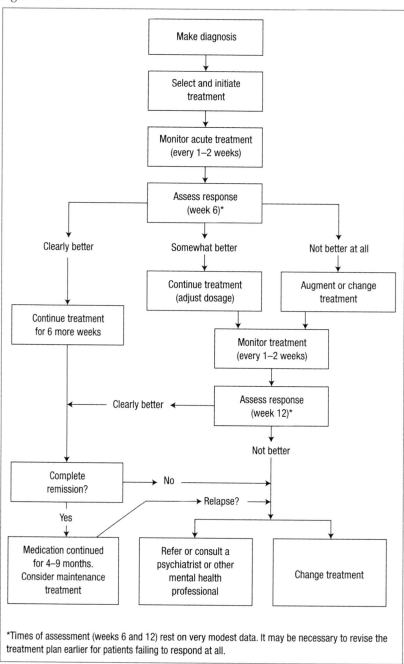

*Times of assessment (weeks 6 and 12) rest on very modest data. It may be necessary to revise the treatment plan earlier for patients failing to respond at all.

Overview of management of depression. *(Reproduced with permission from Depression Guideline Panel: Depression in Primary Care, Volume 1: Detection and Diagnosis and Volume 2: Treatment of Major Depression. Clinical Practice Guideline no. 5, AHCPR publication nos. 93-0550 and 93-0551; Rockville, MD, US Department of Health and Human Services, Public Health Service, Agency for Health Care Policy and Research, 1993.)*

and diminished social resources, so psychosocial intervention would seem particularly appropriate. Finally, counseling bolsters coping skills among physically ill older adults with depression through improving self-esteem and self-efficacy in the management of daily activities and disease-related tasks.

Although the primary care physician may not provide formal psychotherapy, the techniques of cognitive-behavioral therapy (CBT), problem-solving therapy, and interpersonal therapy may be useful adjuncts to clinical management. They are discussed in more detail by Brody and colleagues and by Shearer and Adams.

COGNITIVE-BEHAVIORAL THERAPY

The basic notion underlying CBT is that thinking and actions affect emotions. Depressed persons hold negative beliefs and expectations about themselves, the world, and the future and may misinterpret events because of underlying negative assumptions (cognitive distortions). For example, an older man may feel that his family will no longer love him if he becomes a burden when in fact there is no evidence for this belief. Another example is an older woman who is criticized by her supervisor. The woman focuses on the criticism and believes the supervisor is ready to fire her. CBT works by exposing and addressing these underlying beliefs.

In primary care practice, statements patients make may reveal their underlying negative assumptions. Leading questions such as "When you felt that way, what was going through your mind?" can help expose cognitive distortions. The distortion then can be discussed to cast a more positive light on the situation. A number of cognitions related to medical illness and actual or threatened functional impairment are salient for older adults. Examples include a sense of giving up, poor self-esteem in relation to declining physical health, inability to manage health care expenses, fear of being neglected or abandoned by family, lack of a confidante, worry about becoming dependent on others, and concern that nothing can be done to mitigate the effects of physical illness or functional impairment.

Another component of CBT concerns behaviors. The concept of this component is that engaging in pleasurable activities may lift depression, so specific activities that are enjoyable should be scheduled.

PROBLEM-SOLVING THERAPY

Problem-solving therapy involves helping a patient think through potential solutions to a problem to increase feelings of mastery and control. When problems can be potentially resolved, this technique helps to explore ways to reduce or eliminate the problem. Depressed patients often end their problem-solving activities too soon, and a solution that may be obvious to an outsider is not obvious to a depressed person. Patients can be assisted in breaking the problem into smaller, more manageable steps. When problems do not seem solvable, the practitioner can provide empathy and support and help the patient reframe the problem by identifying and modifying unrealistic expectations and inappropriate negative thoughts about self or situation. The patient should be encouraged to focus on the positive aspects of life, such as family and friends, and the resources available.

INTERPERSONAL THERAPY

Interpersonal therapy involves encouraging the patient to sustain and develop social ties and to maintain involvement in pleasurable activities. Many depressed patients isolate themselves from family and friends. Patients can be encouraged to reconnect with friends. Senior citizen centers and support groups for the newly widowed are two examples whereby depressed persons can develop social ties.

Psychotherapy such as CBT or interpersonal therapy can be administered in a group. Group therapy gives older adults dealing with depression or bereavement the opportunity to obtain feedback from peers and to observe the responses of persons with similar problems. There is little

Table 11-5

Antidepressant Medications

MEDICATION	HOW SUPPLIED	STARTING DOSE	USUAL TOTAL DAILY DOSE	SIDE EFFECTS	INTERACTIONS: MEDICATION AND MEDICAL CONDITIONS
Selective serotonin reuptake inhibitors					
Fluoxetine (Prozac)	10 mg 20 mg 20 mg per 5cc	10 mg qod	qd, 10–60 mg	Nausea, headache, insomnia, dysfunction, weight loss	Cardiac effects usually limited to tachycardia; inhibition of P450 system means that levels of other drugs may be increased
				Anxiety, agitation, anorexia, insomnia	Long half-life; minimum 5-week washout for patients starting an MAOI; at least 2 weeks between stopping an MAOI and starting fluoxetine
Paroxetine (Paxil)	10 mg 20 mg 30 mg 40 mg	10 mg qd	qd, 10–50 mg	Sedation, dry mouth	Minimum 2-week washout for patients starting an MAOI
Sertraline (Zoloft)	50 mg scored 100 mg scored	25 mg qd	qd, 25–200 mg	Loose stools, diarrhea, dizziness	Minimum 2-week washout for patients starting an MAOI
Citalopram (Celexa)	20 mg scored 40 mg scored	10 mg qd	qd, 20–40 mg	Sedation, dry mouth, nausea	Minimum 2-week washout for patients starting an MAOI; possibly less interaction with P450
Tricyclics (secondary amines)					
Desipramine (Norpramin)	10 mg 25 mg 50 mg 75 mg 100 mg 150 mg	10–25 mg qd	bid, 75–300 mg	Dry mouth, blurry vision, constipation	Arrhythmias possible; anticholinergic side effects; inhibition of P450 system means that levels of other drugs may be increased
					—
Nortriptyline (Pamelor; Aventyl)	10 mg 25 mg 50 mg 75 mg 10 mg per 5cc	10 mg qd	bid, 40–200 mg	Dry mouth, blurry vision constipation	—

Table 11-5

Antidepressant Medications (*continued*)

MEDICATION	HOW SUPPLIED	STARTING DOSE	USUAL TOTAL DAILY DOSE	SIDE EFFECTS	INTERACTIONS: MEDICATION AND MEDICAL CONDITIONS
Other antidepressants					
Venlafaxine (Effexor)	25 mg scored 37.5 mg scored 50 mg scored 75 mg scored 100 mg scored	25 mg qd	bid, 75–300 mg	Nausea, headache, sexual dysfunction, drowsiness, dizziness, anorexia, nervousness, dry mouth	Diastolic hypertension (doses greater than 275 mg)
Nefazodone (Serzone)	100 mg scored 150 mg scored 200 mg 250 mg	50 mg qd	bid, 300–500 mg	Sedation, nausea, dizziness, dry mouth, constipation	Increased levels of triazolam, alprazolam, astemizole, cisapride, terfenadine, ketoconazole, erythromycin when administered concurrently with nefazodone due to P450 interaction, which may result in prolonged QT interval; no interaction with lorazepam
Trazodone (Desyrel)	50 mg scored 100 mg scored 150 mg scored 300 mg scored	50 mg qd	bid, 150–400 mg	Sedation, nausea, priapism	Increased levels of digoxin, phenytoin
Mirtazapine (Remeron)	15 mg 30 mg	7.5 mg qhs	qd, 15–45 mg	Sedation, dry mouth, constipation, increased appetite	Agranulocytosis rarely (discontinue if fever, sore throat, or other signs of infection and obtain CBC)
Bupropion (Wellbutrin)	75 mg 100 mg	50 mg qd	tid, 225–450 mg	Anxiety, agitation, nausea, insomnia, weight loss	Contraindicated in seizure disorder, focal CNS disease, known abnormalities on EEG
Doxepin (Sinequan)	10 mg 25 mg 50 mg 75 mg 100 mg 150 mg	50 mg qd	bid, 150–300 mg	Sedation, nausea, dizziness, dry mouth, constipation	Metabolized by P450 system

NOTE: Starting doses are those recommended for older persons, but some frail older persons should be prescribed doses one-half of the starting doses shown here.

ABBREVIATIONS: P450, cytochrome P450; MAOI, monoamine oxidase inhibitor; CBC, complete blood cell count; CNS, central nervous system; EEG, electroencephalogram.

evidence that a particular orientation is more effective than another for managing depression among older patients, and these therapies have overlapping features and strategies. The power of counseling from the clinician and others for older adults with depression should not be underestimated. Although time may be limited, a strategy that emphasizes the need to empathize, encourage, and educate can enhance the effectiveness of treatment of older patients for depression.

Antidepressant Medications

Antidepressant medications appear to be as effective in the care of older adults as in the care of younger adults. General principles of pharmacotherapy for older patients apply to drug therapy for depression: start low, go slow, and observe the patient as you go. Older patients may metabolize medications more slowly and may be more sensitive to side effects than are younger persons. Dosage of medications should be increased a small amount once a week to limit side effects. Age-related declines in the function of the kidney and the liver make older persons more susceptible to toxicity. The patient should be reassessed regularly for effectiveness of treatment and the development of side effects.

Antidepressants have been grouped into three categories: (1) selective serotonin reuptake inhibitors (SSRIs), (2) tricyclic antidepressants (TCAs), and (3) all other antidepressant drugs. The primary care physician should become familiar with the use of at least one agent from each category. Information on specific medications is summarized in Table 11-5.

No one antidepressant medication is clearly more effective than another. The efficacy rate is about 70 percent for all medications (about 30 percent of persons are not helped in the first trial of medication). No single medication results in remission for all patients. The selection of antidepressant medication should be based on the side-effect profile of the medication, prior response to a specific medication, concurrent medical ill-

nesses, and concomitant use of nonpsychotropic medications. A medication that has resulted in a remission of depression in the past should be considered for first-line therapy, as should medications that have resulted in remission for a first-degree relative.

SELECTIVE SEROTONIN REUPTAKE INHIBITORS

The SSRIs have come into widespread use since the National Institutes of Health Depression Consensus Conference on Depression in Late Life was held in 1991. The new SSRI agents include sertraline (Zoloft), paroxetine (Paxil), fluoxetine (Prozac) and citalopram (Celexa). The SSRIs have revolutionized the management of depression in primary care because these drugs appear to be easier to dose (easier to reach a therapeutic dose) and are better tolerated than TCAs. SSRIs are generally thought to be advantageous for use in the care of older persons because compared with TCAs they have fewer anticholinergic side effects, do not appear to markedly affect cognitive functioning, and have fewer and less severe effects on the cardiovascular system, such as orthostatic hypotension. Evidence of tolerability of SSRIs over TCAs is that dropout rates for older patients taking SSRIs are substantially lower than those for persons taking TCAs.

Sexual dysfunction, especially loss of erectile function and problems with orgasm, is one of the more common side effects of SSRIs. One strategy calls for scheduled missing of a dose of the SSRI in the day or two before sexual activity. Sometimes adding cyproheptadine (4 to 12 mg qd), bupropion (75 mg qd), or buspirone (5 to 25 mg qd) to the medication regimen restores sexual function. Because loss of libido and sexual dysfunction can be a symptom of depression, it is important to ask about sexual activity before an SSRI or other medication is prescribed.

TRICYCLIC ANTIDEPRESSANTS

TCAs have been available for decades and are as effective as newer agents in the management of depression. However, the tertiary amines, amitriptyline and imipramine, may cause serious anticholinergic side effects. Anticholinergic activity can cause potentially serious side effects such as confusion, drowsiness, orthostatic hypotension, cardiac conduction disturbances, constipation, urinary retention, dry mouth, and blurry vision.

The risk of intraventricular cardiac conduction delay increases among patients with preexisting conduction defects, so a baseline electrocardiogram is needed before TCA begins. Patients taking medications for hypertension or compromised left-ventricular function or who are deconditioned may be at increased risk of orthostatic hypotension when they take TCAs.

If a TCA is chosen, a secondary amine, such as desipramine (Norpramin) or nortriptyline (Pamelor, Aventyl) often is effective and is associated with fewer of these side effects. TCA blood levels, available for desipramine, nortriptyline, and imipramine, can be helpful to address adherence, to assess whether a dose is therapeutic or toxic, and to evaluate drug-drug interactions. Nortriptyline has the best established therapeutic window (50 to 150 ng/mL).

OTHER ANTIDEPRESSANT MEDICATIONS

Medications other than TCAs or SSRIs may be useful in treating patients with depression. These drugs affect neurotransmitter systems in ways that differ somewhat from the ways that TCAs (norepinephrine) or SSRIs (serotonin) do. For example, medications such as venlafaxine (Effexor) have effects on both the norepinephrine and serotonin neurotransmitter systems whereas bupropion (Wellbutrin) acts on the dopamine system. More detailed information about these drugs is provided in Table 11-5.

PROBLEMS WITH ANTIDEPRESSANT MEDICATIONS

DRUG-DRUG INTERACTIONS: THE CYTOCHROME P450 SYSTEM   The cytochrome P450 enzyme system

metabolizes drugs to allow excretion in the urine or bile. Many medications can inhibit enzyme activity by competing for enzyme sites and resulting in increasing levels of another medication. Other medications can increase production of the enzymes and decrease levels of a second drug. Several SSRIs and other antidepressants inhibit the action of these enzymes, potentially causing toxicity.

Because older adults frequently take multiple medications, it is important to carefully review for possible drug-drug interactions before prescribing an antidepressant. However, the need for doing so should not discourage clinicians from prescribing effective antidepressant therapy when it is indicated.

SEROTONIN SYNDROME   Augmented serotonin activity due to therapeutic use, overdose, or combined use of a number of medications, especially SSRIs, monoamine oxidase inhibitor (MAOI) antidepressants, and selegiline (Eldepryl), can cause serotonin syndrome. Serotonin syndrome can be erroneously interpreted as a need for increasing the dose of the offending drug. Meperidine (Demerol) and dextromethorphan are inhibitors of serotonin uptake and can precipitate serotonin syndrome among patients taking SSRIs or MAOIs. TCAs may be associated with serotonin syndrome, especially when used in combination with SSRIs.

Serotonin syndrome causes cognitive symptoms, autonomic nervous system overactivity, and neuromuscular signs. Cognitive symptoms range from confusion, agitation, anxiety, and irritability to drowsiness and unresponsiveness. Hyperthermia, diaphoresis, tachycardia, tachypnea, hypertension, dilated or unreactive pupils, and gastrointestinal symptoms reflect overactivity of the autonomic nervous system. Neuromuscular signs include myoclonus, hyperreflexia, muscular rigidity, tremor, ataxia, clonus, and nystagmus. The manifestations of serotonin syndrome may evolve over a short time. No laboratory tests are available for the diagnosis of serotonin syndrome, but the prognosis is good if the syndrome is recognized. In severe cases sero- tonin receptor blockade may be appropriate (cyproheptadine [Periactin] 4 to 8 mg initially fol- lowed by 4 mg every 2 to 4 h up to 0.5 mg/kg a day or methysergide [Sansert] 2 to 6 mg), but the mainstay of treatment is to discontinue all sero- tonergic drugs.

WITHDRAWAL SYNDROMES When antidepressant medications are withdrawn, patients sometimes have uncomfortable symptoms. For example, dis- continuing TCAs can cause gastrointestinal dis- tress, sleeplessness, movement disturbances, and anxiety. SSRIs and venlafaxine also are associated with a withdrawal syndrome characterized by dizziness, paresthesias, nervousness, nausea, and sleep disturbance. Symptoms similar to with- drawal from tricyclics also may occur.

Patients with reactions that are mild and tol- erable can be treated with watchful waiting because symptoms generally resolve over a few days. More severe reactions may be addressed by means of restarting the antidepressant and tapering the dose over several weeks. An alter- native is to obtain symptomatic relief with lor- azepam for anxiety, meclizine for dizziness, or antihistamines for dystonia. Withdrawal symp- toms can best be prevented by means of gradual tapering of the dose when medication is to be discontinued (e.g., taper by 10 to 20 percent of the dose each week).

LONG-TERM THERAPY WITH ANTIDEPRESSANTS Maintenance therapy, that is, medication use longer than the 4 to 9 months often recom- mended for an episode of depression, may be considered for persons with three or more episodes of major depression. For persons with two or more episodes, maintenance therapy may be recommended when there is a family history of recurrent major depression or of bipo- lar disorder, when past episodes have been severe, sudden, and life-threatening, or when there is a history of recurrent major depression within 1 year of discontinuing effective medica- tion treatment.

Anxiolytics and Other Medications

Other medications that are not typically consid- ered antidepressants sometimes are used to man- age depression. Anxiety symptoms sometimes accompany depression and may be even more prominent than depressive symptoms at initial presentation. In addition, treatment with SSRIs sometimes can increase anxiety early in the course of therapy. For these reasons, benzodi- azepines such as lorazepam (Ativan) may be appropriately prescribed to depressed patients. These agents should be given only in a time- limited manner (for example, for the first 2 to 3 weeks of taking an antidepressant). Benzodi- azepines should not be prescribed as the sole therapy for depression, and they may exacerbate depression in some older persons.

Methylphenidate (Ritalin) sometimes is used to treat medically ill, depressed older patients who do not tolerate or respond to typical antidepres- sants. If tried, methylphenidate may be given in a dose of 5 to 15 mg/d on a time-limited basis (2 to 3 weeks). Careful attention must be paid to devel- opment of adverse effects of the drug, such as tachycardia or delirium. Specialists sometimes prescribe lithium, carbamazepine (Tegretol), an MAOI, or a thyroid supplement to depressed older patients who are resistant or do not respond to other therapeutic interventions.

Electroconvulsive Therapy

Electroconvulsive therapy (ECT) can be life sav- ing, but many myths continue to surround the use of ECT. ECT is safe and effective and should be considered for older patients who have severe or psychotic depression, who have not responded to trials of antidepressant medication in appropriate doses, who have medical contraindications to med- ications, or who need a rapid response because they are in imminent danger from inanition or sui- cide. The main contraindication to ECT relates to the fitness of the patient for anesthesia. Particular attention must be paid to the cardiovascular and respiratory systems in evaluating a patient for ECT. The primary side effects of ECT are memory loss and confusion, which are generally temporary. Preexisting dementia is not a contraindication to ECT.

Referral

When treatment does not diminish depressive symptoms or improve functional status and socialization within 6 to 12 weeks (e.g., the patient has failed a therapeutic trial of adequate doses of medication), the patient may need specialized treatment. Patients who are actively suicidal or psychotic or have a clinical course that suggests a complex diagnostic or therapeutic dilemma should be referred, often as an emergency, and admitted to a hospital if necessary. Older patients with serious substance abuse problems due to alcohol or other drugs may benefit from specialized programs for substance abuse.

Making a successful referral consists of more than giving the patient a telephone number or referral form. The reason for the referral should be clearly stated and discussed with the patient. Most older persons have no experience with mental health professionals and may have outmoded ideas about what the encounter will be like. Patients should be advised that most consultations will require only one or two visits and will not lead to hospitalization. Clinicians need to reassure the patient that the referral does not reflect rejection or abandonment of care. They should emphasize that postconsultation follow-up care will be arranged with the primary health care team. Patients should be encouraged to involve a family member in the consultation visit, if possible.

For some patients, it is necessary to introduce the idea of a referral to a specialist in mental health over several visits rather than presenting the referral as a decision that must be made immediately. Older patients benefit most from a referral when the clinician has a good working relationship with the psychiatrist or other mental health professional, although in the era of managed care, this is sometimes difficult to establish.

Follow-Up Care of Older Patients with Depression

Patients should be observed closely during the first 6 to 12 weeks of therapy for an episode of major depression. If patients show only minimal response at an adequate dose of an antidepressant medication at the end of that time, the diagnosis should be reconsidered and special attention paid to the presence of medical or psychiatric comorbidity. Consideration should be given to switching medications or obtaining a psychiatric consultation. When a patient has a partial response (the patient is better but symptoms or functional impairment persists), medications should be reassessed to ensure they are being administered at appropriate therapeutic dosages. Again, a deficiency that commonly arises in the management of depression in primary care is failure to attain an adequate therapeutic dose for an adequate duration of time. The use of depression assessment scales may assist in evaluating response to therapy. Even among older patients who have recovered from an episode of depression, vigilance can mean early intervention of recurrent episodes. It also is important to be mindful of the possibility that concurrent medical conditions can interfere with symptom resolution.

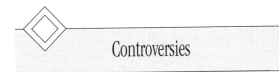

Controversies

We need to learn more about making the primary care setting more effective in detecting and managing depression among older adults. For example, screening for depression frequently is espoused by clinicians, but neither the U.S. Preventive Services Task Force nor the Canadian Task Force on Preventive Health Care recommends screening for depression. Instead, the Guidelines state that clinicians should be alert for signs and symptoms that might stem from depression.

Another controversial issue concerns who should be referred for specialized mental health services assessment and treatment, and at what point in the course of illness the referral should take place. In an era of managed care and carve-outs for mental health, new ways to structure primary health care are needed to improve the management of depression and other mental conditions of older adults.

Clinicians may believe that medical illness is a contraindication to treatment with antidepressants, but older adults with physical illness appear to be just as likely to respond to antidepressant medications, especially an SSRI, as are older patients without physical illness. The presence of somatic symptoms is predictive of a favorable response to fluoxetine among older adults. Randomized controlled trials of paroxetine and of sertraline have shown that these SSRIs are as effective as TCAs and more effective than placebo in the management of depression in late life.

Errors

Older adults are more likely to experience losses than are younger persons—loss of friends and family, loss of social roles, and loss of health and functioning. Most clinicians assume that losses experienced by older adults can explain depression. Although it is important to consider the relation of life events to the onset of depression, it is incorrect to assume that depression is understandable because of these losses. A recent life event should not in itself deter therapy for depression if depression syndrome is present.

Practitioners may be less likely to move from recognition to treatment in the care of older adults than in that of younger adults. Because older patients, clinicians, and families often can find a "reason" for the older person to be depressed, treatment often is delayed or not forthcoming.

Clinicians may focus on anxiety symptoms and may not consider that depression syndrome also is present. In this case patients with both anxiety and depressive symptoms are more likely to receive a benzodiazepine than they are therapy for depression. Benzodiazepines are associated with the potential for dependence, falls, and exacerbation of depression. They should not be used as sole therapy when depression is present.

Family Approach

Family members often bring an older adult into the clinician's office because they are concerned about the behavior of the patient. Family members can provide useful historical information regarding behavior for which the patient is an unreliable informant, such as the occurrence of hallucinations or cognitive impairment. The prescription for increasing pleasurable activities may be more likely to result in change in behavior if the family takes an active role and understands the nature of the illness. Follow-up visits and adherence to pharmacotherapy are more likely to occur when the family is actively involved in the therapeutic plan.

Depressed older adults may be difficult to deal with. Attention to the stresses of the caregiving role, including providing the opportunity for periodic respite from caregiving tasks, is an essential feature of the family approach to care. Some families may try to shield the patient by compensating for or overlooking behavioral difficulties. When it seems necessary, clinicians should broach the subject of elder abuse by asking patients whether they are afraid of anyone or whether someone has hurt them.

Patient Education

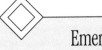

Emerging Concepts

Accepting the diagnosis of depression can be facilitated with several strategies. The patient's problems should not be considered to be all depression or all medical. It is sometimes useful to explain that although the patient has physical conditions or life events that may be related to how the patient is doing, depression may be contributing. Persons whose depression is adequately controlled may deal with their physical problems more effectively.

It is important to emphasize that an evaluation for medical causes of complex symptoms can be concurrent with therapy for depression and that it is important to maintain a positive and hopeful attitude. This may make therapy for depression more effective and assist in the patient's recovery.

If medications are prescribed, the patient should be told that antidepressant medicines are not addictive and that they are not tranquilizers. It may be useful to inform patients that depression is a disorder of altered brain chemistry for which medications are often helpful.

Educating patients in the following three points has been shown to markedly increase the proportion of patients who continue to take medication for an appropriate interval: (1) that the medication will take at least 2 to 4 weeks to work; (2) that side effects may occur but generally resolve with continued treatment; and (3) that the medication has to be continued even if the patient is feeling better.

Refusal to accept the diagnosis of depression should not be taken as a now or never proposition. These issues may have to be readdressed at subsequent visits. A handout providing information about depression and antidepressant medications can assist in this educational process, as can recommended self-help materials (Tables 11-6 and 11-7).

Subsyndromal Depression

Many older adults with clinically significant depression do not meet standard criteria for having major depression, perhaps because it is difficult to assess symptoms such as sleep disturbance in the context of medical illness. In other cases, because older persons convincingly deny having depression, clinicians may not ask about additional symptoms that may suggest depression is present. Subsyndromal, or minor depression frequently exists among patients with marked functional loss that does not fulfill the criteria for major depression or dysthymia. Subsyndromal depression is an active area of investigation, and little is known about treatment implications. Several studies addressing the management of so-called minor depression among older primary care patients are underway or planned.

Vascular Depression

There may be a vascular disease–associated depression that occurs in late life. It is characterized by cognitive deficits and psychomotor retardation with parallels to disease such as Parkinson's disease that involve subcortical brain structures. Lesions in frontocaudate circuits appear to be associated with anhedonia, cognitive dysfunction, and psychomotor retardation—a depression-like syndrome but without mood disturbance. Similar lesions have been reported to occur among older patients with minor depression. This evolving set of observations emphasizes the heterogeneity of the depression syndrome. It suggests the elderly may be prone to a form of depression that falls outside standard sets of criteria but that may be closely associated with vascular lesions in the central nervous system.

Table 11-6
Handout for Older Adults

DEPRESSION: A SERIOUS BUT TREATABLE ILLNESS
Everyone gets the blues now and then. It's part of life. But when there is little joy or pleasure after visiting with friends or seeing a good movie, there may be a more serious problem. Being depressed for a while, without letup, can change the way a person thinks or feels. Doctors call this "clinical depression." Being "down in the dumps" over a period of time is not a normal part of growing old. But it is a common problem, and medical help may be needed. For most people, depression can be treated successfully. "Talk" therapies, medications, or other methods of treatment can ease the pain of depression. There is no reason to suffer. There are many reasons why depression in older people often is missed or untreated. As a person ages, the signs of depression are much more likely to be dismissed as crankiness or grumpiness. Depression can also be tricky to recognize. Confusion or attention problems caused by depression can sometimes look like Alzheimer's disease or other brain disorders. Mood changes and signs of depression can be caused by medicines older people may take for high blood pressure or heart disease. Depression can happen at the same time as other chronic diseases. It can be hard for a doctor to diagnose depression, but the good news is that people who are depressed can get better with the right treatment.
WHAT TO LOOK FOR
How do you know when help is needed? After all, older people may have to face the kinds of problems that could cause anyone to feel "depressed." Many older people have to deal with the death of loved ones or friends. Some may have a tough time getting used to retirement. Others are trying to deal with chronic illness. But after a period of grieving or feeling troubled, most older people do get back to their daily lives. A person who is clinically depressed continues to have trouble coping both mentally and physically and may not feel better for weeks, months, or even years. Here is a list of the most common signs of depression. If these last for more than 2 weeks, tell your doctor about them: • An "empty" feeling, ongoing sadness, and anxiety • Tiredness, lack of energy • Loss of interest or pleasure in everyday activities, including sex • Sleep problems, including very early morning waking • Problems with eating and weight (gain or loss) • A lot of crying • Aches and pains that just won't go away • A hard time focusing, remembering, or making decisions • Feeling that the future looks grim; feeling guilty, helpless, or worthless • Being irritable • Thoughts of death or suicide; a suicide attempt Families, friends, and health workers should watch for clues of depression in older people. Sometimes depression can hide behind a smiling face. A depressed person who lives alone may briefly feel better when someone stops by to say hello or during a visit to the doctor. Symptoms may seem to go away, but when someone is very depressed, the signs come right back. Don't ignore the warning signs. Serious depression can lead to suicide. Listen carefully if someone complains about being depressed or says people don't care.

Table 11-6
Handout for Older Adults (*continued*)

WHAT CAUSES DEPRESSION?
There is no one cause of depression. Depression often strikes people who felt fine but who are struggling with a death in the family or a sudden illness. Sometimes differences in brain chemistry can affect mood and cause depression. Sometimes people become depressed for no clear reason. Depression is sometimes linked to prescription drugs or certain illnesses. Studies show that depression may run in families.
TREATING DEPRESSION
Depression can be treated successfully. Support groups or other social activities can improve mood. Several kinds of "talk" therapies may be useful as well. One method helps people change negative thinking patterns that might have led to depression. Antidepressant medications can also help by improving mood, sleep, appetite, and concentration. Most antidepressant medicines take 6 to 12 weeks before there are real signs of progress, and medicines may have to be used for 6 months or more after symptoms disappear. Older people often take many drugs, and it is important for your doctor to know about all prescribed and over-the-counter medicines being taken.
GETTING HELP
The first step to getting help is to accept that help is needed. The subject of depression and mental illness still makes some people uncomfortable. Some feel that getting help is a sign of weakness. Once you have decided to get help, start with your family doctor. The doctor should check to see if there are medical reasons for the depression. If a depressed older person won't go to a doctor for treatment, relatives or friends can help. They can explain how treatment may help the person feel better. Sometimes a phone call or home visit by the family doctor can break the ice.
PREVENTION
There are some practical steps you can take to prevent depression. One way to prepare for major changes in life, such as retirement, is to keep and maintain friendships over the years. You can also develop interests or hobbies, keep the mind and body active, and stay in touch with family to help limit the effects of depression. Being physically fit and eating a balanced diet are ways to help avoid illnesses that can bring on depression.

SOURCE: Adapted with permission from the National Institute on Aging: *Depression: A Serious but Treatable Illness.* Age Page. Bethesda, MD, US Department of Health and Human Services, Public Health Service, National Institutes of Health, 1998.

Depression as a Chronic Illness

The concept of depression as a chronic illness such as diabetes, as opposed to an episodic illness, has emerged from follow-up studies that have shown that persons who have had an episode of major depression are prone to have additional episodes. Older adults may take longer to recover from depression and have shorter times to relapse than do younger persons. Implications for health care delivery of casting depression in the framework of a chronic illness may lead to the development of disease management models for depression in primary care. This might include development of guidelines, more involvement by nurse or case managers, regular telephone follow-

Table 11-7

Self-Help Materials Related to Depression That May Be Helpful to Older Adults

WRITTEN MATERIAL
Bloomfield HH, McWilliams P: *How to Heal Depression*. Los Angeles: Prelude Press; 1994.
Mathiasen P, Levert S: *Late Life Depression*. New York: Dell Publishing; 1997.
Agency for Health Care Policy and Research: *Depression Is a Treatable Illness: A Patient's Guide*. Washington, DC: US Government Printing Office; 1993 (available from AHCPR, below).

OTHER SOURCES
National Institute of Mental Health, (800) 421-4211 *www.nimh.nih.gov/dart/index.htm*
National Depressive and Manic-depressive Association, (800) 826-3632 *www.ndmda.org*
National Mental Health Association, (800) 969-NMHA or 800-433-5959 (TTY) *www.nmha.org*
Agency for Health Care Policy and Research, (800) 358-9295 *www.ahcpr.gov*

up sessions to monitor the patient's condition, and long-term drug treatment.

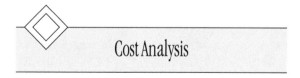

Cost Analysis

TCAs are as effective as SSRIs in the management of depression among patients who can reach and maintain a therapeutic dose. The response rate is 60 to 70 percent with either class of drug. However, SSRIs appear to offer advantages over TCAs that are related to tolerance of side effects, ease of dosing, and diminished danger of toxicity in the event of a suicide attempt.

There have been no economic studies of the cost-effectiveness of antidepressant drugs that focus specifically on the elderly. Although SSRIs may have a higher initial cost, there is evidence in the care of younger persons that these medications are better tolerated than are TCAs, leading to better outcomes with fewer contacts with the health care system. For example, studying more than 13,000 cases in which clinicians reported starting, changing, or discontinuing a prescription for an SSRI or TCA, Martin and colleagues found that general practitioners were less likely to discontinue SSRIs than they were TCAs, even after adjustment for age, sex, and severity of depression. For patients who must pay for their own medications, such as the elderly under Medicare, the cost of the antidepressant itself may be the primary consideration, offsetting any potential savings to the health care system.

Summary

Primary care will continue to occupy a strategic position in the evaluation and treatment of older persons with depression and other mental conditions. Given the demographic changes in the population of the United States, to minimize disability caused by depression, it will be necessary to make primary care of patients with depression as effective as possible. It can be rewarding to clinicians to treat patients with depression. The challenge is to integrate the physical and mental health care of older persons.

Bibliography

Adams WL: Alcohol use in retirement communities. *J Am Geriatr Soc* 44:1082, 1996.

Adams WL, Barry KL, Fleming MF: Screening for problem drinking in older primary care patients. *JAMA* 276:1964,1996.

Alexopoulos GS, Meyers BS, Young RC, et al: "Vascular depression" hypothesis. *Arch Gen Psychiatry* 54:915, 1997.

American Psychiatric Association: *Diagnostic and Statistical Manual of Mental Disorders, DSM-IV*, 4th ed. Washington, DC: American Psychiatric Association; 1994.

American Psychiatric Association Work Group on Major Depressive Disorder: *Practice Guideline for Major Depressive Disorder in Adults.* Washington, DC: American Psychiatric Association; 1993.

Anthony JC, Aboraya A: The epidemiology of selected mental disorders in later life. In: Birren JE, Sloane RB, Cohen GD (eds): *Handbook of Mental Health and Aging,* 2d ed. New York: Academic Press; 1992;27.

Bassuk SS, Berkman LF, Wypij D: Depressive symptomatology and incident cognitive decline in an elderly community sample. *Arch Gen Psychiatry* 55:1073, 1998.

Beck AT, Rush AJ, Shaw BF, Emery G: *Cognitive Therapy of Depression.* New York: Guilford Press; 1979.

Beresford T, Gomberg E: *Alcohol and Aging.* New York: Oxford University Press; 1995.

Brody DS, Thompson TL, Larson DB, et al: Strategies for counseling depressed patients by primary care physicians. *J Gen Intern Med* 9:569, 1994.

Burgio LD, Sinnott J: Behavioral treatments and pharmacotherapy: acceptability ratings by elderly individuals in residential settings. *Gerontologist* 30:811, 1990.

Caine ED: Pseudodementia. *Arch Gen Psychiatry* 38: 1359, 1981.

Callahan CM, Hendrie HC, Nienaber NA, Tierney WM: Suicidal ideation among older primary care patients. *J Am Geriatr Soc* 44:1205, 1996.

Callahan CM, Hui SL, Nienaber NA, et al: Longitudinal study of depression and health services use among elderly primary care patients. *J Am Geriatr Soc* 42:833, 1994.

Canadian Task Force on Preventive Health Care: *The Canadian Guide to Clinical Preventive Health Care.* Ottawa, Ontario, Canada: Canadian Government Publishing; 1994.

Cole MG, Bellavance F: The prognosis of depression in old age. *Am J Geriatr Psychiatry* 5:4, 1997.

Cupp MJ, Tracy TS: Cytochrome P450: new nomenclature and clinical implications. *Am Fam Physician* 57:107,1998.

Depression Guideline Panel: *Depression in Primary Care, Volume 1: Detection and Diagnosis.* Clinical Practice Guideline no. 5, AHCPR publication no. 93-0550; Rockville, MD, US Department of Health and Human Services, Public Health Service, Agency for Health Care Policy and Research, 1993.

Depression Guideline Panel: *Depression in Primary Care, Volume 2: Treatment of Major Depression.* Clinical Practice Guideline no. 5, AHCPR Publication Number 93-0551. Rockville, MD, US Department of Health and Human Services, Public Health Service, Agency for Health Care Policy and Research; 1993.

Devanand DP, Sano M, Tang MX, et al: Depressed mood and the incidence of Alzheimer's disease in the elderly living in the community. *Arch Gen Psychiatry* 53:175, 1996.

Flint AJ, Rifat SL: Anxious depression in elderly patients: response to antidepressant treatment. *Am J Geriatr Psychiatry* 5:107, 1997.

Flint AJ, Rifat SJ: Two-year outcome of elderly patients with anxious depression. *Psychiatry Res* 66:23, 1997.

Gallo JJ: TCAs vs. SSRIs: same bang for whose buck? *Arch Fam Med* 8:326, 1999.

Gallo JJ, Marino S, Ford D, Anthony JC: Filters on the pathway to mental health care: II. sociodemographic factors. *Psychol Med* 25:1149, 1995.

Gallo JJ, Rabins PV, Iliffe S: The "research magnificent" in late life: psychiatric epidemiology and the primary health care of older adults. *Int J Psychiatry Med* 27:185, 1997.

Gallo JJ, Rabins PV, Lyketsos CG, et al: Depression without sadness: functional outcomes of nondysphoric depression in later life. *J Am Geriatr Soc* 45:570, 1997.

Gallo JJ, Fulmer T, Paveza GJ, Reichel W: *Handbook of Geriatric Assessment,* 3rd ed. Gaithersburg, MD: Aspen Publishers, 2000.

Hirschfield RMA, Keller MB, Panico S, et al: The National Depressive and Manic-Depressive Association consensus statement on the undertreatment of depression. *JAMA* 277:333, 1997.

Hughes D, Morris S, McGuire A: The cost of depression in the elderly: effects of drug therapy. *Drugs Aging* 10:59, 1997.

Iliffe S, Tai SS, Haines A, et al: Assessment of elderly people in general practice: 4. depression, functional ability and contact with services. *Br J Gen Pract* 43:371, 1993.

Kivela SL, Pahkala K, Eronen P: Depressive symptoms and signs that differentiate major and atypical depression from dysthymic disorder in elderly Finns. *Int J Geriatr Psychiatry* 4:79, 1988.

Klerman GL, Weissman MM, Rounsaville BJ, Chevron ES: *Interpersonal Psychotherapy of Depression.* London, UK: Jason Aronson; 1997.

Klinkman MS, Schwenk TL, Coyne JC: Depression in primary care—more like asthma than appendicitis: the Michigan Depression Project. *Can J Psychiatry* 42:966, 1997.

Krishnan KRR, Hays JC, Blazer DG: MRI-defined vascular depression. *Am J Psychiatry* 157:497, 1997.

Kumar A, Schweitzer E, Zhisong J, et al: Neuroanatomical substrates of late-life minor depression. *Arch Neurol* 54:613, 1997.

Lebowitz BD, Pearson JL, Schneider LS, et al: Diagnosis and treatment of depression in late life: consensus statement update. *JAMA* 278:1186, 1997.

Lehmann SW, Rabins PV: Clinical geropsychiatry,in: Gallo JJ, Busby-Whitehead J, Rabins PV, et al (eds): *Reichel's Care of the Elderly: Clinical Aspects of Aging,* 5th ed. Baltimore: Lippincott Williams & Wilkins; 1999;179.

Lin EH, Von Korff M, Katon W, et al: The role of the primary care physician in patients' adherence to antidepressant therapy. *Med Care* 33:67, 1995.

Lundervold D, Lewin LM: Older adults' acceptability of pharmacotherapy and behavior therapy for depression: initial results. *J Appl Gerontol* 9:211, 1990.

Lyketsos CG, Steele CD, Steinberg M: Behavioral disturbances in dementia, In: Gallo JJ, Busby-Whitehead J, Rabins PV, Silliman R, Murphy J (eds): *Reichel's Care of the Elderly: Clinical Aspects of Aging,* 5th ed. Baltimore: Lippincott Williams & Wilkins; 1999:214.

Martin RM, Hilton SR, Kerry SM, Richards NM: General practitioners' perceptions of the tolerability of antidepressant drugs: a comparison of selective serotonin reuptake inhibitors and tricyclic antidepressants. *BMJ* 314:646, 1997.

Mills KC: Serotonin syndrome. *Am Fam Physician* 52:1475, 1995.

Nezu AM, Nezu CM, Perri MG: *Problem-solving Therapy for Depression: Theory, Research, and Clinical Guidelines.* New York: Wiley; 1989.

Niederehe G: Psychosocial treatments with depressed older adults. *Am J Geriatr Psychiatry* 4 (suppl 1):S66, 1996.

Penninx WJH, Guralnik JM, Ferrucci L, et al: Depressive symptoms and physical decline in community-dwelling older persons. *JAMA* 279:1720, 1998.

Rabins PV, Merchant A, Nestadt G: Criteria for diagnosing reversible dementia caused by depression: validation by 2-year follow-up. *Br J Psychiatry* 144:488, 1984.

Radloff LS: The CES-D scale: a self-report depression scale for research in the general population. *Appl Psychol Meas* 1:385, 1977.

Reynolds CF, Frank E, Kupfer DJ, et al: Treatment outcome in recurrent major depression: post hoc comparison of elderly ("young old") and midline patients. *Am J Psychiatry* 153:1288, 1996.

Reynolds CF, Frank E, Perel JM, et al: High relapse rate after discontinuation of adjunctive medication for elderly patients with recurrent major depression. *Am J Psychiatry* 153:1418, 1996.

Reynolds CF, Frank E, Perel JM, et al: Nortriptyline and interpersonal psychotherapy as maintenance therapies for recurrent major depression: a randomized controlled trial in patients older than 59 years. *JAMA* 281:39, 1999.

Reynolds CF, Kupfer DJ, Hoch CC, et al: Two-year follow-up of elderly patients with mixed depression and dementia: clinical and electroencephalographic sleep findings. *J Am Geriatr Soc* 34:793, 1986.

Reynolds CF, Schneider LS, Lebowitz BD, Kupfer DJ: Treatment of depression in elderly patients: guidelines for primary care. In: Schneider LS, Reynolds CF, Lebowitz BD, Friedhoff AJ (eds): *Diagnosis and Treatment of Depression in Late Life: Results of the NIH Consensus Development Conference.* Wasington, DC: American Psychiatric Association; 1994:463.

Robertson MM, Katona CLE: *Depression and Physical Illness.* New York: John Wiley & Sons; 1997.

Robins LN, Regier DA: *Psychiatric Disorders in America: The Epidemiologic Catchment Area Study.* New York: Free Press; 1991.

Rovner B, Broadhead J, Spencer M: Depression in Alzheimer's disease. *Am J Psychiatry* 146:350, 1989.

Schneider LS: Pharmacologic considerations in the treatment of late-life depression. *Am J Geriatr Psychiatry* 4 (suppl 1):S51, 1996.

Schneider LS, Olin JT: Efficacy of acute treatment for geriatric depression. *Int Psychogeriatr* 7 (suppl):7, 1995.

Schulberg HC, Block MR, Madonia MJ, et al: Treating major depression in primary care practice: eight-month clinical outcomes. *Arch Gen Psychiatry* 53:913, 1996.

Schulberg HC, Mulsant B, Schulz R, et al: Major depression in older primary care patients. Presented at Spotlight on the Elderly: Eleventh Annual NIMH International Research Conference on Mental Health Problems in the General Health Care Sector; Washington, D.C., 1997.

Shearer SL, Adams GK: Nonpharmacologic aids in the treatment of depression. *Am Fam Physician* 47:435, 1993.

Simon GE, VonKorff M, Heiligenstein JH, et al: Initial antidepressant choice in primary care: effectiveness and cost of fluoxetine vs. tricyclic antidepressants. *JAMA* 275:1897, 1996.

Skoog I: The prevalence of psychotic, depressive, and anxiety syndromes in demented and non-demented 85-year olds. *Int J Geriatr Psychiatry* 8:247, 1993.

Skoog I, Aevarsson O, Beskow J: Suicidal feelings in a population sample of 85 year olds. *Am J Psychiatry* 153:1015, 1996.

Small GW, Hamilton SH, Bystritsky A, et al: Fluoxetine Collaborative Study Group A: Clinical response predictors in a double-blind, placebo-controlled trial of fluoxetine for geriatric major depression. *Int Psychogeriatr* 7:41, 1995.

Unutzer J, Patrick DL, Simon G, et al: Depressive symptoms and the cost of health services in HMO patients aged 65 years and older: a 4-year prospective study. *JAMA* 277:1618, 1997.

US Preventive Services Task Force: *Guide to Clinical Preventive Services: An Assessment of the Effectiveness of 169 Interventions,* 2d ed. Baltimore: Williams & Wilkins; 1996.

Wagner EH, Austin BT, Von Korff M: Organizing care for patients with chronic illness. *Milbank Q* 74:511, 1996.

Wells KB, Stewart A, Hays RD, et al: The functioning and well-being of depressed patients: results from the Medical Outcomes Study. *JAMA* 262:914, 1989.

Wolfe RM: Antidepressant withdrawal reactions. *Am Fam Physician* 56:455, 1997.

Wragg RE, Jeste DV: Overview of depression and psychosis in Alzheimer's disease. *Am J Psychiatry* 146:577, 1989.

Yesavage JA, Brink TL: Development and validation of a geriatric depression screening scale: a preliminary report. *J Psychiatr Res* 17:37, 1983.

Mel P. Daly

Dementia

Dementia is a condition characterized by impairments in higher cognitive function in patients who have a clear sensorium. This contrasts with delirium, in which the sensorium is also impaired. Memory loss often occurs, but many other domains of higher cognitive functioning (concentration, abstract reasoning, calculation, language functioning, praxis, visuospatial orientation, decision-making abilities, etc.) can also be affected, depending on the underlying causes. These impairments result in the reduced ability of patients with dementia to perform tasks (paying bills, making decisions about health and finances, etc.) that require integration and processing of information necessary to live independently. Frequently, patients with dementia may not present with memory loss, as it may not be the most disabling cognitive impairment among patients presenting with dementing illnesses. Therefore, a high index of suspicion that this disorder exists should be entertained for patients who present with changes in behavior,

orientation, language, and ability to perform normal activities of daily living (ADLs).

Overview: How Common Are Memory Problems in the Office Practice?

Dementia is by far the most common age-associated neurologic diagnosis. The incidence of dementia doubles every 5 years after the age of 65. The prevalence of dementia is approximately 1 percent in 60-year-olds; however, by the age of 85, 30 to 45 percent are affected. Over 65 percent of persons residing in nursing homes have some form of dementia. As the population of the United States over the age of 65 years increases, the prevalence and incidence of memory problems related to dementia will likely increase. This will place a substantial burden on the health care system, with estimated annualized costs exceeding $100 billion.

Principal Diagnoses

What Are the Most Likely Diagnoses Based on the Prevalence of Disease in Different Age Groups?

NORMAL AGING

Normal cognitive aging is a heterogeneous process. Most elderly persons perform as well, if not better, on formal cognitive testing than younger persons tested; however, performance on these tests can be influenced by motivation, educational background, concomitant medical and/or psychiatric or psychological illness, and personality (Table 12-1).

Table 12-1

Causes of Memory Loss and Dementia

Age-associated memory loss/benign
    senile forgetfulness
Alzheimer's disease
Multi-infarct dementia
    Embolic events
    Atherosclerosis
    Vasculitis
    Mixed etiologies
Frontal lobe dementia (Pick's disease)
Diffuse Lewy body dementia
Dementia associated with Parkinson's disease
Alcohol-related dementia
Normal pressure hydrocephalus
    Communicating
    Noncommunicating
Huntington's disease
Jakob-Creutzfeldt disease or other slow viruses

Most studies suggest that short-term (working memory) does not change with normal aging. The rate at which new information can be stored in learned memory, however, is variable. In general, the total amount of memory that can be stored continues to grow well into late old age.

Process-oriented memory can decline with aging. This can affect an older individual's ability to derive conclusions from newly integrated information that may require integration and action based on the information provided. This can affect how older persons adjust to changing information demands, yet in most instances, these changes do not meet the criteria for a dementing illness.

Benign senescent forgetfulness can occur in "normal" older persons, but it is usually not associated with other aspects of cognitive impairment and rarely affects daily functioning. It can be difficult to distinguish normal forgetfulness associated with aging from the early manifestations of impaired cognitive functioning associated with a dementing illness.

ALZHEIMER'S DISEASE

Alzheimer's disease (AD) is the most common cause for dementia. It is a progressive disorder characterized by impairment in higher neuropsychiatric and cognitive functioning, manifested by changes in behavior, personality, and reduced ability to perform normal daily activities. In most clinical settings in which patients present with signs and symptoms of memory loss, 50 to 70 percent of patients will be ultimately diagnosed with "probable AD" or AD coexisting with another condition, such as multi-infarct dementia.

Although a definitive diagnosis of AD can only be determined by autopsy, it is estimated that the diagnosis can be made with 80 to 85 percent accuracy using clinical and laboratory and radiologic testing.

AD is a true "cortical dementia," in that patients are frequently active, disinhibited, and often childlike in their behavior. Only in the later stages of AD do patients frequently become apathetic and lose motor functioning.

MULTI-INFARCT DEMENTIA

The next most common cause of dementia is multi-infarct vascular disease. Multi-infarct dementia (MID) frequently occurs as a result of vascular ischemic events. These take place in both the cortical and subcortical areas of the brain. Cerebral amyloid angiopathy can occur concomitantly and confuse the clinical presentation, probably because amyloid deposition can also occur in AD (causing similar symptoms). Atherothrombotic stroke, cardiogenic (embolic), and lacunar (secondary to hypertensive hyalinosis) disease most often account for vascular mechanisms causing dementia. This combination of pathologies constitutes approximately 15 to 30 percent of patients with full-blown dementia. Widespread vascular events related to underlying hypertensive disease is the most frequent cause.

FRONTAL-LOBE DEMENTIA

Another common cause of cortical dementia syndrome is the so-called frontal-type dementia, of which Pick's disease is the most common example. Frontal-type dementia is characteristically associated with significant behavioral and personality changes, such as disinhibited sexual behaviors, hyperorality, and incontinence in inappropriate settings.

DIFFUSE LEWY BODY DEMENTIA

Diffuse Lewy body dementia (DLB) is a disorder that is characterized by extrapyramidal motor symptoms (that are often indistinguishable from patients with Parkinson's disease) that frequently occur at the same time that symptoms of dementia occur. Patients with DLB dementia also often have fluctuations in alertness and can have hallucinations and delusions. Cognitive functioning may be variable. Recent studies suggest that DLB dementia may be far more common than previously appreciated.

DEMENTIA ASSOCIATED WITH PARKINSON'S DISEASE

After a number of years, up to 40 percent of patients with Parkinson's disease (PD) develop dementing illness that is frequently indistinguishable from AD. Patients with PD typically display symptoms that reflect a general slowing of cognition and an inability to perform higher executive function tasks, in conjunction with the typical progressive motor signs and symptoms of PD (bradykinesia, rigidity, and tremor).

NORMAL PRESSURE HYDROCEPHALUS

The dementia associated with normal pressure hydrocephalus (NPH) is characterized by a clinical triad of gait apraxia, dementia, and urinary incontinence. These symptoms can occur at any time during the illness; however, the full triad of symptoms may only be present when the patient develops dementia. The mechanism that causes brain dysfunction in patients with NPH is unknown, but it may relate to changes in cerebrospinal fluid composition and to changes in how the cerebrospinal fluid (CSF) is absorbed.

ALCOHOL-RELATED DEMENTIA

Dementia frequently occurs in the context of chronic alcohol abuse. This dementia should be distinguished from the amnesia and characteristic pathology of the Wernicke-Korsakoff syndrome (confabulation, lack of awareness, and normal motor activity). Often, patients with chronic alcohol abuse have other underlying etiologies for their cognitive impairment (AD, MID, etc.).

RARE CAUSES OF IRREVERSIBLE DEMENTIA

Other, very rare, causes of dementia exist. These should be considered in the differential diagnosis for patients with atypical presentations. Examples include Jakob-Creutzfeldt disease (a slow viral encephalopathy, that presents with dementia associated with myoclonus), Huntington's chorea (a genetic, autosomal dominant disorder characterized by choreoform movements and behavioral disturbances), dementia pugilistica, progressive supranuclear palsy, cortical basal degeneration, primary progressive aphasia, and the ALS/parkinsonian/dementia complex of Guam.

REVERSIBLE CAUSES OF DEMENTIA

Many older persons with changes in cognition have potentially reversible causes that can often be readily identified (Table 12-2). These include the following.

DEMENTIA ASSOCIATED WITH DEPRESSION It is estimated that up to 15 percent of patients who present with memory impairment or who are unable to perform higher cognitive functioning tasks may have some degree of underlying depression. This depression can be difficult to distinguish from other causes of dementia and may require a trial of treatment for depression that in some cases, reverses impairments in cognitive functioning.

THYROID DISEASE There is well-documented evidence that under- or overactive thyroid functioning can contribute to impairments in higher cognitive functioning. Older patients with thyroid disease can present atypically (e.g., apathetic hyperthyroidism), and dementia can be a clue that impairments of thyroid functioning exist.

OTHER CAUSES Vitamin B_{12} and folic acid deficiency has been associated with changes in higher cognitive functioning resulting in a dementing illness. Tertiary syphilis can also cause a dementia-like illness and should always be considered in the differential diagnosis, especially among older persons who may have been exposed to syphilis during war-time years. Systemic illnesses, including infectious diseases (HIV virus, tuberculosis, hepatitis, and chronic fatigue syndrome), have been implicated. HIV-associated dementia is rare in older persons. It should be considered, however, among persons who have signs and symptoms of dementia and received a blood transfusion in the years between 1978 and 1985 or who had unprotected sexual intercourse with prostitutes.

Delirium can cause acute and subacute cognitive impairment in older persons. An inability to concentrate and a reduced attention span characterize this syndrome. Patients often fail to register new information or engage in sustained levels of cognitive activity. There are many causes for delirium. Patients who present with acute or subacute changes in cognitive functioning should always be investigated for delirium. Elderly patients with dementia are particularly vulnerable to delirium when acute illness (infection, ischemia, hypoxemia, dehydration, blood loss, etc) occurs. Patients with dementia who undergo general anesthesia are especially susceptible to developing postoperative delirium.

MEDICATION-RELATED DEMENTIA Medications can be a potential cause of changes (including chronic changes) in levels of higher cognitive functioning. Typically, this can occur with sedating agents such as benzodiazepines, major tranquilizers, sedating antihistamines, sedating antihypertensive medications, and beta-blockers. Older persons can be more prone to side effects of these classes of drugs and to the toxicity associated with their use. This is because age-associated changes in

Table 12-2

Potentially Reversible Causes of Memory Loss and Dementia

Prescription drug toxicities
Delirium (multiple potential causes)
Pseudodementia (dementia associated with
   depression)
Hypothyroidism or hyperthyroidism
Vitamin B_{12} deficiency
Folic acid deficiency
Tertiary syphilis
Other nutritional deficiencies
Central nervous system space-occupying
   lesions
   Subdural hematoma
   Brain tumors (primary or metastatic)
   Abscess
   Meningioma
Systemic illnesses
   Chronic fatigue syndrome
   HIV disease
   Tuberculosis
   Other bacterial and viral encephalitides

total body fat accumulation and impaired abilities to metabolize and excrete drugs can result in higher serum and central nervous system levels of many medications.

What Are Serious or Life-Threatening Diagnoses to Consider?

Most patients with dementia have a chronic and relapsing form of dementia (e.g., AD, MID). Memory loss as a presenting symptom and dementia as an illness typically present insidiously and require careful diagnostic evaluation and ongoing therapeutic interventions over time. Occasionally, patients present with an acute and subacute clinical presentation that can suggest a condition that is life-threatening. This clinical situation most commonly occurs in patients with acute reversible causes for dementia or delirium. Intracerebral abscesses, subdural hematomas, and any condition (that may be reversible) causing delirium should prompt an immediate evaluation to identify potentially life-threatening causes. Meningitis and encephalitis should also be considered if a patient develops an acute or subacute relapsing clinical presentation. Very rarely, patients with brain tumors can present with a clinical picture suggestive of a dementing illness. These patients require an aggressive approach to diagnosing and treating the condition, but rarely (except in the context of an acute presentation) do these conditions require an emergency intervention or treatment to reverse a life-threatening condition.

Typical Presentation

How Do Different Symptoms Suggest One Diagnosis or Another?

Although complaints of memory disturbance and slowing of cognition are commonly ascribed to

the aging process, there is little evidence to suggest that this is so. The only consistent finding in studies assessing cognitive functioning with advancing years is a general slowing of processing. Thus, when memory loss occurs in older persons, it should never be considered a normal concomitant of aging until potential causes are ruled out.

There are many reversible causes for changes in higher cognitive functioning, including delirium (and its myriad of causes), depression, and comorbid medical illnesses. Each of these disorders has its own disorder-specific presentation and should always be considered. It is important to remember that older individuals presenting with any of these disorders can do so atypically.

Nonreversible dementias can often be distinguished based on the patient's presenting symptoms and symptoms that can occur as part of the natural history of the disorder.

ALZHEIMER'S DISEASE

Alzheimer's disease typically presents with impairment of higher cognitive functioning that interferes with a person's ability to perform basic and instrumental activities of daily living (IADLs). Early in the course of the disease, forgetfulness and difficulties with higher executive functioning are typical. In the early stages of AD, the ability to accomplish familiar tasks (planning meals, using a telephone, driving, and self-care activities) is usually preserved. Persons with mild to moderate AD have difficulties learning new information. When patients become unable to perform these activities, they or family members usually become concerned and present for evaluation. Patients with mild to moderate AD are generally active, disinhibited, and unconcerned. Occasionally, patients with AD exhibit "catastrophic" reactions reflecting an awareness on their part that they are unable to perform familiar tasks. A characteristic feature of patients with early to middle AD is a lack of insight that can, in later stages of AD, translate into apathy and abulia (an inability to act, initiate, or decide).

As the disease progresses, patients can develop behavioral changes, such as asking the same question repeatedly, getting lost and wandering, and ultimately, being unable to perform usual tasks. Other symptoms that can manifest in the middle to later phases of the disease include irritability, apathy, psychosis, disorientation, and agitation. Eventually, patients with AD become completely dependent on others for all of their physical and self-care activities.

VASCULAR DEMENTIA

Features suggestive of a vascular dementia include abrupt or step-wise onset of cognitive deficits that are often temporally associated with an acute cerebrovascular event. There are often associated abnormalities on neurologic examination. The diagnosis, however, is often difficult to make because many patients with vascular dementias present with signs and symptoms that only by a process of exclusion can be ascribed to a vascular dementia. Patients with vascular dementias can have coexisting AD, and often it is impossible to distinguish between these conditions.

Vascular dementia is a heterogeneous condition with symptoms and signs such as sudden onset of aphasia, amnesia, or agnosia. Lacunar infarcts can result in a dementia that is step-wise or progressive, yet may be associated with focal deficits, or can cause symptoms of subcortical dementia: apathy, bradyphrenia, rigidity, and bradykinesia. This presentation of dementia may be indistinguishable from the presentation of a dementia syndrome associated with depression (pseudodementia). Diffuse cortical atherosclerosis can result in dementia associated with a variety of motor and behavioral symptoms.

FRONTOTEMPORAL DEMENTIA

These disorders are much less common than either AD or MID. The diagnosis is suggested by clinical symptoms of dementia associated with disproportionate impairments in reasoning and judgment. Patients with frontotemporal dementia can have impairments in memory, characteristically they have grossly disturbed judgment, decreased mental flexibility, and behavioral disturbances, such as inappropriate social behavior (aggression, hyperactivity, ebullience, and hypersexuality). In the later phases of these disorders, patients ultimately progress to apathy and abulia.

DEMENTIA ASSOCIATED WITH PARKINSON'S DISEASE

Among patients with PD, approximately 30 to 40 percent will develop dementia. Dementia is frequently underdiagnosed in these patients since motor functioning is the overwhelming clinical presentation. The characteristic physical findings of PD usually precede symptoms of cognitive impairment by a number of years. Patients who present with motor symptoms relatively contemporaneous with cognitive symptoms frequently have DLB disease. Pathologic features of AD, PD, and DLB frequently coexist. Patients with dementia associated with PD usually have more preserved recent memory but more impaired higher executive functioning than a typical patient with AD. Apathy, lack of initiative, and impaired executive level functioning are characteristic. Unlike most other dementing illnesses, patients with dementia associated with PD can have concomitant (often graphic and disturbing) visual hallucinations.

OTHER CAUSES OF DEMENTIA

NPH is a rare disorder that is characterized by a triad of dementia, urinary incontinence, and gait apraxia. The memory disturbance is usually mild, and urinary incontinence is not universally present. The gait disorder, however, is distinctive, characterized by an inability to initiate gait (magnetic gait). This gait is different to the gait of PD in that patients with NPH have no difficulty in initiating movement; however, each step is deliberately taken and is as if each foot is magnetically attached to the ground. Patients with PD, once they "get going," typically have a festinating gait and have difficulty stopping on command.

Patients with alcohol-related dementia usually are apathetic and often irritable, especially when questioned about cognitive functioning. Memory, orientation, and attention are variably involved. Although both hyper- and hypothyroidism can cause dementia, older persons with hyperthyroidism can present with a dementia associated with apathy. Psychosis can occur in either condition. Vitamin B_{12} deficiency can be associated with a dementia that is characterized by slowness, confusion, irritability, and apathy. Dementia can occur coexistently with other systemic disorders, such as diabetes mellitus, chronic fatigue syndrome, and HIV infection. These disorders characteristically cause noncortical dementia that presents with apathy, chronic fatigue, and slowing in cognition (in the context of systemic illness).

Are Any Symptoms Suggestive of a Serious or Life-Threatening Condition?

Memory loss should always be considered an important symptom requiring investigation and treatment. It rarely is the presenting symptom of a life-threatening illness. In patients who have had a history of memory loss associated with new-onset headaches or seizures, however, the possibility of a space-occupying lesion, such as a subdural hematoma, brain tumor, or abscess, should be considered. The possibility of chronic meningitis or encephalitis should also be considered.

The possibility of delirium should always be entertained in patients presenting with acute or subacute symptoms of memory loss. Patients with delirium frequently have symptoms of psychomotor agitation or retardation, reversal of the day and night cycle, and a fluctuating course. Mentation is usually clouded. The presentation is usually acute or subacute in onset. Delirium, depending upon its underlying etiology, can be a potentially life-threatening condition.

Physical Examination

How Do Specific Examination Findings Suggest One Diagnosis or Another?

All patients who present with symptoms of memory loss should have a complete physical examination, focusing specifically on a detailed neurologic and mental status examination. The general physical examination should focus on identifying potentially reversible causes of dementia or delirium. Dementia associated with physical illness, such as advanced cardiac or pulmonary disease, can occur because of reduced cerebral oxygen perfusion, hence a careful cardiopulmonary examination is always indicated.

The remainder of the examination should focus on a comprehensive neurologic and neuropsychological examination. Findings on neurologic examination can help differentiate MID from dementia associated with PD. Focal neurologic deficits, such as hemiparesis, dysarthria, hyperreflexia, hemianopsia, and hemisensory loss, are suggestive of central nervous system vascular pathology. Rigidity, bradykinesia, shuffling gait, and tremor can suggest the possibility of PD/DLB.

Standardized mental status assessment instruments, such as the Mini-Mental State examination, should be administered to all patients who present with memory loss. Whereas these scales are relatively specific for diagnosing cognitive impairment in clinical settings, they may not be sensitive enough when compared to comprehensive neuropsychological evaluations among patients who are well educated. In general, screening testing instruments should be used to identify abnormalities in cognitive functioning from which clinical decision making can identify a potential need for more comprehensive neuropsychological testing.

Several mental status questionnaires have been developed. The most commonly used is the 30-item Mini-Mental State examination and the 26-item

Blessed Information-Memory-Concentration test. These instruments are a structured set of questions, can be easily administered by trained professionals, and are well accepted by patients. Unfortunately, these tests often fail to identify mild cognitive impairment, particularly in well-educated persons. In addition, although these scales provide a global assessment of cognitive functioning, they do not provide specific enough information about causes of mental status changes. Nonetheless, they can be used to document the progress of a dementing illness.

Neuropsychological testing can be useful early in the course of the disease and when patients present with signs or symptoms of a dementia, yet have normal scores on screening testing. Neuropsychological testing involves a comprehensive battery of tests (usually it takes about 2 h to complete) that evaluates multiple domains of higher cognitive functioning (memory, intelligence, abstract reasoning, language, calculation abilities, conceptual abilities, visuospatial orientation, etc.). Neuropsychological testing may prove useful in differentiating patients with unusual presentations. It can also help identify if an affective disorder may be contributing to causing signs and symptoms suggestive of a dementing illness. Neuropsychological testing can also help in differentiating AD from depression, delirium, or vascular dementias. Formal neuropsychological testing can define a baseline level of functioning for a patient and then be used to monitor the rate of progression of change, to evaluate the effectiveness of interventions, and to provide information for patients and caregivers.

Do Particular Examination Findings Suggest a Serious or Life-Threatening Condition?

Findings on physical or neurologic examination that suggest the presence of a central nervous system space-occupying lesion (abscess, tumor, or hemorrhage), an acute intracerebral infectious process (meningitis, encephalitis), or an acute systemic illness (sepsis, arrhythmia, hypoxia) warrant immediate intervention to prevent potential life-threatening adverse consequences. Findings such as papilledema, hypertension, and bradycardia occuring together are suggestive of raised intracranial pressure. Neck rigidity can be suggestive of meningitis or a subarachnoid hemorrhage. Focal neurologic signs result from cerebral damage. Other findings on examination can point to an underlying systemic illness (septic shock, congestive heart failure, cardiac arrhythmia, etc.).

Can Dementia Be Accurately Identified On Physical Examination and How?

Although specific findings on physical examination can help suggest a diagnostic etiology, in general, findings on physical examination are not sensitive or specific enough to be helpful. Dementia associated with PD and DLB usually occurs in the setting of typical clinical signs (tremor, rigidity, and bradykinesia); however, even among these patients, coexistent AD or MID should be considered. Focal neurologic signs are usually found in patients with MID. Frequently, the diagnosis of dementia is one of exclusion and often can only be definitive on postmortem examination.

Laboratory Tests

What Laboratory Tests, If Any, Should Always Be Ordered in a Patient with Memory Loss?

ROUTINE TESTS

The American Academy of Neurology's guidelines for the diagnosis of dementia make specific recommendations about "required" laboratory studies (Table 12-3). According to these guidelines,

Table 12-3

Diagnostic Approach to Memory Loss and Dementia

History
    Patient and/or family report
    Review of medications
    Risk factor assessment (alcohol and drug
    abuse, cardiovascular disease, family history,
    trauma, or falls)
    Caregiver assessment
    Psychosocial assessment
Examination
    Comprehensive physical examination
    Neurologic examination
    Mental status testing
    Neuropsychological testing
    Functional assessment
Laboratory studies
    Complete blood count
    Metabolic profile (liver, kidney, calcium,
    glucose)
    Thyroid function tests
    Vitamin B_{12} level
    Folic acid level
    Syphilis serology
    Other (Lyme testing, toxicology, HIV
    antibody tests, etc., when indicated)
Neuroimaging
    CT Scan
    MRI Scan
    Functional neuroimaging (PET/SPECT,
    functional MRI scanning)
    EEG
Lumbar puncture
    (Neurosyphilis encephalitis, meningitis,
    multiple sclerosis)

patients with suspected dementia should have laboratory studies including: complete blood count, serum electrolytes (including calcium), glucose, creatinine, blood urea nitrogen, liver function tests, thyroid function tests, serum vitamin B_{12} level, and syphilis serology. Selected patients should also have testing for HIV, undergo toxicology screening, and be tested with serum folate levels, chest x-ray, and urinalysis. If a diagnosis of central

nervous system vasculitis is suspected, an erythrocyte sedimentation rate should be obtained. In selected patients, a serum cortisol level, Lyme antibody testing, and heavy metal screening may be indicated. In general, laboratory testing is indicated to rule out potential reversible causes for signs and symptoms of dementia.

LUMBAR PUNCTURE

Lumbar puncture is not a routine diagnostic test for persons with dementia. Lumbar puncture should be done if metastatic cancer, meningitis, tertiary syphilis, hydrocephalus, encephalitis, demyelinating disease, HIV-associated meningitis or encephalitis, or inflammatory disease is suspected.

NEUROIMAGING

Neuroimaging studies are not required if the cause of dementia is obvious from the history, examination, or laboratory studies. Indications for neuroimaging studies include: recent onset of symptoms, dementia with focal symptoms, and dementia with atypical signs or symptoms (e.g., headache or seizures). Other indications for neuroimaging studies are early age of onset of symptoms (under 60 years) or when the cause of the cognitive changes is not obvious.

CT scanning is the most frequently used neuroimaging study. Although CT scanning is well-tolerated by patients, it is less sensitive to detecting cerebrovascular disease and ischemic white matter changes than magnetic resonance imaging (MRI). MRI is more expensive and is less well-tolerated by patients.

The role of "functional" neuroimaging studies in the evaluation of patients with dementia has not been fully determined. Single photon emission computed tomography (SPECT) and positron emission tomography (PET) are used to evaluate regional blood flow (SPECT) and glucose metabolism (PET). Some dementias produce characteristic SPECT or PET patterns. Vascular dementias are associated with focal changes in blood flow in many areas of the cerebral cortex, whereas AD is typically associated with reduced blood flow or glucose metabolism in the temporoparietal area. Frontotemporal dementia produces abnormalities in either the frontal or temporal lobes. The general usefulness of SPECT and PET scanning in patients who present with memory loss or other symptoms suggesting a dementing illness is not well-established. Ultimately, functional neuroimaging may have its greatest usefulness when imaging occurs at the same time that a patient is performing a mental or physical task. The ability to perform a task may potentially be correlated with focal abnormalities detectable on brain scanning.

ELECTROPHYSIOLOGY TESTS

Electroencephalography (EEG) is indicated in certain instances. If the diagnosis of Jakob-Creutzfeldt disease is being considered, then EEG is diagnostic. This condition and other viral encephalopathies produce characteristic sharp-wave complexes superimposed upon a slow background rhythm on EEG testing. EEG testing can also distinguish dementia from other encephalopathies (diffuse slow-wave slowing), seizures (focal activity), and normal aging.

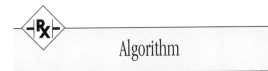

Algorithm

The diagnosis of Alzheimer's dementia can be made with up to 90 percent accuracy from a careful review of a patient's presenting symptoms and diagnostic testing. It is, however, important to exclude the approximately 15 percent of patients who have a potentially reversible cause for their memory loss.

The United States Department of Veterans Affairs published an algorithm (Fig. 12-1) guiding the differential diagnosis of dementia. By following a step-wise, logical, and sequential approach, a specific diagnosis can usually be determined. In some cases, no diagnosis can be confidently made despite a comprehensive evaluation. These patients should be frequently reassessed.

The assessment process should always include a comprehensive evaluation of symptoms, a neurologic examination, a mental status examination, and testing of neuropsychological functioning. Frequently, by comparing findings over time, the diagnosis can be made.

Although most primary care practitioners can evaluate and manage most patients with dementia, the help of members of a multidisciplinary team of individuals with expertise in diagnosis and treatment can be invaluable. When primary care practitioners require additional assistance about diagnosis testing or treatment, specialty consultation is always indicated. This consultation can involve assistance from practitioners in: neurology, neuropsychology, geriatric psychiatry, nursing, rehabilitation, or social services. A referral to a neurologist should be made for all patients with early-onset dementia (before age 60 years), patients with rapidly progressive disorders, and patients with dementia associated with unusual physical signs. A neurosurgeon can be especially helpful in managing patients with hydrocephalus, subdural hematomas, and patients with other intracranial space-occupying lesions (neoplasm, abscesses).

Neuropsychologists can be of special help when a patient's underlying intellectual level is high or low, and when there is a question about whether depression is contributing to the cognitive decline. Geropsychiatrists are especially helpful in diagnosing depression in the context of dementia and in making suggestions about the pharmacologic approach to managing patients with dementia who have behavioral disturbances.

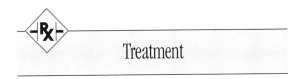

Treatment

General Approach

The goal of treating a patient with memory loss and dementing illness is to maintain the person at the highest possible level of functioning and to minimize consequences of the illness in the least

Figure 12-1

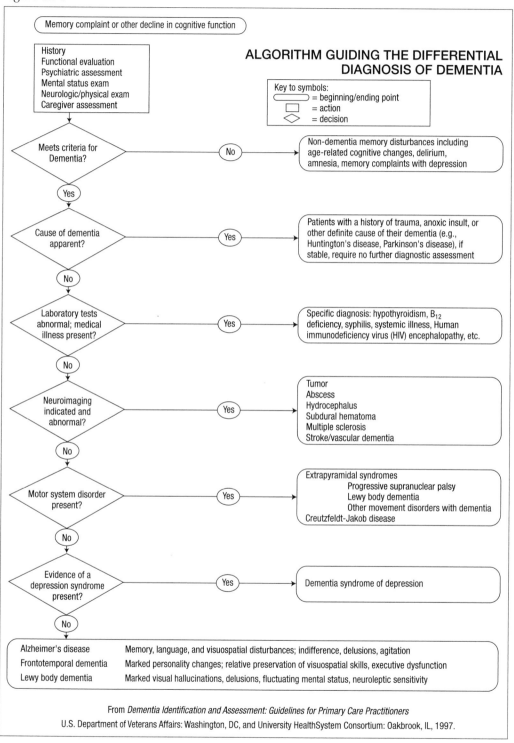

Algorithm guiding the differential diagnosis of dementia.

restrictive environment. At different stages of the disorder, primary care practitioners may call upon the expertise of practitioners from many varying disciplines. The ongoing care of a patient with a dementing illness often requires a multidisciplinary approach, drawing on the expertise of professionals from many disciplines (Table 12-4). This team can include, but not be be limited to, physical and occupational therapists, social workers, legal aid experts, financial aid experts, home health care specialists, audiologists, ophthalmologists, podiatrists, registered dieticians, and more formalized services, such as adult medical daycare, respite, personal care, homemaker services, and caregiver support services. The role of the primary care clinician is to coordinate and oversee the delivery of these services when they are indicated.

Treating patients with memory loss includes regular evaluations, education, frequent contact with family members and caregivers, and careful attention to general health. The optimal approach to caring for patients with dementia involves a comprehensive medical, psychological, and social intervention strategy. In most cases, symptoms of the underlying disorder are progressive, and the needs of patients and their caregivers change over time. Therefore care must be longitudinal and, by definition, can be optimally provided in a primary care setting.

Clinicians need to be aware that the caregiver of a patient with a progressive dementing illness is a key resource and that optimal care can only be delivered if the caregiver is included as an integral part of the decision-making process. Caring for patients with dementia is frequently physically and emotionally stressful and has been shown to result in more health-related problems among caregivers. Caregivers to patients with dementia are also more likely to engage in harmful coping mechanisms (e.g., smoking, drinking alcohol, and using medications to calm down). A major determinant of decisions to institutionalize a patient with dementia is the willingness and ability of caregivers to provide assistance to care recipients when it is required. Caregivers are particularly more likely to experience burden and stress when caring for a patient with dementia who is incontinent of feces or urine and for patients who have significant behavioral outbursts (for further discussion about caregiver issues, see Chap. 4).

Primary care clinicians should schedule regular office or home visits that should include the presence of the caregiver. At these visits, primary care clinicians need to address concerns of the caregiver and make suggestions about strategies to help manage them. This can include giving advice about establishing familiar routines, distracting and redirecting preservative behaviors, establishing a toileting schedule, or establishing an exercise program. Caregivers will often have questions about the disease and the likely progression. Only by partnering with caregivers can optimal care be delivered over the course of a dementing illness.

Table 12-4

Multidisciplinary Team Approach to Memory Loss and Alzheimer's Disease

Primary care practitioners
Neuropsychology
Geriatric psychology
Nursing
Physical and occupational therapy
Social services
Legal aid
Financial aid
Home health care agencies
Audiology
Podiatry
Nutrition
Formalized services
Daycare
Respite
Personal care
Homemaker support
Caregiver support

Drug Therapy

Drug treatment is summarized in Table 12-5.

Table 12-5

Treatment

Drugs used to treat Alzheimer's disease
  Cholinomimetic agents
    Tacrine
    Donepezil
    Metrifonate
    Eptastigmine
Potentially beneficial agents
    Nonsteroidal anti-inflammatory drugs
    Estrogens
    Antioxidants (vitamin E, vitamin C,
      ginkgo biloba, selegiline)
    Antiamyloid interventions
Drugs used to treat behavioral sequelae of
    dementia
  Psychosis
    Haloperidol
    Thioridazine
    Risperidone
    Others (divalproex, onlazapine)
  Agitation
    Lorazepam
    Trazodone
    Carbamazepine
  Anxiety
    Lorazepam
    Buspirone
    Propranolol
    Others (SSRIs, trazodone)
  Insomnia
    Lorazepam
    Temazepam
    Zolpidem
    Trazodone
  Depression
    SSRIs
    Tricyclic antidepressants (nortriptyline,
      desipramine)
  Aggression
    Trazodone
    Risperidone
    Others (buspirone, olanzapine,
      carbamazepine, SSRIs)

ALZHEIMER'S DISEASE

Two pharmacotherapeutic agents are currently available for treating cognitive impairment associated with AD. Tacrine was the first acetylcholinesterase inhibitor (AChE) available to treat patients with mild to moderate AD. Tacrine is a centrally acting agent with reversible AChE inhibitory activity that augments central nervous system acetylcholine concentrations.

TACRINE   Cognitive dysfunction in patients with AD is directly associated with loss of cholinergic neurons. In clinical trials, patients treated with tacrine showed improvements in cognition when compared to placebo. This agent must be administered four times a day because of its short half-life and requires titrating of dosing to usually effective doses (160 mg/day) over a period of 18 to 20 weeks. Up to one third of patients treated with tacrine experienced significant adverse reactions, including cholinergic effects (gastrointestinal distress, insomnia) and elevations of liver enzymes, frequently requiring discontinuing the medication. Although tacrine appears to reduce declines in cognitive performance and can increase global clinical performance in patients with AD, its effectiveness over the long term is controversial.

DONEPEZIL   Tacrine has largely been superseded by a second-generation AChE inhibitor, donepezil, now available for treating patients with cognitive impairments related to AD. In clinical trials, donepezil enhanced cognitive functioning in most patients (rated by formal testing scales). Patients who discontinued donepezil demonstrated a loss of benefit. Donepezil is usually well tolerated, especially at the lower starting dose (5 mg/day). The higher (10 mg/day) dose requires a 4-week titration period and may be more likely to cause cholinergic-mediated side effects (nausea, diarrhea, and insomnia). The advantages of donepezil over tacrine are that it can be given once a day, it does not require as long an introductory dosing period, and there is no need for monitoring of liver function. Donepezil is metabolized by the cytochrome p450 system, so caution should be used when medications metabolized by this system are prescribed. This agent is usually worth trying in patients with mild to moderate AD (MMSE scores of > 18). It can be effective in slowing the progression of decline in cognitive functioning, and in some patients, early improvements in memory may be noted.

VASCULAR DEMENTIA

The focus of treating patients with vascular dementia includes modifying and treating potential risk factors, such as hypercholesterolemia, cigarette smoking, hypertension, sedentary lifestyle, and obesity. Exercise, control of diet, and stopping cigarettes are indicated for all patients with these risk factors. Aspirin is most appropriate for prophylaxis for patients at risk for MID, and should disease progression occur in patients who have been treated with aspirin, using agents such as ticlopidine or clopidogrel should be considered. Among patients with atrial fibrillation, anticoagulation therapy should be instituted unless contraindicated.

DEMENTIA ASSOCIATED WITH PARKINSON'S DISEASE

In general, patients with PD who develop dementia do not improve when their underlying parkinsonian symptoms are treated with agents such as dopaminergic drugs or selegiline. Symptoms of Parkinson's disease can worsen if these patients are treated with cholinergic agents (tacrine or donepezil).

DRUG THERAPY FOR BEHAVIORAL SYMPTOMS

Behavioral and neuropsychiatric symptoms are common and frequently distressing to patients and caregivers of patients with dementing illnesses. These symptoms usually manifest as agitation, anxiety, insomnia, psychotic outbursts, or depression. Many approaches have been used to manage behavioral problems associated with dementia. Most frequently, nonpharmacologic

interventions, including redirecting a patient's focus, modifying the environment, reducing choices, and modifying external entrainers (day/night, changes of settings) are effective. For recalcitrant behaviors, pharmacologic interventions may be indicated. As in all elderly patients, drugs should be used carefully, started in low doses, and titrated gradually, observing for side effects and deleterious drug interactions. Pharmacologic interventions for treating behavioral outbursts can reduce distress, decrease caregiver burden, and potentially, delay institutionalization.

Antipsychotic medications are most effective for patients who have a predominance of psychotic symptomatology (delusions, hallucinations, and disordered thinking). These agents have similar efficacies but differ in their side-effect profiles. How they are used should depend on the type and frequency of symptoms and the side-effect profile. Haloperidol is a high-potency agent that frequently causes extrapyramidal side effects, such as rigidity, akathisia, and occasionally, tardive dyskinesia. Lower-potency agents, such as chlorpromazine and thioridazine, are more likely to cause side effects of sedation (this can be a potentially beneficial effect), postural hypotension, and anticholinergic effects. More recent evidence suggests that agents such as risperidone and clozapine are effective in treating agitation and psychosis in elderly patients and are associated with few or absent extrapyramidal effects. Clozapine, although effective, can cause serious agranulocytosis, so white blood cell count needs to be checked on a monthly basis.

Benzodiazepines are most effective for treating anxiety or agitation. In general, these agents are less effective than antipsychotics for treating more severe symptoms or mixed symptoms of agitation, anxiety, and psychosis. Agents with short half-lives, such as lorazepam or oxazepam, are preferred for treating anxiety associated with dementia. Long-acting agents, such as flurazepam and diazepam, should be avoided as they are likely to be associated with a greater likelihood of falling.

Many patients with dementing illnesses also have symptoms of depression, including dysthymia, loss of appetite, insomnia, and irritability. Selective serotonin reuptake inhibitors (SSRIs), including fluoxetine, paroxetine, and sertraline, are highly effective for treating patients with depression associated with dementia. These agents have, in general, a safer side-effect profile than traditionally used tricyclic antidepressant agents. Nortriptyline or desipramine is the safest among the tricyclic antidepressants for older persons. Other antidepressant agents, including trazodone (especially effective for older persons with insomnia), nefazodone, and bupropion, can be useful in treating depressive symptoms associated with AD.

Insomnia associated with dementia is best treated with first attending to nonpharmacologic interventions, such as modifying the environment and involving the older person in activities during the day, so that they are tired when retiring for sleep (see Chap. 10). Short-acting benzodiazepines, zolpidem, and sedating antidepressants (trazodone) are often effective.

For patients with behavioral symptoms not responding to these interventions, anticonvulsants, beta blockers, carbamazepine, buspirone, or sodium valproate may be worth trying.

Treatment of Other Conditions

Occasionally, patients with normal pressure hydrocephalus can derive some benefit by having their cerebral spinal fluid diverted via a ventriculoperitoneal shunting procedure. Symptoms related to dementia, however, rarely are improved by this procedure. Patients with toxic or metabolic encephalopathies are often treated effectively by eliminating the offending agent and treating the underlying cause. For patients with infectious-related changes in cognition (syphilis, tuberculosis, infectious meningitis), treatment with antibiotics can potentially reverse their symptoms.

While vitamin B_{12} deficiency is a well-documented cause of dementia, the treatment of this disorder infrequently results in a reversing of

symptoms. Similarly, patients with dementia associated with long-standing hyperthyroidism or hypothyroidism rarely improve with treatment of the underlying disorder. Similarly, the dementia associated with chronic alcohol abuse can rarely be improved by treatment. All patients with suspected alcohol-related dementia should discontinue alcohol ingestion, however, and some may experience an improvement in cognition. If any of these disorders are identified in the assessment process, specific treatment interventions may at least help arrest or delay progression of cognitive symptoms that can be associated with the underlying condition.

Controversies

Up to 15 percent to patients with dementia can have a potentially reversible cause for their illness (of which polypharmacy is one of the most common causes). While there is no direct evidence that a dementia workup consisting of laboratory testing and medication review improves outcomes for patients who present with symptoms and signs of dementia, it makes intuitive sense to address these issues when evaluating and treating a patient with dementia. There are no clinical trials addressing the utility of diagnostic neuroimaging for improving diagnostic accuracy or patient outcomes. Much of the approach to diagnosis and treatment of patients with dementing illnesses is derived from expert opinions and consensus practice guidelines. Furthermore, there is no direct evidence to support how frequently a patient with dementia should be seen by a clinician. Intuitively, these patients are at high risk for comorbidity and progression of their illnesses and, therefore, should be seen on a regular basis (probably every 3 months). This is especially true for patients being treated with AChE inhibitors.

Other controversies in treating patients with AD surround the duration of treatment. Studies of the effectiveness of pharmacotherapeutic agents for treating patients with AD have been relatively short-lived (6 months). There are no data supporting the long-term effectiveness of these agents.

There is good evidence that when interventions designed to enhance support (psychological and physical) for caregivers of patients with dementia are instituted, institutionalization can be delayed, patient behavior improved, and caregivers self-reported well-being enhanced. The type of intervention that is of benefit is controversial. For example, there is inconsistent evidence that respite care is of benefit in reducing caregiver burden and depression. Other types of interventions such as support groups may be equally efficacious.

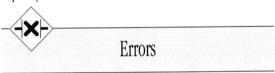

Errors

Failure to Differentiate Normal from Disease

The vast majority of older individuals have preserved cognitive abilities even into advanced age. Temporary lapses in memory occur commonly in older individuals, and "benign senescent forgetfulness," a condition that refers to memory loss that is greater than expected, frequently occurs in healthy older individuals. These age-associated abnormalities in cognitive functioning are usually not severe enough to interfere grossly in daily functioning, yet can be frequently confused with dementia. It is important for practitioners to differentiate normal "age-related" memory changes from the impairments associated with dementing illnesses. Although it is important to reassure patients and family members about memory complaints that do not constitute sufficient severity to suggest a dementing illness, it is equally

important to identify a potential dementing disease early in its course.

Failure to Recognize Comorbid Conditions in a Patient with Underlying Dementia

If the rate of cognitive decline exceeds that expected for an older person's diagnosis, it is important to consider the possibility of comorbid illnesses. Delirium can often be overlooked in older persons with cognitive impairment. Older persons with dementia are at greater risk for undetected comorbid illnesses that can worsen cognitive and functional status and increase morbidity and mortality.

Many patients with an underlying dementing illness, such as Alzheimer's disease, frequently have coexisting cerebrovascular disease. These patients can also have many vascular risk factors, including hypertension, diabetes mellitus, coronary artery disease, atrial fibrillation, a sedentary lifestyle, and tobacco abuse. There are no specific clinical trials that prove an additional benefit of adding stroke prevention (aspirin, clopidogrel, ticlopidine) to the medication regimen of a person with AD. It makes plausible sense, however, that preventing a vascular disease as a potential second cause of dementia (especially if there are risk factors) should be included as part of the therapeutic regimen.

Even among patients without dementia, prophylaxis with anticoagulation medications among patients with atrial fibrillation who are at risk for cerebrovascular disease is underused. The use of aspirin for high-risk patients is also not emphasized, particularly among older patients with dementia. All patients with or without dementia should be counseled about risk factors for cerebrovascular disease and treated, should risk factors exist. Interventions, such as controlling blood pressure, encouraging exercise, dietary modification, recommending discontinuing cigarette smoking, and instituting treatment with agents such as aspirin, ticlopidine, clopidogrel, Coumadin, or vitamin E, may be indicated.

Failure to Recognize Depression

There is good evidence that depression worsens cognitive functioning in older individuals. Also, treatment of older patients with depression results in reductions in symptoms of agitation, aggression, and physical performance. There is good evidence that depression occurring in patients with dementia is a risk factor for suicide in the elderly. Primary care practitioners often underestimate the impact of depression on cognitive functioning and behavior. Depression should always be considered as a significant comorbid illness among patients with dementia because it can exacerbate disability due to the primary illness or mask diagnosing a reason for changes in cognitive performance.

Missing the Diagnosis of Diffuse Lewy Body Dementia

Another area of error that can occur in treating patients with cognitive impairment includes treating older persons with dementia associated with DLB with neuroleptic medications. In many patients with DLB dementia, treatment with neuroleptic medications can result in severe irreversible extrapyramidal side effects or the neuroleptic malignant syndrome. DLB dementia should always be considered as a potential cause if symptoms of dementia occur contemporaneously with extrapyramidal motor signs. This is unlike the dementia associated with PD, where motor signs precede symptoms of dementia by many years.

Other Errors

Currently, there is no evidence to suggest that patients with dementing illnesses other than AD derive any benefit from treatment with cholinesterase inhibitors. Controversies about when and how to treat patients with presumed dementia associated with normal pressure hydrocephalus reflect an uncertainty among published studies about the effectiveness of intervention and timing

of interventions. In general, among patients with NPH, symptoms of dementia are most likely to improve if they have been of short duration, and the diagnosis of NPH has been confirmed by radionuclide cisternography.

Family Approach

What to Do with Family Members

Family members are most critical in successfully formulating a comprehensive plan of care for a patient with progressive memory impairment. Family members often have questions about the diagnosis. Persons who care for patients with progressive cognitive impairment often become burdened both physically and psychologically in caring for their loved one.

The primary care practitioner needs to address issues related to caregiving from the outset. Early on, loved ones and caregivers have many questions related to diagnosis, treatment, and support services. Questions often surround issues related to independence, driving, travel, finances, and appropriate living arrangements.

Practitioners caring for patients and caregivers of patients with progressive cognitive decline must recognize the importance of the patient-caregiver dyad in determining physical and psychological outcomes for both patients and caregivers. It is important for practitioners to recognize that family members and other caregivers must be included in the comprehensive plan of care. Goals for patients with progressive dementing illnesses must include the caregiving family so that patients and caregivers can be apprised of the appropriateness and effectiveness of care interventions over time. This will frequently involve increasing caregiving demands on the part of family members and loved ones over time.

Caregiver Resources

There are many resources available to help a caregiver provide assistance for a patient with a progressive dementing illness. Loved ones and caregivers are often best able to identify appropriate community resources and the most appropriate service for an individual in need of care. Social workers are often useful resources in identifying and helping with access to these services. Many programs exist, such as the Alzheimer's Association, adult social and medical daycare centers, day hospitals, and eating-together programs. These programs often provide information about the underlying illness while enhancing socialization, coping skills, and providing emotional support.

Other Services

There are many other kinds of services available for caring for patients with progressive memory and cognitive declines. Case management service, either through a private service or agency-based service, can help patients or their caregivers in day-to-day activities. They can also suggest appropriate supports, such as respite service, adult day care, in-home service, temporary placement, and caregiver support resource services (groups, counseling, and referrals to appropriate health care providers). For employed caregivers, it can also be important that health care professionals provide information about work-related plans that may incorporate a flexible arrangement. Therefore, a balance can be achieved between work-related responsibilities and caring for an older impaired individual. This can involve developing a routine that incorporates work and caring for the elder individual, respite care, and adult daycare. Legal advice about advanced directives, financial issues, and complex placement-related issues can often best be obtained from lawyers who have a special interest in elder-care related issues. Anticipatory guidance about how to finance care, ranging from long-term home care to residential care, may be best provided by elder law and financial specialists.

Internet Information

The Internet is an excellent source of information about caring for older individuals with progressive memory disorders and their potential needs. For patients with memory problems, the Alzheimer's Association is an excellent resource and can be accessed at 1-800-272-3900 or its disease educational referral center at 1-800-438-4380. The Web site, *http://www.alz.org*, links the Alzheimer's Association page to local sites and presents a step-by-step approach to obtaining a thorough assessment of this disorder. The *www.adrc.wustl.edu\ alzheimer* provides useful information about frequently asked questions about AD and provides excellent descriptions of the progression of the disorder.

For patients with progressive memory loss and physical disability, the *www.medque.com* is an excellent online service that provides information about medical supply equipment for patients with impairments of activities of daily living. For family members who wish to obtain health care information about issues related to AD and other illnesses relating to aging, the *www.healthfinder. gov* site is an excellent resource. For information about caregiving, the Internet provides many sites for accessing useful information. The *www.care-giver.com* site provides a linkage to many information sites related to caregiving. The *www.iog. wayne.edu\GeroWebd\GeroWeb.html* provides an excellent resource center for all aspects of aging, including aging with cognitive impairments. Other sites provide information about more restrictive kinds of living arrangements for older individuals with cognitive impairment, including assistive living settings and continuing care facilities (*www.ncal.org* and *www.newlife styles.com*) (Table 12-6).

Table 12-6
Web Site Resources

Alzheimer's Association	*http://www.alz.org*
	www.adrc.wustl.edu\alzheimer
Medical equipment	*www.medque.com*
Caregiving information	*www.caregiver.com*
General information	*www.iog.wayne.edu\GeroWebd\GeroWeb.html*
Living arrangements	*www.ncal.org*
	www.newlifestyles.com; 1.800.869.9549

Patient Education

What Should Patients Be Told About Their Memory Loss?

In the early phases of a dementing illness, patients are frequently aware that their level of higher cognitive functioning is becoming progressively impaired. They may experience a "catastrophic reaction," recognizing that they should be better able to perform in cognitive testing. At this stage of the disorder, it is important that patients recognize that every effort is being made to identify potentially reversible causes for their symptoms. They must also recognize that appropriate interventions are being instituted to, at least potentially, reverse or attenuate the rate of decline of their symptoms. At this stage of a progressive dementing illness, it is important that patients identify surrogate decision makers and become involved in anticipatory guidance-type planning, including writing a will, living will, and determining or declaring a durable power of attorney.

In the middle to later phases of dementing illnesses, patients are less aware of information that may be delivered by practitioners. It is, however, important that patients and caregivers feel comfortable around practitioners providing their medical and nursing care. At this stage of the disorder, it is particularly important that family members and potential caregivers recognize the symptoms and signs of progression in the disease.

In advanced stages of dementia, patients become increasingly physically dependent and require assistance with even the most basic activities of daily living. At this stage of the disorder, formal caregiving and institutionalization is often indicated. Comfort and palliative care issues are also important.

Should Patients Drive?

There is excellent evidence that patients with dementia, even at mild stages, are more likely to exhibit hazardous driving behaviors and have a greater likelihood of being involved in motor vehicle crashes. There is also evidence that the rate of motor vehicle crashes in demented patients significantly increases with each year after diagnosis. In studies examining performance of older individuals with dementia on road testing when compared to patients who do not have dementia, up to 50 percent of patients with even mild AD did not pass these tests. There are no studies that definitively describe or quantify fatalities linked to drivers diagnosed with AD. There is, however, enough evidence to suggest that patients with memory loss and cognitive impairment have a more significant risk of motor vehicle crashes. Thus, driving privileges for patients with dementia should be carefully evaluated. This can be done by formal testing by the department of motor vehicles or by simulated testing available through most occupational therapy departments. The AARP can also provide useful information about driving testing resources.

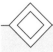

Emerging Concepts

Genetic Testing

Mutations on three chromosomes have been linked to AD and other neurodegenerative conditions. While genetics has no clinical application at present, this is a burgeoning field of research, and it is possible that in the near future testing may be available that is useful in the clinical setting.

Mutations associated with AD (on chromosomes 1, 14, and 21) account for less than 10 percent of all cases but are linked to early onset of the disease (before the age of 55 years). A mutation in the gene for the amyloid precursor protein has been found, resulting in an increased production of beta-amyloid leading to a fibrillar aggregation that is toxic to neurons. The locus for this gene is on chromosome 21. A second locus, found on chromosome 14, is estimated to account for up to 50 percent of early-onset cases of AD. This locus encodes for a protein called presenilin-1. Many mutations in the gene for presenilin-1 have been identified in patients with early-onset Alzheimer's disease.

Persons with the apolipoprotein E-4 (Apo E-4) genotype are at risk for developing late-onset AD. The allele coding for this genotype is located on chromosome 19. The presence of Apo E-4 occurs in up to 40 percent of patients with AD who present at a late age and may ultimately become a marker for early detection. The specificity for Apo E-4 genotype is low, and many individuals, even those homozygous for the allele, do not develop the disease. Other patients with late-onset AD may have mutations on chromosome 1, and a second locus has been identified on chromosome 12.

In the future, cerebrospinal fluid testing may become more useful in diagnosing AD. There is a growing body of evidence to suggest that measuring cerebrospinal fluid beta-amyloid, tau concentrations, and presence of neuronal thread proteins can help in making an early diagnosis of AD.

New Treatments

NONSTEROIDAL ANTI-INFLAMMATORY DRUGS (NSAIDs)

There is recent evidence that suggests that NSAIDs (ibuprofen, aspirin) may delay the onset and slow the progression of AD among patients who have AD. There is even evidence to suggest that they may have consumed fewer NSAIDs than a comparative group of elderly individuals without AD. The neuroprotective mechanism of NSAIDs may be mediated by a reduction in brain inflammation resulting in amyloid protein deposition. A potential vascular platelet aggregation effect may also be implicated. The beneficial effect of NSAIDs is small, and gastrointestinal side effects are common in elderly patients who take NSAIDs.

ESTROGENS

There is evidence from case-controlled studies that estrogen replacement therapy can be associated with a reduced likelihood of patients developing AD. The protective effects of estrogens may be mediated through many mechanisms including neuroprotective and neurotrophic effects. Animal studies suggest that estrogen may enhance learning and neurotransmitter uptake levels. There is further evidence to suggest that estrogen may improve cognitive functioning among patients with AD who are treated with cholinomimetic agents (tacrine). Prospective studies are ongoing to evaluate the efficacy of estrogens as a therapeutic agent for postmenopausal women. Neurologic functioning is being assessed in these studies. If a benefit is shown and estrogens are found to have long-term safety, estrogen therapy may be recommended as a neuroprotective agent for post-menopausal women.

VITAMIN E, SELEGILINE, AND ANTIOXIDANTS

Vitamin E and selective monoamine oxidase-B inhibitors (selegiline) may be protective against neurotoxicity and may be useful in treating patients with AD by potentially modifying or attenuating rates of degeneration of cholinergic-producing cells. Any agent that may protect against oxidative damage may potentially attenuate nerve damage that can be associated with progression of dementing illnesses. Antioxidants, such as vitamin E, vitamin C, and ginkgo biloba extract, and monoamine oxidase-B inhibitors can be important agents in delaying symptoms and progression of symptoms in patients with dementing illnesses mediated through antioxidant effects. Little is known about their long-term efficacy, and future study is indicated.

ANTIAMYLOID INTERVENTIONS

One of the important potential neuropathologic features in patients with AD is deposition of amyloid in the association cortex and other areas of importance related to cognitive functioning. Amyloid deposition can be an early marker for AD, and there is evidence that genetic mutations that allow for premature deposition of amyloid can be associated with familial early-onset AD. This has prompted research to suggest strategies for modifying amyloid deposition that can be associated with AD. The goal of interventions is to attenuate toxicity from amyloid deposition. Medications designed at reducing amyloid deposition are currently under investigation. One such agent is JTP-4819, a protease that cleaves the amyloid precursor protein, thereby reducing pathologic amyloid deposition. The drug also increases acetylcholine release and enhances neuropeptide function. This agent is currently being studied in humans.

OTHER CHOLINOMIMETIC AGENTS

Clinical trials of other agents to improve cognitive functioning are ongoing, including trials of metrifonate, physostigmine, rivastigmine, and others. The most recently studied has been metrifonate, an agent that has no intrinsic anti-AChE activity. It is, however, a potent inhibitor of AChE. This agent achieves high levels of inhibition of AChE and, in studies, has a favorable side-effect profile and a long duration of activity. Significant improvements in cognitive scoring have also been shown. Other cholinergic agents, such as eptastigmine, are also being studied and may be potentially important agents in treating patients with AD. Many other agents are under investigation.

FOLIC ACID AND HOMOCYSTEINE

Recent evidence suggests that high serum homocysteine levels and low folic acid levels are associated with dementia. These findings have also been shown in patients with coronary artery disease and colon cancer. Folic acid intake has been shown to be associated with a reduced incidence of heart disease. Ingesting folic acid reduces homocysteine levels. Prospective trials are required to evaluate if taking a multivitamin (containing folic acid, vitamin C, and vitamin E) can prevent dementia.

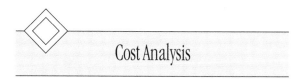

Cost Analysis

Alzheimer's disease usually begins after age 70 years; however, it can occur in an early-onset familial form. The disease now affects 4 to 8 million people in the United States and is estimated to cost the nation $100 billion annually. This makes it the nation's third most costly disease after cancer and heart disease. As the number of older Americans increases, and among those over the age of 65, the number of old old persons will climb at the most rapid rate. Among this group of older persons (the oldest old), persons with cognitive impairment commonly require the most health care resources (supervision, attention, pharmacologic interventions, and institutionalization).

Bibliography

Aevarsson O, Svanborg A, Skoog I: Seven-year survival rate after age 85 years. Relation to Alzheimer disease and vascular dementia. *Arch Neurol* 55:1226, 1998.

Agency for Health Care Policy and Research: *Recognition and Initial Assessment of Alzheimer's Disease and Related Dementias*. Clinical Practice Guideline No. 19. AHCPR Publication No. 97-0702. U.S. Department of Health and Human Services. Public Health Service. Rockville, MD: Agency for Health Care Policy and Research; November 1996.

American Academy of Neurology: Practice parameters for diagnosis and evaluation of dementia. *Neurology* 44:2203, 1994.

American College of Medical Genetics: Statement on use of apolipoprotein E testing for Alzheimer disease. *JAMA* 274:1627, 1995.

American College of Physicians: Magnetic resonance imaging of the brain and spine: a revised statement. *Ann Intern Med* 120:872, 1994.

American Medical Directors Association: *Dementia, Clinical Practice Guideline*. Columbia, MD: American Medical Directors Association; 1998.

American Psychiatric Association: *Practice Guideline for the Treatment of Patients with Alzheimer's Disease and Other Dementias of Late Life*. Washington, DC: American Psychiatric Press, Inc; 1996.

American Psychiatric Association: *Practice Guideline for the Treatment of Patients with Alzheimer's Disease and Other Dementias of Late Life*. American Psychiatric Association; May, 1997.

American Psychological Association, Presidential Task Force on the Assessment of Age-Consistent Memory Decline and Dementia: *Guidelines for the Evaluation of Dementia and Age-Related Cognitive Decline*. Washington, DC: American Psychological Association; February 1998.

Bourgeois MS, Schulz R, Burgio L: Interventions for caregivers of patients with Alzheimer's disease: a review and analysis of content, process, and outcomes. *Int J Aging Hum Dev* 43:35, 1996.

Chui H, Zhang Q: Evaluation of dementia: a systematic study of the usefulness of the American Academy of Neurology's Practice Parameters. *Neurology* 49:925, 1997.

Clarfield AM: The reversible dementias: do they reverse? *Ann Intern Med* 109:476, 1988.

Clarke R, Smith AD, Jobst KA, et al: Folate, vitamin B_{12}, and serum total homocysteine levels in confirmed Alzheimer disease. *Arch Neurol* 55:1449, 1998.

Coffey CE, Cummings JL, Duffy JD, et al: Assessment of treatment outcomes in neuropsychiatry: a report from the Committee on Research of the American Neuropsychiatric Association. *J Neuropsychiatry Clin Neurosci* 7:287, 1995..

Corey-Bloom J, Thal LJ, Galasko D, et al: Diagnosis and evaluation of dementia. *Neurology* 45:211, 1995.

Eccles M, Clark J, Livingstone M, et al: North of England Evidence Based Guidelines Developmental Project: guideline for the primary care management of dementia. *BMJ* 317:802, 1998.

Folstein MF, Folstein SE, McHugh PR: Mini-Mental State. A practical method for grading the cognitive state of patients for the clinician. *J Psychiatr Res* 12:189, 1975.

Geldmacher DS: Clinical experience with donepezil hydrochloride: a case study perspective. *Adv Therapy* 14:305, 1997.

Grasel E: Temporary institutional respite in dementia cases: who utilizes this form of respite care and what effect does it have? *Int Psychogeriatr* 9:437, 1997.

Janicki MP, Heller T, Seltzer GB, et al: Practice guidelines for the clinical assessment and care management of Alzheimer's and other dementias among adults with intellectual disability. AAMR-IASSID Workgroup on Practice Guidelines for Care Management of Alzheimer's Disease among Adults with Intellectual Disability. *J Intellect Disabil Res* 40(Pt 4):374, 1996.

Juva K, Makela M, Erkinjuntti T, et al: Functional assessment scales in detecting dementia. *Age Aging* 26:393, 1997.

Katz PR, Ouslander JG: Clinical practice guidelines and position statements: the American Geriatrics Society Approach. *J Am Geriatr Soc* 44:1123, 1996.

Kaufer DI: Dementia with Lewy bodies. *Mediguide Geriatr Neurol* 1:1, 1997.

Kaufer DI, Cumings JL, Christine D: Effect of tacrine on behavioral symptoms in Alzheimer's disease: an open-label study. *J Geriatr Psychiatry Neurol* 9:1, 1996.

Keady J, Nolan M: A stitch in time. Facilitation of proactive interventions with dementia caregivers: the role of community practitioners. *J Psychiatr Ment Health Nurs* 2:33, 1995.

Knight BG, Lutsky SM, Macofsky-Urban F: A meta-analytic review of interventions for caregiver distress: recommendations for future research. *Gerontologist* 33:240, 1993.

Launer LJ, Andersen K, Dewey ME, et al: Rates and risk factors for dementia and Alzheimer's disease: results from EURODEM pooled analyses. EURODEM Incidence Research Group and Work Groups. European Studies of Dementia. *Neurology* 52:78, 1999.

Mittelman MS, Ferris SH, Shulman E, et al: A family intervention to delay nursing home placement of patients with Alzheimer disease. A randomized controlled trial. *JAMA* 276:1725, 1996.

National Institute on Aging: Apolipoprotein E genotyping in Alzheimer's disease. *Lancet* 347:1091, 1996.

Penninx BW, Guralnik JM, Ferrucci L, et al: Depressive symptoms and physical decline in community-dwelling older persons. *JAMA* 279:1720, 1998.

Rogers SL, Doody RS, Mohs RC, et al: Donepezil improves cognition and global function in Alzheimer's disease: a 15-week, double-blind, placebo-controlled study. Donepezil Study Group. *Arch Intern Med* 158:1021, 1998.

Rogers SL, Farlow MR, Doody RS, et al: A 24-week, double-blind, placebo-controlled trial of donepezil in patients with Alzheimer's disease. Donepezil Study Group. *Neurology* 50:136, 1998.

Roman GC, Tatemichi TK, Erkinjuntti T, et al: Vascular dementia: diagnostic criteria for research studies. Report of the NINDS-AIREN International Workshop. *Neurology* 43:250, 1993.

Sano M, Ernesto C, Thomas RG, et al: A controlled trial of selegiline, alpha-tocopherol, or both as treatment for Alzheimer's disease. The Alzheimer's Disease Cooperative Study. *N Engl J Med* 336:1216, 1997.

Screening for Dementia. U.S. Preventive Services Task Force. *Guide to Clinical Preventive Services.* 2nd ed. Alexandria, VA: International Medical Publishing, 1996.

Small GW, Rabins PV, Barry PB, et al: Diagnosis and treatment of Alzheimer's Disease and related disorders. *JAMA* 278:1363, 1997.

Snowdon DA, Greiner LH, Mortimer, et al: Brain infarction and the critical expression of Alzheimer disease. The Nun Study. *JAMA* 277:813, 1997.

Teunisse S, Bollen AE, van Gool WA, et al: Dementia and subnormal levels of vitamin B_{12}: effects of replacement therapy on dementia. *J Neurol* 243:522, 1996.

U.S. Department of Veteran Affairs, University Health System Consortium. Dementia Identification and Assessment: Guidelines for Primary Care Practitioners. University Health System Consortium. March 1997:1–103.

Urrutia L, Read S, Swartz R, et al: Differentiation of Alzheimer's disease, frontotemporal dementia and parkinsonian-dementias. Facts and Research in Gerontology (Alzheimer's disease). 1996.

Weytingh MD, Bossuyt PM, van Crevel H: Reversible dementia: more than 10% or less than 1%? A quantitative review. *J Neurol* 242:466, 1995.

Alan M. Adelman

Chapter
13

Hearing and Visual Impairment

Hearing and visual impairment are both common disorders in the elderly. Both of these sensory deficits are predictive of subsequent functional impairment, as well as cognitive impairment and social isolation. Thus, it is important for the primary care clinician to identify individuals with hearing and/or visual impairment, identify the cause, and initiate appropriate therapies.

HEARING IMPAIRMENT

Hearing impairment can lead to a number of problems including depression and social isolation. Individuals with hearing loss may be at greater risk for cognitive impairment and dementia. Patients with hearing loss rate their self-health poorer than those without hearing loss.

Although hearing amplification may not benefit all with hearing loss, those for whom it is appropriate will benefit if they use it. The use of hearing amplification can prevent social isolation and depression. Unfortunately, the prevalence of hearing aid use is low. Only 10 to 20 percent of patients who can benefit from a hearing aid use one, and an additional 5 to 10 percent have previously used a hearing aid, but no longer use one.

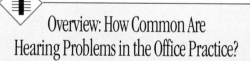

Overview: How Common Are Hearing Problems in the Office Practice?

Hearing impairment is the most common sensory disorder and one of the most common disabilities among the elderly. The prevalence of hearing loss in adults in the United States ranges from approximately 20 to 60 percent. Approximately 30 percent of community-dwelling elderly report hearing

impairment. Some estimates are twice this number. The incidence of hearing problems increases with age. Approximately 20 percent report significant hearing loss defined as hearing loss associated with functional impairment. The prevalence of hearing loss is even greater in nursing home populations and approaches 70 to 90 percent.

Principal Diagnoses

The cause of hearing loss can be divided into three categories: sensorineural, conductive, and mixed (Table 13-1). Sensorineural hearing loss is due to problems in the cochlea or cranial nerve VIII. Presbycusis, ototoxicity due to medica-

Table 13-1

Causes of Hearing Loss in the Elderly

Sensorineural
   Presbycusis
   Ototoxicity
      High-dose loop diuretics
      Chemotherapeutic agents
      Aminoglycosides
   Infections involving cranial nerve VIII
   Injury by vascular events
   Tumors of cranial nerve VIII
   Idiopathic sudden sensorineural hearing loss
Conductive
   Cerumen impaction
   Otosclerosis
   Chronic otitis media
   Tumors
   Degenerative disorders
      Meniere's disease
   Trauma
   Vasculitis
   Hemorrhagic disorders

tions, and Meniere's Disease (see Chap. 20) are common causes of hearing loss due to sensorineural function.

Conductive hearing loss is caused by reduced sound conduction in either the external auditory canal or the middle ear and is the major cause of hearing loss in the elderly. Common causes of conductive hearing loss include cerumen impaction, otosclerosis, and chronic serous otitis media.

Presbycusis

Presbycusis is the most common cause of sensorineural hearing loss in the elderly, affecting more than 30 percent of elderly individuals over the age of 75 years. It is bilateral hearing loss and starts in the higher frequency ranges above 2000 Hz. It usually starts in middle age and progresses with age. Eventually, perception of lower frequencies becomes impaired. Presbycusis interferes with speech discrimination. It affects men more than women.

The exact cause is unknown, but the hearing loss of presbycusis is probably most often caused by cumulative damage to the cochlea over time. In addition, there also appears to be a central auditory processing disorder occurring at the same time, because the difficulty with speech discrimination is more than would be expected resulting from just the hearing loss.

Presbycusis can be worsened by a number of medical conditions including cerebrovascular disease, diabetes mellitus, hypothyroidism, hypertension, and chronic lung disease. It can also be worsened by factors such as chronic alcohol abuse and long-term noise exposure.

Ototoxicity

Medications can cause hearing impairment. The most commonly implicated medications include aminoglycoside antibiotics, high-dose loop diuretics, and chemotherapeutic agents (e.g., cisplatin).

The mechanism of hearing loss is direct damage to the cochlea.

Cerumen

Cerumen impaction in the external auditory canal is the most common cause of reversible hearing impairment in the elderly. Older persons are more likely to overproduce sebaceous material that can accumulate in the external auditory canal.

Otosclerosis

Otosclerosis is the next most common cause of conductive hearing loss in the elderly. The hearing loss results from the immobility of the bony ossicles of the middle ear. It is an autosomal dominant, inheritable disorder.

Chronic Otitis Media

Chronic otitis media is a relatively common condition in the elderly. It refers to chronic or intermittent drainage through a perforation of the tympanic membrane. It can be associated with a cholesteatoma, a mass of squamous cell debris that can cause bony erosion and hearing loss.

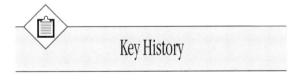

Key History

The onset of hearing loss is usually insidious and is often noted by family and friends before it is noticed by the individual suffering from the hearing loss. Patients with hearing loss can complain of difficulty hearing in the following situations: conversations in a crowded room, listening to the television, and favoring the use of one ear when using the telephone. It is important to ask the patient the timing of the hearing loss (e.g., insidious, progressive, or sudden) and the ears affected (unilateral or bilateral). Presbycusis is characterized by an insidious, progressive onset, whereas hearing loss due to medications is more sudden in onset. Hearing loss due to medications or otosclerosis is typically bilateral, whereas hearing loss due to chronic serous otitis media is usually unilateral.

Physical Examination

Hearing can be grossly evaluated in several ways. A clue to hearing impairment is the patient's request for the examiner to repeat questions during the interview. Another clue is that the patient does not give an answer appropriate for the question asked by the examiner. These two clues must be differentiated from cognitive impairment.

Another crude measure of hearing is the "whisper test," where the examiner softly whispers a series of numbers and has the patient repeat the numbers. Although it is widely used, this test may not be reproducible from examiner to examiner.

An examination of the ears should be performed. The ear canal should be examined for masses or blockages such as cerumen. The tympanic membrane should be visualized and any perforations or other abnormalities noted.

The clinician should perform the Rinne and Weber tests using a 512-mHz tuning fork. Both tests are used to differentiate a conductive hearing loss from a sensorineural hearing loss. The Rinne test compares air conduction and bone conduction of sound. The test is performed by placing the tuning fork on the mastoid process (testing for bone conduction) and then near the external auditory canal (testing for air conduction). Each ear is tested separately. Normally, the patient will hear "air conduction" better than "bone conduc-

tion." Bone-conducted sound that is perceived by the patient to be louder than air conduction usually suggests a conductive hearing loss.

The Weber test is also used to evaluate the cause of hearing loss. To perform the Weber test, the examiner places the tuning fork either on the center of the forehead or the top of the patient's head. "Lateralization" of the sound to one side implies a conductive hearing loss on the side of lateralization or a sensorineural hearing loss on the opposite side.

Ancillary Tests

Screening Tests

There are two reliable screening tests that can be used by an office-based clinician. The Hearing Handicap Inventory in the Elderly-Short Version (HHIE-S) (Table 13-2) and portable audioscopy can be used either individually or in combination to screen for hearing loss.

The HHIE-S is a 10-item questionnaire with scores ranging from 0 to 40, with 0 being no hearing impairment to 40 being maximum hearing impairment. The overall accuracy of the HHIE-S is 75 percent, using a cutoff score of 26.

A portable audioscope is easy to use and has a sensitivity of 87 to 96 percent and specificity of 70 to 90 percent. For screening purposes, the clinician need only test the patient at 1000 and 2000 Hz. These tones are in the speech perception range.

Audiologic Evaluation

Patients who fail either the HHIE-S or portable audioscopy, or both, should be referred for formal audiologic testing. Formal audiologic assessment in a soundproof room is considered the gold

Table 13-2

Hearing Handicap Inventory for the Elderly—Short Version

1. Does a hearing problem cause you to feel embarrassed when you meet new people?
2. Does a hearing problem cause you to feel frustrated when talking to members of your family?
3. Do you have difficulty hearing when someone speaks in a whisper?
4. Do you feel handicapped by a hearing impairment?
5. Does a hearing problem cause you difficulty when visiting friends, relatives, or neighbors?
6. Does a hearing problem cause you to attend religious services less often than you would like?
7. Does a hearing problem cause you to have arguments with family members?
8. Does a hearing problem cause you difficulty when listening to TV or radio?
9. Do you feel that any difficulty with your hearing limits or hampers your personal or social life?
10. Does a hearing problem cause you difficulty when in a restaurant with relatives or friends?

Scoring: yes = 4, no = 0, sometimes = 2.
SOURCE: Reproduced with permission from IM Ventry, B Weinstein: The hearing handicap inventory for the elderly: a new tool. *Ear Hearing*; 3:133, 1986.

frequency at which the individual can understand speech. Bone conduction testing, acoustic reflexes, and tympanometry are used to detect middle ear pathology such as otosclerosis. Audiologic testing can also be useful in identifying patients who may require further diagnostic evaluation to rule out conditions such as acoustic neuromas.

Other Tests

Syphilis is an uncommon, but potentially curable, cause of sensorineural hearing loss. Hearing loss can be the only symptom of late latent syphilis. Therefore, some clinicians recommend serologic testing for syphilis in patients with sensorineural hearing loss.

If a mass lesion is suspected, then computed tomography (CT) can be useful in examining the bony structures surrounding the cochlea. Magnetic resonance imaging (MRI) with gadolinium is useful in examining the acoustic nerve for tumors. If vestibular symptoms are present, vestibular testing can be performed including electronystagmometry and rotational tests.

Treatment

standard for the diagnosis of hearing disorders. Patients with a hearing loss detected on screening testing should undergo a formal audiologic evaluation by a qualified audiologist if they are potential candidates for hearing aids.

Formal testing includes pure tone audiometry, speech reception threshold, bone conduction testing, evaluation of acoustic reflexes, and tympanometry. Speech reception threshold is the lowest

The standard treatment of hearing impairment falls into one of three categories: medical, surgical, and rehabilitative approaches to hearing loss. The choice of treatment depends on the diagnosis. Treatment of hearing loss begins with the referral to the audiologist. Audiologists will not only test the individual, but will develop a treatment plan that can include hearing amplification. They can also instruct the patient in listening strategies and communication techniques. These methods can help to maximize and preserve what hearing the patient has remaining.

Medical

CERUMEN

There are a variety of methods to remove cerumen. In the office, cerumen can be removed with an ear spoon or curette, or by gentle irrigation with lukewarm water or hydrogen peroxide. A variety of over-the-counter remedies for removing cerumen are also available, but the effectiveness of these treatments has not been proven. A solution of sodium bicarbonate (1 tablespoon in 4 oz water; 2 drops in the affected ear, 4 times daily for 1 to 2 weeks) has been shown to be effective in dissolving cerumen. If these treatments fail, irrigation is usually effective in removing cerumen.

OTOTOXIC DRUGS

Potentially ototoxic medications should be discontinued if possible. Altering the dosing schedule can decrease the potential for ototoxicity. For example, once-daily dosing of gentamicin can be just as effective in treating susceptible organisms causing infection, but can be associated with decreased ototoxicity.

Surgery

Hearing amplification can be effective for otosclerosis. If amplification fails, stapedectomy is often effective. Cochlear implantation is indicated in patients with severe sensorineural deafness who are either not candidates for hearing amplification or who have failed attempts at hearing amplification. Age should not be a contraindication for cochlear implantation. When the hearing loss is greater than 80 dB, surgical interventions to amplify hearing are less likely to benefit the patient.

Patients with chronic otitis media can be treated with topical antibiotic drops such as neomycin/polymyxin B solution. If the drainage is chronic and persistent, the patient should be referred to an otolaryngologist.

Table 13-3
Assistive Hearing Devices

Telephone amplifiers
Large-area amplification systems
Television listening systems
Remote microphone systems
Alerting devices

Aural Rehabilitation

Amplification is a mainstay of treatment. A variety of aids to hearing are available.

ASSISTIVE HEARING DEVICES

Many assistive hearing devices are available (Table 13-3). Assistive listening devices that amplify sound across all frequencies include telephone amplifiers and large-area amplifications. The problem with these types of amplifiers is that they amplify all sounds, including background noise. An example of a large-area amplifier is a simple amplification device that can be purchased at most electronic stores. The user wears the amplification device around his or her neck or on a belt. The amplified sound is conveyed to the listener by earphones. This type of device can provide adequate amplification if the user is in a relatively quiet room, listening to television, or carrying on a conversation with one or two persons. In a crowded room, however, with many conversations going on, this type of device may not be helpful because all the sounds in the room will be amplified.

Television listening systems and remote microphone systems transmit the sound from the source directly to the user. An example would be a speaker delivering a speech, where the speech is being directly transmitted to the hearing impaired individual through a remote microphone system. In this situation, only the speaker's voice is being amplified and not the background noise in the room.

Many individuals use both assistive listening devices and hearing aids, tailoring their choice by the situation and amplification needed.

HEARING AIDS

Hearing aids come in two varieties: those placed behind the ear or within the auditory canal. In recent years, behind-the-ear units are becoming less commonly used, as miniaturization and digitalization have made excellent within-the-canal units possible.

Hearing aids are very effective in helping many individuals with sensorineural hearing loss. Studies of hearing impaired elderly persons who received hearing aids have shown improved social, emotional, communication, and cognitive functioning when compared with those waiting for amplification.

One of the most significant problems with hearing aids is that they are often not used. The elderly are less likely to use a hearing aid than a younger individual. Reasons for not wearing the hearing aid include denial of hearing loss as a problem, cost, and the perception that a hearing aid calls attention to the hearing impairment. Many individuals find it difficult to manipulate the controls and are annoyed by the buzzing sound that occasionally occurs. The presence of an auditory processing disorder that prevents the patient from recognizing sound despite adequate amplification can be another factor that accounts for dissatisfaction with hearing aids.

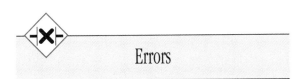

Errors

Primary care practitioners often fail to recognize and screen for signs and symptoms of hearing loss. The problem is often overlooked and not discussed. The estimated average duration of hearing impairment before it is either brought to the attention of or uncovered by the clinician is around 10 years. Although many patients decline to be formally evaluated and decline to wear hearing aids once purchased, the initial identification of the problem must be the first step.

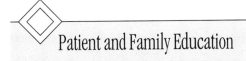

Patient and Family Education

Patients and family members should be educated about the signs and symptoms of hearing loss. The cause and prognosis of the hearing impairment should be reviewed. There are several behavioral techniques that can be of help to the hearing impaired patients. Family members should speak slowly and distinctly and directly face the individual when speaking, since lip reading can be an important aid to the hearing impaired person.

When a hearing aid has been prescribed, family members and friends can help encourage the individual to use the device. The patient and family should be informed that hearing aids are not a panacea. Hearing can be improved, but cannot be returned to normal. Patients should also be warned that an adjustment period occurs during which the user becomes accustomed to amplified sounds and learns to tune out unwanted sounds.

The Americans with Disabilities Act of 1990 has improved access to devices for the hearing impaired. There are professional groups and support groups whose primary focus is on the hearing impaired (Table 13-4).

Table 13-4

Resources for the Hearing Impaired

Self-Help for Hard of Hearing People, Inc.
    7910 Woodmont Ave, Suite 1200
    Bethesda, Maryland 20814
    Voice: 301-657-2248
    TTY: 301-657-2249
    FAX: 301-913-9413
    http://www.shhh.org/

American Speech-Language-Hearing
    Association
    http://www.asha.org/

American Academy of Audiology
    http://www.audiology.com

VISUAL IMPAIRMENT

Overview: How Common Is Visual Impairment in the Office Practice?

Functional blindness (low vision or blindness) is defined as vision worse than 20/200 in one or both eyes. The prevalence of functional blindness varies from 1 percent at age 70 years to almost 20 percent by age 90. Age-related macular degeneration, cataracts, and glaucoma account for 50 percent of all causes of blindness. These and other common causes of visual impairment are listed in Table 13-5.

Visual impairment has been implicated as a risk factor for a number of problems including hip fractures, falls, and poor mobility. Some studies have also linked increased mortality with visual impairment. In addition, visual impairment can lead to social isolation.

Principal Diagnoses

Cataracts

A cataract is an opacification of the lens. The prevalence of cataracts increases with advancing years and approaches 100 percent by age 90. Cataracts can develop in one or both lenses. There are multiple risk factors for developing cataracts (Table 13-6). The single greatest risk factor is

Table 13-5

Common Causes of Visual Impairment in the Elderly

PROGRESSIVE CAUSES	ACUTE CAUSES
Cataract	Retinal hemorrhage
Age-related macular degeneration	Corneal abrasion
Primary open-angle glaucoma	Vitreous hemorrhage
Diabetic retinopathy	Vitreous floaters
	Acute closed-angle glaucoma
	Corneal ulceration
	Herpetic eye disease
	Inflammatory eye disease
	Retinal detachment
	Choroidal neovascularization
	Central retinal artery occlusion
	Temporal arteritis

Table 13-6

Risk Factors for the Development of Cataracts

Normal aging
Diabetes mellitus
Ultraviolet B radiation
Corticosteriods
Smoking
Alcohol
Deficiency of vitamin C or E

normal aging. In general, cataracts are thought to develop because of an alteration in the lens metabolism.

Age-Related Macular Degeneration

Age-related macular degeneration (AMD) is one of the leading causes of vision loss in the elderly and is the leading cause of untreatable blindness. It can be either unilateral or bilateral. The prevalence of AMD is estimated to be approximately 20 percent in 75- to 85-year-olds to almost 40 percent in those individuals greater than 85 years of age.

AMD is divided into two types: nonexudative (dry) and exudative (wet). The two common features of both types are drusen (an amorphous material that accumulates in the retina) and degeneration in the area of the macula, which results in decreased central vision. Eighty percent of individuals have nonexudative AMD. Although exudative AMD occurs less frequently, it causes more severe vision loss.

Nonexudative AMD is marked by the accumulation of drusen throughout the retina. It has a yellowish appearance on funduscopic examination. Exudative, or wet, AMD is characterized by the appearance of choroidal neovascularization and hemorrhage. It is these two characteristics that lead to the severe vision loss seen in wet AMD.

Glaucoma

Glaucoma is an optic neuropathy that is usually associated with increased intraocular pressure (IOP). It is one of most common causes of blindness in the United States and the most common cause among African-Americans. There are two types of glaucoma: primary open-angle, or idiopathic, and angle-closure.

PRIMARY OPEN-ANGLE GLAUCOMA

Primary open-angle glaucoma is the most common form, accounting for approximately 60 to 70 percent of the cases. The cause of idiopathic glaucoma is resistance to outflow of the aqueous humor through the trabecular system of the eye. In the past, it was thought that this increased resistance lead to increased IOP, but now it is known that glaucoma can occur in the absence of increased IOP. Damage to the optic nerve can occur without increased IOP. In approximately 10 percent of cases, IOP is normal.

Although it is usually bilateral, glaucoma can be unilateral. Risk factors for the development of primary open-angle glaucoma include African-American race, increasing age, hypertension, diabetes, severe myopia, and family history of glaucoma.

PRIMARY ANGLE-CLOSURE GLAUCOMA

Primary angle-closure glaucoma occurs in individuals with a narrow anterior chamber. When there is closure of this chamber, as occurs when the pupil is dilated, the pressure within the eye builds rapidly. Damage to the optic nerve can quickly occur if this problem is not promptly addressed. Often, the patient develops symptoms such as eye pain and nausea very quickly. Risk factors for the development of angle-closure glaucoma include elderly women and hyperopia (far-sightedness). Anticholinergic medications (antidepressants, antipsychotics) can precipitate an acute episode of primary angle-closure glaucoma.

What Are Serious or Life-Threatening Diagnoses?

There are several conditions that can cause sudden visual impairment (Table 13–5). These conditions must be diagnosed and treated immediately to avoid permanent or severe visual loss.

Giant cell arteritis is an inflammatory process that involves the temporal artery and can lead to unilateral or bilateral sudden visual loss. This condition is discussed in Chap. 9.

Cerebrovascular disease can also cause acute vision loss by several different mechanisms. Amaurosis fugax refers to a sudden unilateral loss of vision that is usually transient. The underlying cause is a transient ischemic attack (TIA) of the retina by an embolus or plaque. Cerebrovascular accidents in the distribution of the posterior cerebral artery can also cause visual loss. Central retinal artery occlusion caused by an embolus can lead to permanent visual loss. Occasionally, a cholesterol plaque (Hollenhorst plaque) can be visualized in the retinal artery.

Retinal detachment usually begins as a tear in the peripheral retina. As it progresses, the visual loss becomes greater. Patients at greatest risk are those with severe myopia, eye trauma, or a history of cataract extraction.

Retinal vein occlusion can also lead to sudden visual loss. Hypertension, glaucoma, and diabetes are risk factors for venous occlusion.

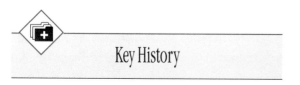

Key History

Common symptoms of visual impairment are shown in Table 13-7. Early symptoms of glaucoma include glare and poor contrast differentiation. Glare is most troublesome to patients in bright sunlight or at nighttime. Poor contrast differentiation is the difficulty or inability to distinguish shapes in a poorly illuminated environment. The

Table 13-7

Common Symptoms of Visual Impairment

Decreased visual acuity
Glare
Poor night vision
Image distortion
Central scotoma
Difficulty reading
Monocular diplopia
Visual loss
Pain
Redness
Discharge
Blurred vision
Floaters

combination of glare and poor contrast differentiation makes nighttime driving particularly troublesome for patients with early cataracts.

An early symptom of open-angle glaucoma is decreased visual acuity, particularly in peripheral fields of vision. Only in the later phases of the disease does central visual acuity become affected. Symptoms of primary angle-closure glaucoma include eye or brow pain, blurred vision, and colored halos around lights. The patient can also complain of a reddened eye. All of these symptoms usually developed rapidly, over a short period of time.

In contrast to open-angle glaucoma, AMD is characterized by the gradual deterioration of central vision with the preservation of peripheral vision. Patients can also complain of light sensitivity.

Sudden visual impairment is a medical emergency and should be immediately evaluated by an ophthalmologist. Associated symptoms can include eye pain, redness, eye discharge, flashes of light, and floaters. Systemic symptoms such as nausea, vomiting, dizziness, and vertigo can also suggest more serious pathology.

Physical Examination

General Vision Screening

The U.S. Preventive Services Task Force recommends vision screening, but does not specify a frequency (see Chap. 3). The American Academy of Ophthalmology recommends a complete eye examination every 1 to 2 years after 65 years of age. The examination should include: complete eye history; measurement of visual acuity; refraction, if appropriate; dilated eye examination; measurement of intraocular pressure; and a slit lamp examination.

This examination should be conducted by either an optometrist or ophthalmologist since the comprehensiveness of the examination is beyond the scope of most primary care clinicians. Patients with acute visual impairment should be evaluated promptly by primary care practitioners and referral made to an ophthalmologist, when indicated.

Screening for Glaucoma

Screening for glaucoma is not recommended. In the past, Schiotz tonometry was used to screen for glaucoma in the primary care setting. This instrument is inaccurate and its use is associated with an increased risk of corneal abrasion. The yield for general screening is low. Detecting glaucoma requires accurate measurement of the IOP, careful funduscopic examination of the optic cup by an experienced examiner, and a thorough assessment of visual field.

Treatment

Cataracts

For prevention, patients should wear UV protective lenses when exposed to sunlight. The treatment of early cataracts includes corrective lenses, magnification, visual aids, enhanced illumination, or sunglasses. Although these interventions can limit the severity of visual impairment, eventually, most patients will require a more definitive treatment for their cataract(s).

Cataract surgery remains the principal treatment for cataracts. The most important indication for cataract removal is decreased patient quality of life due to the cataract. Other indications for surgery include: (1) visual impairment with Snellen acuity of 20/50 or worse; and (2) visual disability of a one-eyed patient. Contraindications to surgery include: the patient's vision can be corrected with glasses or other visual aid; there is no impairment in the patient's functioning; or the patient is not medically fit. Once surgery is decided upon, phacoemulsification and extracapsular surgery are equally effective. An intraocular lens is frequently implanted, obviating the need for corrective glasses in most cases.

Age-Related Macular Degeneration

There is no effective treatment for AMD that restores vision. The results of laser therapy to halt the progression of the disease have been mixed. Even when initially successful, most individuals continue to have progressive disease. The purpose of laser therapy is to either prevent choroidal neovascularization by treating drusen or to halt the progression of established neovascularization. The use of laser therapy remains experimental (see "Emerging Concepts").

All patients with AMD should screen their central vision on a daily basis using an Amsler grid. A change in their central vision can indicate progressive disease.

Glaucoma

PRIMARY OPEN-ANGLE GLAUCOMA

Treatment of idiopathic glaucoma falls into three categories: medical, laser, and surgery. Medical therapy is most commonly prescribed initially with the goal of decreasing IOP. There are six categories of either topically applied or orally administered medications currently available for the treatment of open-angle glaucoma. Although primary care clinicians generally do not prescribe these medications, they need to be aware of potential systemic side effects of the medications (Table 13-8).

If medical therapy fails to halt the progression of glaucoma, laser or surgical interventions can be considered. Laser trabeculoplasty or surgical trabeculectomy are both aimed at increasing aqueous flow and subsequent decreases in the IOP.

PRIMARY CLOSED-ANGLE GLAUCOMA

Closed-angle glaucoma is treated in a similar fashion as open-angle glaucoma. Medical therapy is tried first to lower the IOP. If the pressure is successfully lowered, then a laser iridotomy or incisional iridectomy can be performed as a definitive therapy. If the IOP cannot be lowered by medical therapy, then laser or surgical therapy is usually performed. Prophylactic iridotomy is recommended if the unaffected eye is similar anatomically to the affected eye. This is due to the fact that approximately 50 percent of individuals will have an episode of closed-angle glaucoma in the opposite eye within 5 years.

Errors

Similar to hearing impairment, visual impairment can have adverse social and medical effects. Patients tend to attribute visual impairment to normal aging, and clinicians often do not ask specifically about visual impairment. In open-angle glaucoma, there can be a delay between the onset of the disease and subsequent symptoms. At a minimum, clinicians should inquire whether the patient has noted any visual changes. If so, they should be encouraged to have a complete eye examination.

Family Approach

As in hearing impairment, family members can be the first to note that the patient is experiencing visual difficulties. Family members should encourage the patient to obtain a thorough eye evaluation when there is a visual problem.

Patient and Family Education

In the early stages of cataract formation, patients should be reassured about the cause of their visual impairment and that there is potential for an excellent prognosis. Patients should also be counseled regarding potential problems with nighttime driving such as glare.

All patients with visual impairment should be instructed in the use of low vision aids or referred to an individual who can provide such instruction. Visual impairment from many causes can be partially alleviated with the use of low vision aids (Table 13-9). Low vision aids are very effective and inexpensive. In addition to proper illumination and appropriate prescription lenses, there are a variety of different commercially available magnifying devices including handheld magnifying lenses, microscopes, and telescopes. Leat and colleagues reported that the ability to read went from 20 percent of those referred to a low vision clinic to almost 90 percent, after attendance. Although not a cure, low vision aids can improve the patient's ability to perform activities of daily living including reading.

Table 13-8

Drugs for Glaucoma

Category	Examples of Drugs	Systemic Side Effects
Beta-adrenergic antagonists (topically applied)	Timolol (Timoptic) Carteolol (Ocupress) Betaxolol (Betoptic)	Bronchospasm, bradycardia, depression, confusion, impotence, congestive heart failure
Adrenergic agonists (topically applied)	Epinephrine (Glaucon) Dipivefrin (Propine) Brimonidine (Alphagan) Apraclonidine (Iodipine)	Elevated blood pressure, headache, palpitations, insomnia
Cholinergic agonists (topically applied)	Pilocarpine (Pilopine HS, Ocusert-Pilo) Carbachol (Miostat)	Bronchospasm, diaphoresis, change in vision, diarrhea, nausea
Carbonic anhydrase inhibitors (systemic)	Acetazolamide (Diamox) Methazolamide (Neptazane)	Anorexia, confusion, drowsiness, depression, malaise, GI distress, renal calculi, acidosis
Carbonic anhydrase inhibitors (topically applied)	Dorzolamide (Trusopt) Brinzolamide (Azopt)	Fewer systemic side effects than systemically administered
Prostaglandin receptor agonist (topically applied)	Latanoprost (Xalatan)	Rash, angina, muscle and joint pain

Table 13-9

Low Vision Aids

Magnifying devices
Proper illumination
Appropriate prescription lenses
Large print books

For the patient that enjoys reading, there are several options for the visually impaired. There are books and magazines published with large print. Books on tape are available at most bookstores and at public libraries. For more resources for the visually impaired, see Table 13-10.

Emerging Concepts

Age-Related Macular Degeneration

Since choroidal neovascularization (CN) is the main cause of loss of vision in AMD, treatments to either prevent or halt the progress of CN are being examined. A number of different laser treatments are being examined, including diode, argon green, and angiography guided laser therapies. Photodynamic therapy is being investigated. This treatment involves the use of photosensitizing drugs that accumulate in the diseased tissues. Activation of these drugs with specific wavelengths of light causes destruction of the CN. External beam radiation therapy is also being examined.

Pharmacologic approaches to the management of AMD are also under investigation. These treatments involve the use of drugs that either slow or halt neovascularization. Another approach is the use of neuroprotective agents that can be effective against both dry and wet AMD.

A diet high in antioxidants can lower the risk of AMD. There is speculation that antioxidants can protect the retina. Clinical studies are underway that should determine the protective role of dietary antioxidants.

Table 13-10

Resources for Individuals with Visual Impairment

National Association for the Visually Handicapped (NAVH)
NAVH New York City
22 West 21st Street
New York, NY 10010
Voice: 212-889-3141
Fax: 212-727-2931
NAVH San Francisco
3201 Balboa Street
San Francisco, CA 94121
Voice: 415-221-3201
Fax: 415-221-8754
http://www.navb.org/
American Academy of Ophthalmology
http://www.eyenet.org/public/pi/
(This website has numerous links to support groups and other resources.)
Glaucoma Service Foundation to Prevent Blindness
Wills Eye Hospital, 3rd Floor
900 Walnut Street
Philadelphia, PA 19107-5598
http://wills-glaucoma.org/
Prevent Blindness America
500 E. Remington Rd.
Schaumburg, IL 60173
847-843-2020
800-331-2020
http://www.prevent-blindness.org

Glaucoma

Traditionally, it has been postulated that open-angle glaucoma is caused by the effects of IOP. Since IOP is not universally present in all patients with open-angle glaucoma, the exact mechanism is still unclear. Some have postulated a vascular component as part of the cause of open-angle glaucoma. As the cause is further elucidated, new treatments and approaches will become available.

Bibliography

American Academy of Ophthalmology: *American Academy of Ophthalmology Preferred Practice Patterns: Comprehensive Adult Eye Evaluation.* San Francisco; 1996.

American Academy of Ophthalmology: *American Academy of Ophthalmology Preferred Practice Patterns: Glaucoma.* San Francisco; 1996.

Bressler NM, Bressler SB: Preventative ophthalmology: age-related macular degeneration. *Ophthalmology* 102:1206, 1995.

D'Amico DJ: Diseases of the retina. *N Eng J Med* 331:95, 1994.

Freeman WR, Blumenkranz MS: Age-related macular degeneration: is help on the way (editorial)? *Ophthamology* 105:1585, 1998.

Jerger J, Chmiel R, Wilson N, Luchi R: Hearing impairment in older adults: new concepts. *J Am Geriatr Soc* 43:928, 1995.

Leat SJ, Fryer A, Rumney NJ: Outcome of low vision aid provision: the effectiveness of a low vision clinic. *Optom Vis Sci* 71:199, 1994.

Liesegang TJ: Glaucoma: changing concepts and future directions. *Mayo Clin Proc* 71:689, 1996.

Maggi S, Minicuci N, Marini A, et al: Prevalence rates of hearing impairment and comorbid conditions in older people: the Veneto study. *J Am Geriatr Soc* 46:1069, 1998.

Margrain TH: Minimising the impact of visual impairment (editorial). *BMJ* 318:1504, 1999.

Mulrow CD, Lichtenstein MJ: Screening for hearing impairment in the elderly. Rationale and strategy. *J Gen Int Med* 6:249, 1991.

Nadol JB: Hearing loss. *N Eng J Med* 1092, 1993.

Popelka MM, Cruickshanks KJ, Wiley TL, et al: Low prevalence of hearing aid use among older adults with hearing loss: the Epidemiology of Hearing Loss Study. *J Am Geriatr Soc* 46:1075, 1998.

Quillen DA: Common causes of vision loss in elderly patients. *Am Fam Physician* 60:99, 1999.

Reuben DB, Mui S, Damesyn M, et al: The prognostic value of sensory impairment in older persons. *J Am Geriatr Soc* 47:930, 1999.

United States Preventive Services Task Force. *Clinician's Handbook of Preventive Services*, 2nd ed. Baltimore: Williams & Wilkins; 1998.

Ventry IM, Weinstein B: The hearing handicap inventory for the elderly: a new tool. *Ear Hearing* 3:133, 1986.

Barbara Resnick
Michael Corcoran
Ann Marie Spellbring

Chapter

Gait and
Balance Disorders

WALKERS Medications for Spasticity **Errors**	**Family Approach and Patient Education** Handouts for Patient and Families Regarding Fall Prevention

Overview: How Common Are Gait and Balance and Movement Problems in the Office Practice?

Changes in gait and balance commonly accompany aging and can be indicative of the health and biologic age of the older individual. Although up to 85 percent of older adults (age 65 to 69 years) report no difficulty in walking, the prevalence decreases to 66 percent of individuals between 80 to 84 years of age. In addition, 51 percent of those who are over 85 years of age report no difficulty in walking. Thirteen percent of older adults age 65 to 69 years living in the community complain of balance problems or unsteadiness when walking or changing positions, and about 46 percent of those 85 years of age or older report balance problems. From 8 to 19 percent of community dwelling older adults have difficulty walking or require the assistance of another person and/or special equipment to facilitate ambulation.

Not only are gait and balance issues prevalent in the older population, but also the implications of alterations in either gait or balance can be devastating. Gait and balance disorders put older individuals at an increased risk of falling, which frequently results in injury, and it can also cause psychosocial sequelae such as a loss of self-esteem, autonomy, depression, anxiety, fear of falling that influences activity, and social isolation. Unfortunately, many older adults and health care providers accept gait disorders and decreased mobility as a normal age change. Older adults especially, may assume that slowing down and stiffening of joints is inevitable. Gait disorders,

however, are often a symptom of underlying diseases that can be treatable. The office practitioner must aggressively evaluate older adults for these problems, identify potentially treatable conditions, and provide the patient and family with appropriate therapeutic interventions.

Principal Diagnoses

Diseases and their associated impairments play a more important role in gait, balance, and movement disorders than age-related changes. Nevertheless, to evaluate and treat older adults, it is essential to be familiar with the common physiologic and physical changes that occur with age and how these changes influence gait and balance (Table 14-1). Moreover, normal changes must be recognized so that they are not attributed to specific disease states and inappropriate treatment instituted.

With age, there is a decline in gait speed of 0.2 percent per year up to age 63, and this decline increases up to 1.6 percent per year after age 63. Other characteristics of gait that change with aging include a decline in step length, stride length, ankle range of motion, decreased vertical and increased horizontal head excursions, decrease in spinal rotation, decrease arm swing, increased length of double support phase of walking, and a reduction in propulsive force generated at the push off phase.

With age, there is a decrease in sensory input (proprioception, vision), slowing of motor responses, and other musculoskeletal limitations.

Table 14-1

Common Age-Related Musculoskeletal and Neurologic Changes that Influence Gait and Balance

SYSTEM	COMMON CHANGES
Muscle	Decreased aerobic and anaerobic capacity
	Decreased muscle bulk
	Loss of muscle fibers (Type II-fast twitch)
	Quadriceps most likely to atrophy
	Decreased oxygen delivery to muscles
Neurologic	Reduced effectiveness of neurotransmitters
	Changes in nerve cells (decreased effectiveness of synaptic connections)
	Decreased number of nerve cells
	Increased reaction time
	Decreased number of motor units
	Reduced sensory capacity
	Thresholds for sensory information increases
Skeletal	Loss of bone mass
	Decreased elasticity of connective tissue and muscle
	Degenerative changes
	Increased thoracic kyphosis
	Flattening of the lumbar curve
	Posterior pelvic tilt and/or lumbar lordosis
	Flexed hip and knee joints
	Dorsiflexion of the ankle joint

The combination of these changes results in an increase in unsteadiness or postural sway under both static and dynamic conditions. Most older adults will compensate for these changes. For example, visual input can be used to augment proprioceptive loss, and older individuals will look down to view the correct placement of their feet when ambulating.

There are a number of common pathologic gait disorders in the older adult (Table 14-2) that can occur alone or in combination. The abnormal pattern of movement can occur because: (1) the patient has no choice, that is, the movement is caused by spasticity, weakness, or deformity; or (2) the abnormal movement is compensating for another problem such as dizziness or pain. Gait and balance can be compromised by cardiovascu-lar, arthritic, and orthopedic conditions. They are probably most commonly influenced by neurologic disorders.

Neurologic Problems

STROKE

Strokes affect 731,000 Americans annually, with most strokes (80 percent) being ischemic, 66 percent of which result in chronic neurologic deficits that impair gait and balance. Approximately 30 percent of older persons with abnormal gait patterns have evidence of cerebral infarcts on CT scan, but no known history of hemiparesis or other motor deficits from the stroke.

Table 14-2

Gait Disorders

TYPE OF GAIT	DESCRIPTION OF GAIT
Frontal lobe gait	Wide base of support
	Slightly flexed posture
	Small shuffling hesitant steps
	Poor initiation of gait—"slipping clutch syndrome"
	Turns by pivoting both feet in a small circle
	Cannot control changes in base of support
Sensory ataxic gait	Wide based stance—"foot stamping walk"
	High step and stamping walk
	Heel touches first then foot stamps
	Visual input used to ambulate
	Positive Romberg's sign
Cerebellar ataxic gait	Wide-based stance
	Small irregular unsteady steps
	Drunken veering and lurching
	Impaired trunk control
	Difficulty with tandem gait
	Turns en bloc
Spastic gait	Swings affected leg slowly in outward arc—circumduction of the leg
	Legs trace a semicircle when walking
	Feet scrape the ground
	Scissoring occurs
	Short steps
	Narrow base
Spastic paraparesis	Legs move slowly in a stiff manner
	Short labored steps with decreased hip and knee movement (bilateral circumduction)
	Toes scrape the ground
	Scissoring occurs
	Short steps
	Narrow base
Steppage gait	Feet are lifted high off the ground to prevent scrapping toes
	Toes hit first then heels
	Head down to observe foot placement
Peripheral vestibular imbalance	Unsteady gait
Antalgic and gonalgic gait	Reluctant to put weight on the joint
	Heel strike avoided on affected foot
	Push off avoided
	Decreased stance and swing phases of gait
	Decreased walking velocity
	Knee and foot flexed
	Decreased hip and knee extension
	Limp due to leg length discrepancies

Table 14-2

Gait Disorders (*continued*)

TYPE OF GAIT	DESCRIPTION OF GAIT
Podalgic gait	Pain with ambulation
	Toe contact occurs for three-fourths of the gait cycle
Dementia related gait	Decreased walking speed
	Decreased step length
	Increased double support time
	Increase step to step variability
	Increased postural sway
	Flexed posture
	Apraxic gait
Festinating gait	Symmetric rapid shuffling of feet
	Trunk bent forward hips and knees flexed
	Difficulty stepping
Parkinsonian gait	Festination
	"Marche á petits pas"—short flat footed shuffles
	Delayed gait initiation
	Body moves forward before feet
	Freezing
	Wide stance
	"En bloc" turning
	Loss of postural control
	Retropulsion—falls back "in one piece" like a log
	Propulsion
Waddling gait	Lateral trunk movement away from the foot with exaggerated rotation of the pelvis and rolling of hips
	Difficulty with stairs and chair rise
Vestibular ataxic gait	Broad based with frequent side stepping
	Drift toward the sound of vestibular impairment
	Unsteady
Cautious gait	Flexed posture
	Decreased stride length
	Decreased walking speed
	Low center of gravity
	Wide based
	Short steps
	Turning "en bloc"

Impairment depends on the size, location, and nature of the offending lesion. A stroke can result in a hemiplegia, hemiparesis, or paraparesis, which results in a loss of muscle strength and frequently, proprioceptive input on the affected side. In hemi-plegia, the affected leg is often stiff, slightly flexed at the hip and extended at the knee, and the foot is plantar-flexed. The affected arm is often maintained in a position of flexion at the elbow. All of this influences gait and balance. There is also an alteration in the sequence of postural muscle activation on the affected side. Instead of the normal sequence of distal to proximal muscle activation, the proximal muscles of the hemiplegic or paretic extremity are activated first. This impairs the individual's ability to initiate a quick postural response. Poor postural control has also been attributed to vestibular dysfunction and visuospatial impairment (hemi-inattention) or neglect (hemianopsia) following a stroke.

Cerebral infarcts include état lacunaire, a syndrome that results from multiple small cerebral infarcts secondary to hypertensive cerebrovascular disease. Specific infarcts that involve only the cerebellar area result in cerebellar ataxia.

PARKINSONISM

Parkinson's disease is very common in the older adult, with 1 to 2 percent of those older than 60 years of age having the disease. The age-specific incidence and the prevalence increase with age. Males are affected slightly more often than females.

The common form of Parkinson's disease in the older adults is idiopathic Parkinson's disease. This disease is characterized by the disruption in synthesis of dopamine from pigmented neurons in the substantia nigra and locus ceruleus. The deficiency of dopamine, which functions as a neurotransmitter in the striatum and in other related brain centers, results in the vast array of physical changes, cognitive dysfunction, and depressive symptoms that characterize Parkinson's disease.

PERIPHERAL NEUROPATHIES

Peripheral neuropathy is a serious complication of many common problems found in older adults. Table 14-3 describes common types of neuropathies and associated diseases and causes. There are three components of the peripheral nervous system (PNS): the nerve cell body (neuron), the axon, and the myelin sheath enveloping the axon. Diseases of these components are described as neuronopathies, axonopathies, and myelinopa-

thies, respectively. Peripheral neuropathies are classified as focal or multifocal, and can influence a single nerve (mononeuropathy) or multiple nerves (mononeuritis multiplex). Small myelineated and unmyelineated fibers can be involved, resulting in decreased pain and temperature sensation. Conversely, large myelineated fibers can be involved resulting in areflexia and reduction in vibration and position sense.

NORMAL PRESSURE HYDROCEPHALUS

Normal pressure hydrocephalus occurs when the lateral and third ventricles are enlarged out of proportion to generalized cerebral atrophy. Classically, normal pressure hydrocephalus (NPH) is characterized by the triad of dementia, urinary incontinence, and several different gait disturbances, as described in Table 14-4. The prevalence of NPH is not as common as once believed, occurring in only 1 percent of a population of older adults with dementia.

SPINAL CORD INVOLVEMENT

The degenerative changes of cervical spondylosis, which is the most frequent cause of cord compression in the elderly, begin with desiccation and fragmentation of the intervertebral discs. There is a decrease in elasticity of the annulus, and the disk height diminishes. Osteophytic spurs can develop around the disk, and there can be parallel degeneration of the hypophyseal joints to reduce the size of the neural foraminae. The changes all result in a decrease in movement of the spinal cord and nerve roots within the cord, and influence lower extremity function. Vitamin B_{12} deficiency, in addition to causing peripheral neuropathies, can result in cord degeneration and myelopathy.

PERIPHERAL VESTIBULAR DYSFUNCTION

Vestibular dysfunction can be either peripheral (involve end organs including the semicircular canals, utricle or saccule, the vestibular nerve and

Table 14-3
Diagnostic Categories of Peripheral Neuropathies

DIAGNOSTIC CATEGORIES OF PERIPHERAL NEUROPATHIES	SPECIFIC DISEASES WITHIN EACH CATEGORY	SIGNS AND SYMPTOMS
Distal symmetrical sensorimotor neuropathy (glove and stocking)	Hereditary neuropathies	Distal muscle wasting
	Metabolic and Endocrine disorders	Decreased/absent tendon reflexes
	Drugs and toxins	Loss of sensation
	Vitamin deficiencies	
	Alcohol	
	Neoplasms	
	Infections	
	Acromegaly	
	Hypothyroidism	
	Paraproteinemia	
Polyradiculoneuropathy	Acute inflammatory demyelination	Weakness is more prominent than sensory complaints
	Chronic inflammatory demyelination	Proximal limb, trunk, and cranial nerve involvement
		Hypoactive/absent reflexes
Mononeuritis multiplex	Mononeuritis multiplex of gradual onset	Asymmetrical limb involvement
	Mononeuritis multiplex of abrupt onset	Symptoms determined by nerves involved
Large-fiber sensory neuropathy	Neoplastic sensory neuropathy	Loss of proprioceptive sense
	Drug-associated sensory neuropathy	Severe sensory ataxia
		Loss of vibration and joint position sense
		Preserved pain, temperature and touch
Small-fiber sensory and autonomic neuropathy	Diabetes	Pain
	Amyloidoses	Pricking and burning sensations
		Impaired pain and temperature
		Preserved vibration and position sense
Motor neuropathy	Lead intoxication	Fasciculations
	Hepatic porphyrias	Severe proximal and distal wasting and weakness
	Diphtheria	

nuclei), or central (involve brain stem and cerebellum). Episodes of vertigo can be due to age-related changes occurring in the vestibular portion of the inner ear, such as degeneration in the ampullary mechanism of the semicircular canal, labyrinthitis or vestibular neuronitis from infection, Meniere's disease, medications, head trauma, or degeneration of the cervical spine.

Table 14-4

Diseases and Common Abnormal Gait and Balance Presentations

DISEASE	GAIT AND BALANCE PRESENTATION
Stroke	Frontal lobe gait
	Cerebellar ataxic gait
Lacunar infarcts	Spastic paraparesis
Late stage Alzheimer's disease	Frontal lobe gait
Normal pressure hydrocephalus	Frontal lobe gait
	Gait apraxia
	Parkinsonian gait
	Festinating gait
Spinal cord compression	Spastic paraparesis
Hyperthyroidism	Spastic paraparesis
	Waddling gait
Parkinson's disease	Festinating gait
	Parkinsonian gait
Labyrinthine disease	Vestibular ataxic gait
Degenerative joint disease	Antalgic gait (hip)
	Gonalgic gait (knee)
Foot disorders	Podalgic gait
B_{12} and thiamine deficiency	Steppage gait
	Sensory ataxic gait
	Cerebellar gait
	Spastic paraparesis
Diabetic neuropathy	Sensory ataxic gait
	Steppage gait
Vestibular damage	Cerebellar ataxic gait
Spinocerebellar degeneration	Cerebellar ataxic gait
Chronic alcohol abuse	Cerebellar ataxic gait
	Steppage gait
Supranuclear palsy	Cerebellar ataxic gait
Hypothyroidism	Cerebellar ataxic gait
	Waddling gait
Cervical spondylitic myelopathy	Spastic paraparesis

MOVEMENT DISORDERS

TREMOR   By definition, a tremor refers to rhythmic oscillations produced by involuntary contractions of reciprocally innervated antagonistic muscles. Tremor is categorized by the activity that maximizes the tremor. A postural or action tremor is most evident when antigravity posture is being maintained. A rest tremor is one that is most evident when the limb is inactive. Kinetic or intention tremor is a rhythmic movement present in a limb as it approaches a goal.

Tremor can be due a variety of conditions, both physical and pathologic. Table 14-5 lists the common metabolic and toxic, physical, and emotional

Table 14-5

Causes of Tremor

Hyperthryoidism
Uremia
Liver failure
Alcohol withdrawal
Lithium
Tricyclic antidepressants
Caffeine, theophylline
Isoproterenol
Valproate sodium
Steroids
Narcotics
Emotions
Fatigue and exercise
Hypoglycemia
Pathologic disease (parkinsonism, demyelinating disease, vascular insult, neuropathies, tumors, and trauma)
Infections

causes of tremor. The majority of tremors in older adults are parkinsonism tremors, benign essential tremors, and metabolic and toxic tremors.

CHOREOATHETOSIS Choreiform movements are spontaneous or involuntary brief muscle contrac-tions that produce simple movements, such as flexion or extension of a finger, or complex semi-purposeful movements, such as raising the hand to the face. These movements can occur at rest or with voluntary movements, and are irregular. Com-mon causes of choreiform movements are listed in Table 14-6, with tardive dyskinesia from medica-tions being the disorder most frequently seen in older adults.

MYOCLONUS Myoclonic movements are brief, shock-like contractions of muscle that can lead to almost undetectable movement, or produce large movements of the limbs or trunk. They are also irregular, and can be initiated by touch, inten-tional movement, or noise. Myoclonus can arise from disorders of the spinal cord, brain stem, and cerebral hemispheres. It is most often a benign disorder described as "sleep jerks."

DYSTONIA Dystonic movements are characterized by slow protracted muscle contractions that pro-duce abnormal postures of limbs and axial struc-tures. The dystonic contractures can be bizarre. Meige's syndrome (cranial dystonia) is the most common dystonia in the older adult. Meige's syn-drome affects the face, causing forceful involun-tary contractures. It occurs commonly in the 6th and 7th decades, with women being more often affected than men.

Table 14-6

Causes of Choreiform Movement

CAUSE	FEATURES
Drugs: neuroleptics; reserpine; levodopa	Drug use Facial and oral motor movements
Metabolic: hyperthyroidism and hypocalcemia	Altered thyroid tests and calcium levels
Vascular: vasculitis, polycythemia	Sudden onset of hemichorea Altered CBC, ANA, ESR
Infections: encephalitis, Creutzfeldt-Jakob	Dementia, additional neurologic symptoms/signs
AIDS	HIV positive
Genetic: Huntington's disease	Chorea, dementia, personality changes

ABBREVIATIONS: CBC, complete blood count; ANA, antinuclear antibody; ESR, erythrocyte sedimentation rate.

TICS   Tics are repetitive, stereotyped movements that generally involve the face, respiratory muscles, neck, and shoulder. The movements can be voluntarily repressed or initiated. Generally, tics are benign and not indicative of central nervous system disease.

Orthopedic Problems

The most common orthopedic disease in the older adult is degenerative joint disease. Osteoarthritis is due to a series of degenerative processes that affect the articular structures of the bones and result in pain and diminished function. The incidence of osteoarthritis increases with age and the majority include the hands, hips, knees, spine, and midfoot. Other arthritic disorders that commonly influence gait and balance include gout and rheumatoid arthritis. Any orthopedic injury, such as a fracture or contusion, can cause pain that can alter balance and gait.

Orthopedic foot problems have a significant effect on gait and balance. Older adults can have atrophy of the plantar pad, which causes a loss in shock absorption, onychogryphosis (overgrown, claw-like toenails), corns, and pressure areas that cause pain and thereby, alter gait.

Endocrine Disorders

Thyroid disease is common in the older adult with 17.5 percent of those 75 years of age or older having evidence of hypothyroidism, and subclinical hyperthyroidism occurring in 1 to 5 percent of the population over 65 years of age. Thyroid hormones affect the function of virtually every organ system, and the major role of the thyroid is to maintain metabolic stability. Hypothyroidism has been reported to cause a sensory polyneuropathy and thus, result in an ataxic gait. A myopathy can also be present causing proximal weakness and myalgias. Hyperthyroidism-associated gait disturbances usually occur due to proximal myopathy, although a related myelopathy and neuropathy have also been reported.

Medications

There are a variety of medications that can influence gait and balance. The major drug groups include sedating psychotropic medications such as benzodiazepines (especially the long-acting agents), tricyclic antidepressants, phenothiazines, anticonvulsants, salicylates, and antivertigo agents (such as Antivert). Moreover, any medications that cause orthostatic hypotension or reduced intravascular volume (antihypertensive agents, diuretics, and antianginal agents) will likewise impair balance and thereby, alter gait.

Idiopathic Senile Gait Disorder

Eighteen percent of those in the community with gait disorders have no specific disease-related cause of their impairment. These individuals are believed to have an "idiopathic senile gait disorder." This is described as a gait pattern that is broad-based with small steps, diminished arm swing, stooped posture, flexion of the hips and knees, uncertainty and stiffness in turning, occasional difficulty initiating steps, and a tendency toward falling. These changes in gait can also be seen in other disease states, but the associated signs and symptoms of these diseases are not present. It is only when clinical and laboratory examination fail to reveal any specific cause of the gait disturbance that the diagnosis of an idiopathic senile gait disorder is made.

What Serious or Life-Threatening Diagnoses Must Always Be Considered, Even If Rare?

Diseases and their associated impairments are often the cause of gait and balance disturbances. Some or all of these conditions can potentially be life-threatening. Falls resulting in hip fracture are associated with a mortality of up to 25 percent in the year after hip fracture. Therefore, aggressive attempts to establish the underlying cause(s) of gait and balance changes are essential. Any of the diagnoses identified previously should be considered, and it is also possible that multiple diagnoses are present. A single diagnosis can be determined in approximately 60 percent of all older adults with a gait disorder; however, anywhere from 28 to 75 percent of gait disorders are caused by multiple diagnoses. Establishing the underlying cause of the problem allows the primary care provider to identify and treat the presenting disorder before it becomes more serious or life-threatening.

Typical Presentation

How Do Different Symptoms Suggest One Diagnosis or Another?

CEREBROVASCULAR DISEASE

Patients with hemiplegia, hemiparesis, or paraparesis secondary to cerebrovascular disease often present with a spastic gait. When walking, arm swing on the affected side is impaired, and the toes of the involved leg scrape against the floor due to decreased ankle dorsiflexion. Patients may have frontal lobe gait disorders, sensory ataxic gait, or cerebellar ataxic gait, depending on the site of the lesion. Descriptions of these gaits are presented in Table 14-2. Moreover, the patient with a stroke may have a severe loss of proprioception and marked lack of muscular coordination. This results in gait disturbances and disturbances of other purposeful movements.

État lacunaire presents with combinations of postural defects, hypertonia, impaired fine movements, impaired facial movements, and dementia. The gait disorder is of the "marche á petit pas type" (small steps, rapid cadence) (see Table 14-2) and pseudobulbar crying (emotional liability) are also common, distinguishing this syndrome from Parkinson's disease. Cerebellar involvement results in a cerebellar ataxia with an ataxic gait that becomes somewhat worse when the eyes are closed. The patient can present with a staggering, unsteady, irregular, wide-based gait.

PARKINSON'S DISEASE

Signs and symptoms that help characterize Parkinson's disease (Table 14-7), and differentiate this disease from others with similar gait presentations, include tremor, rigidity, bradykinesia, and static/kinetic postural abnormalities. The tremor is classically a 4- to 6-Hz tremor and is present when the limb is at rest. The tremor will disappear when the patient is asleep or voluntarily moves the limb. The tremor generally begins in one hand and then spreads to the ipsilateral foot, and the contralateral limbs, and perhaps to the head, tongue and jaw. The presence, however, of tremor alone is not sufficient for the diagnosis of Parkinson's disease.

The second common feature of Parkinson's disease is rigidity. The rigidity is perceived as cogwheeling resistance to passive movement of a joint, and is best appreciated at the wrist and elbow. Rigidity is often first detected in the nuchal musculature.

The third common feature is bradykinesia, or akinesia. Bradykinesia refers to the slowness and imprecision of voluntary movements, the loss of automatic or associated movements, or the inability to initiate any movement. Voluntary movements may be visibly slowed. Repetitive dexterous movements become irregular in tempo and amplitude, leading to scratchy, small handwriting (micrographia) and difficulty with hand tools, eating utensils, and personal care. The blink rate is decreased, facial expression fixed, and the voice can become soft and monotonous. Speech is hurried, a festination of sound production that is similar to the festinating gait (see Table 14-2). There can be an associated inability to swallow and drooling is common.

The fourth feature of Parkinson's disease involves static and kinetic postural abnormalities. Patients often assume a flexed posture (simian posture), with flexion of the knees, trunk, elbows,

Table 14-7

Signs and Symptoms of Parkinson's Disease

CARDINAL AREAS	SPECIFIC SYMPTOMS
Bradykinesia	Progressively smaller handwriting
	Reduced semiautomatic gestures
	Reduced spontaneous facial movements, mask-like stare, and infrequent blinking
	Slowed movements
	Soft voice that trails off
Rigidity	Breathing, eating, swallowing, and speech affected
	Cogwheel rigidity where muscles move in series of short jerks
	Lead-pipe rigidity where muscles move smoothly but stiffly
	Sustained muscle contraction
	Ambulation with arms held stiffly at sides
Postural instability	Difficulty with balance when walking or standing
	Frequent falls
	Stooping forward to maintain center of gravity
Tremor	Resting tremor that involves hands and feet; head, neck, face, lips, tongue, or jaw less often affected
	Often the initial presenting symptom and affects 50%–70% of patients
	Tremor is regular and rhythmic (4–6 beats per second)
	Tremor occurs at rest
	Pill-rolling type-tremor

wrists, and metacarpophalangeal joints. Fixed spinal deformities (scoliosis) can develop. The trunk, when standing, can drift to the side or backward, and retropulsion is common. Dementia and depression frequently occur in patients with Parkinson's disease.

PERIPHERAL NEUROPATHIES

The signs and symptoms of specific neuropathies are described in Table 14-3. Generally, patients with neuropathies will complain of sensory changes, proprioceptive deficits, and may walk with stiff legs, reduced toe clearance, and a tendency toward circumduction. Early paresthesias can give way to full loss of position sense causing sensory ataxia, wide-based "tottering," and weakness. In patients with Vitamin B_{12} deficiency, ataxia of the gait can be the presenting problem.

NORMAL PRESSURE HYDROCEPHALUS

NPH classically presents with a triad of symptoms including dementia, urinary incontinence, and gait disturbances. The gait disturbance, however, sometimes precedes the other features of the disease by as much as 3 or 4 years. The syndrome begins with small-steps and an apraxic gait with marked imbalance. The gait disturbance is usually akinesic or dyskinesic with a tendency toward retropulsion.

SPINAL CORD DISEASE

Spinal cord involvement, including cervical spondylitic myelopathy or a cervical tumor, classically presents with increased tendon reflexes bilaterally in the limbs. In older adults, however, tendon reflexes can be decreased due to normal age-related changes. Patients will more likely present with nonspecific gait changes, increased muscle tone, progressive spasticity, and incontinence.

Orthopedic and foot problems present with complaints of pain, particularly pain with ambulation. With advanced degenerative joint disease, crepitus can be palpable on passive range of motion and suggests cartilage abnormalities. Cartilage damage tends to be asymmetric within each involved joint and the external appearance of the joint is often deformed. With advancing disease, range-of-motion limitations occur. Careful examination of the feet of older adults can reveal pressure areas, corns, calluses, and nail abnormalities that impact comfort and can alter gait patterns.

VESTIBULAR DISORDERS

Older adults can present with a variety of signs and symptoms that indicate vestibular dysfunction (Table 14-8). Vertigo usually occurs suddenly,

Table 14-8
Disorders Resulting in Peripheral Vestibular Imbalance

DISORDER	SIGNS AND SYMPTOMS
Benign paroxysmal positional vertigo	Sudden, intense head spinning for 30 seconds or less following position change
	Mild nausea
	Symptoms worse in AM
	Hearing and neurologic exam WNL
	Rotary nystagmus
Dysequilibrium of aging	Unsteadiness after turning head or changing position
Labyrinthitis and vestibular neuronitis	Sudden onset vertigo
	Nausea and vomiting
	Episodes of unsteadiness
	Vertigo persists for days
	Preceding viral infection common
	Head movement exacerbates vertigo
Meniere's disease	Vertigo lasting 30 min to 12 h
	Hearing loss (low frequency sensorineural)
	Tinnitus
	Feeling of ear fullness
	Sudden unsteadiness of gait
Drugs	
Aminoglycosides	Spinning sensation
Anticonvulsants	Balance worse in the dark
Benzodiazepines	Oscillopsia (objects move back and forth with head movement)
Salicylates	
Head trauma	Vertigo may occur days to weeks post trauma
	May have associated hearing loss
Cervical vertigo	Episodes of disequilibrium
	Induced by positional head and neck movements
	Tendency to stagger

ABBREVIATION: WNL, within normal limits.

lasts briefly, and can be associated with position changes as in benign positional vertigo. Conversely, vertigo can last for days and be associated with a viral infection as in vestibular neuronitis. Meniere's disease presents with vertigo that is associated with tinnitus, hearing loss, and a feeling of fullness in the ears. In all cases of peripheral vestibular imbalance, the gait is affected by the associated sensations and the balance changes.

MOVEMENT DISORDERS

The stereotyped and rhythmic nature of tremors differentiates these disorders from other gait and balance disorders (Table 14-9). Benign essential tremor commonly affects the hands, head, and voice. The tremor occurs during a maintained posture and during kinetic movements, but not at rest. The tremor has a frequency of 5 to 9 Hz. The head tremor can be horizontal (no-no) or vertical (yes-yes), and voice tremor can also occur. Tremors begin insidiously and progress. Patients will note that alcohol reduces the tremor, the effects of which last for 30 min to 1 h. These individuals will also complain of difficulty with handwriting, drinking liquids, fine manipulations, and eating. Patients with cerebellar disease can have both a postural and characteristic kinetic tremor. The kinetic tremors, with frequencies of 3 to 5 Hz, are noted on finger-nose and heel-shin tests. The tremors associated with alcohol withdrawal consist of gross movements involving the entire body.

The presentation of choreiform movements is jerky and irregular, which is what helps to differentiate these disorders from a tic. Comparatively, myoclonic movements are similarly irregular, but are less shock-like than choreiform movements. Dystonia, particularly Meige's syndrome, presents with forceful involuntary closure of the eyelids, involuntary opening of the eye, and tongue protrusion. There can be retraction of the corners of the mouth, contraction of the platysma, jaw clenching, lip pursing, and torticollis. Patients may complain of difficulty driving or doing needle work, and may have dysarthria and dysphagia. These findings may also be noted in patients with tardive dyskinesia, however, the later is associated with the use of neuroleptics.

Are Any Symptoms Suggestive of a Serious or Life-Threatening Condition?

Recognition of the gait change as a symptom of an underlying problem, rather than assuming it is a normal age change, is an important aspect of care of the older adult. The underlying diseases that cause gait disorders have the potential of being serious or life-threatening. It is essential, therefore, to determine the underlying cause of the gait disorder, using the gait pattern as well as associated signs and symptoms. In so doing, the underlying disease can be treated and the gait disorder can resolve or improve.

Table 14-9
Distinguishing Tremor From Involuntary Movement Disorders

CONDITION	CHARACTERISTICS
Tremor	Rhythmic oscillations produced by involuntary contractions of reciprocally innervated antagonistic muscles
Athetosis	Slow writhing movements of the fingers and hands
Chorea	Irregular, purposeless movements of various body parts
Ballismus	Wild, forceful, flinging movements of proximal body parts
Dystonia	Spasmodic twisting movements with relatively sustained postural abnormalities
Tics	Erratic, rapid, repetitive stereotyped movements
Myoclonus	Abrupt, involuntary, single or repetitive jerks of muscle groups

When a sudden change in balance and/or gait occurs, it is particularly important to establish that dizziness or lightheadedness due to cardiac disease is not the cause of the change. A sensation of feeling faint, or dizzy, due to a reduction in cerebral blood flow (usually due to diminished cardiac output) can be life-threatening. In addition to complaints of dizziness these individuals would have abnormal findings on cardiac examination.

Physical Examination

The physical examination must begin with an evaluation of gait and balance. The Get-up and Go test, is a practical assessment tool for elderly patients. The patient is asked to rise from a straight-backed office chair, stand still briefly, walk approximately 10 ft., turn and walk back to the chair, turn around, and sit down. Performance is graded using a 5-point scale: (1) normal; (2) very slightly abnormal; (3) mildly abnormal; (4) moderately abnormal; and (5) severely abnormal. Quality of movement is assessed primarily for impairments in balance. A score of 3 or greater suggests that the patient is at increased risk of falling.

An understanding of normal adult gait is necessary to recognize abnormal patterns of movement. The functional unit of gait, which serves as the basis for evaluation, is the gait cycle.

Assessment of the Gait Cycle

Normal adult gait is a cyclical process that begins when the heel of one extremity strikes the ground. This is termed heel strike, and represents the starting point of the gait cycle. The end of one cycle occurs when that same heel strikes the ground again. Heel strike signals both the beginning and the end of the gait cycle. One complete gait cycle is also called the stride. A step, in con-

trast, is defined as heel strike of one extremity to heel strike of the opposite extremity. There are two steps in every stride or gait cycle. Normal step length is about 78 cm.

There are two distinct phases of a gait cycle: (1) stance; and (2) swing (Fig. 14-1). The stance phase is defined by the period of weight support beginning at heel strike and progressing through foot flat, mid-stance, heel off, and ending at toe off. Stance usually makes up 60 percent of the gait cycle. The swing phase begins at toe off as the foot clears the ground. Swing comprises the remaining 40 percent of the gait cycle.

Gait efficiency is related to movement of a person's center of gravity through space. There are six determinants of gait (Table 14-10) that function to minimize horizontal and vertical displacements in the center of gravity. A loss of one gait determinant can be partially compensated for by the other determinants. As more determinants are lost, the gait becomes less efficient and the energy cost of ambulation becomes higher. In response to increased energy requirements, comfortable walking speed is decreased. Balance is related to the line of gravity passing distally between the base of support formed by the feet.

Muscle Activity in the Gait Cycle

Forward movement is produced by gravity, inertia, and propulsion produced by muscle contraction. Muscle contractions are of three types: concentric,

Table 14-10

Determinants of Gait

Pelvic rotation
Pelvic tilt
Knee flexion in stance phase
Foot mechanisms
Knee mechanisms
Lateral placement of the pelvis

isometric, and eccentric. A concentric contraction shortens the distance between a muscle origin and insertion. In contrast, an eccentric contraction is a lengthening contraction that increases the distance between a muscle's origin and insertion. Isometric contractions result in no change in the length of a muscle. All three types of muscle contraction are seen in normal human gait (see Fig. 14-1).

Muscles, or muscle groups, are only intermittently active during the normal gait cycle. There are variable periods of relative inactivity that allow the muscles to rest. A similarly efficient process occurs with quiet standing. When standing, the major muscle activity is in the plantar flexor group, with relative inactivity in the other major muscle groups. This balance is possible because the line of gravity passes in front of the ankle and knee joints, through the center of gravity behind the hip joint, and cephalad through the spine and head. Distally, the line of gravity passes between the base of support formed by the feet. This base of support is increased when the feet are spread farther apart, and with use of an assist device such as a cane or walker.

How Do Specific Examination Findings Suggest One Diagnosis or Another?

Abnormal gait can result from a variety of pathologic states occurring both centrally and peripherally (see Table 14-2). Muscle weakness, central nervous system disease, sensory changes, structural abnormalities, and pain can profoundly alter the normal pattern of human locomotion. The final gait pattern can be quite specific and diagnostic of a particular disease process.

GAIT ABNORMALITIES ASSOCIATED WITH MUSCULOSKELETAL WEAKNESS

Gait abnormalities associated with focal muscle weakness produce a characteristic pattern of movement during the gait cycle. A weakened ankle dorsiflexor can not only be seen on physical examination but it is often heard as the foot "slaps" to the ground at heel strike. More pronounced weakness in this same muscle group will produce a distinct steppage gait. Similarly, impaired knee extension secondary to weak quadriceps muscles can mani-

Figure 14-1

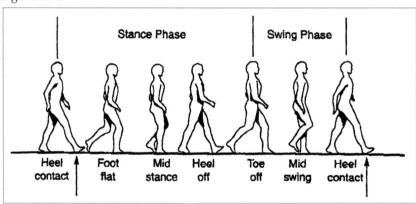

Changing positions of the legs during the phases of a single gait cycle from right heel contact to the next right heel contact. (Adapted with permission from C Norkin, and P Levangie: *Joint Structure and Function: A Comprehensive Analysis, 2nd ed.* Philadelphia: F.A. David; 1992; 451.)

fest as a "back knee" or genu recurvatum movement at the knee. This is followed by a "lurching" forward of the trunk. This keeps the gravity line in front of the knee to prevent buckling. Structural abnormalities like joint ankylosis and leg length discrepancies can be easily identified during the musculoskeletal examination and demonstrate an often predictable gait deficit.

GAIT ABNORMALITIES ASSOCIATED WITH CENTRAL NERVOUS SYSTEM DISEASE AND VASCULAR DISORDERS

Vascular lesions of the central nervous system frequently result in abnormalities in gait. Sequelae of stroke include spasticity and alterations in muscle tone that can produce extensor and flexor synergies, often referred to as spastic hemiplegia. The extension synergy pattern includes hip and knee extension, internal rotation of the hip and plantar flexion, and inversion of the foot (equinovarus). The leg is functionally lengthened requiring circumduction of the limb to clear the toes. Step length is shorter, stance time is longer, and the normal fluid pattern of gait is lost. The flexor synergy presents as a pattern of hip and knee flexion and ankle dorsiflexion making ambulation difficult, if not impossible. Adductor spasticity is sometimes seen and can result in a scissoring gait where the affected extremity is pulled toward midline; although this is more characteristic of the gait associated with cerebral palsy or myelopathy.

Small vessel disease associated with hypertension and multiple white matter lesions of the basal ganglia and periventricular white matter (Binswanger's disease) presents as a frontal gait disorder or gait apraxia. Characteristics of this gait abnormality are a wide base of support, small shuffling steps (marche à petit pas), magnetic floor response or difficulty picking the feet up, and difficulty turning and poor balance.

Vascular and other lesions of the cerebellum can present as a gait ataxia with characteristic incoordination of movement. The gait is broad-based with staggering and lurching. Unilateral hypotonia can cause falling to the side of the lesion, and truncal ataxia is a prominent finding. Cerebellar atrophy can be alcohol related, familial, or idiopathic.

Cervical spondylosis is a degenerative condition of the cervical spine where loss of disk height and osteophyte formation can lead to narrowing of the cervical canal. Subsequent compression of neural tissue can result in a cervical myelopathy with both upper and lower motor neuron findings on examination. The gait is typically spastic with elements of hip adduction resulting in scissoring, plantar flexion manifested by reduced toe clearance with toes scraping the ground and shortened, and stiff-legged steps. Examination findings can include hyperreflexia, hypertonia, extensor plantar responses, and varying degrees of upper and/or lower extremity weakness. Cervical myelopathy is less commonly a complication of rheumatoid arthritis where atlantoaxial (C-1 on C-2) subluxation can produce instability. This is a common cause of neck pain and, in some instances, spinal cord compression. Vitamin B_{12} deficiency has also been associated with a myelopathy producing an ataxic gait pattern and upper motor neuron findings on examination.

Mild dementia can be associated with a non-specific "cautious" gait, with widened base of support, shortened stride length, flexed posture, and slow gait speed. Movement is noted to be "en bloc." More severe dementia typically presents as a frontal lobe gait with poor gait initiation, small shuffling steps, and impaired equilibrium. Frontal release signs can also be present in patients with dementia.

GAIT ABNORMALITIES ASSOCIATED WITH SENSORY CHANGES

Abnormal gait can be the result of impaired visual, vestibular, and proprioceptive function. The gait is ataxic and wide-based as in cerebellar disease; however, steps are high and stamping rather than small and shuffling. Impaired joint proprioception and abnormal sensory feedback can result in forceful knee extension with a sometimes audible heel tap at heel strike followed by a foot "stamp." Romberg test is positive and the gait worsens if visual input is impaired.

Sensory abnormalities are often associated with both focal and generalized peripheral neuropathies (see Table 14-3). A mixed sensory and motor neuropathy with varying degrees of decreased sensation and weakness can be found in a host of disease states. The peripheral neuropathy commonly associated with diabetes mellitus is a symmetric sensory neuropathy that begins distally in the toes and can eventually involve the fingers and hand in what has been termed a "glove-and-stocking" distribution. Vitamin B_{12} deficiency can effect both the central and peripheral nervous systems with involvement of the posterior columns and/or peripheral nerves. With peripheral involvement, examination shows a wide-based gait, depressed or absent deep tendon reflexes, and distal muscle wasting and weakness. Hypothyroidism can also result in a glove-and-stocking symmetric and painful peripheral neuropathy involving the hands and feet; however, it is more commonly associated with a proximal myopathy.

GAIT ABNORMALITIES ASSOCIATED WITH STRUCTURAL CHANGES AND PAIN

Structural abnormalities that can affect gait include limb length discrepancy, joint ankylosis, contractures, and a variety of arthritic conditions. Limb length discrepancies can be true or apparent. A true leg length discrepancy is measured from the anterior superior iliac spine to the medial malleoli. It can result from polio or childhood epiphyseal plate fracture. An apparent leg length discrepancy can be due to pelvic obliquity (e.g., scoliosis) or from a deformity of the hip joint. Measurement is taken from the umbilicus or other nonfixed point to the medial malleoli. A leg length difference of more than 1.5 in. causes a person to walk on the forefoot of the shorter leg to functionally increase its length. If the difference is less than this, the pelvis on the shorter side will drop during stance phase of that limb

and there will be increased hip and knee flexion, and hip hiking or circumduction on the swing side to compensate.

Joint ankylosis, or fusion, results in the use of compensatory mechanisms. In the case of ankle fusion, hip and knee movements increase to help normalize the gait pattern. A familiar example of this occurs with walking in high heels, which functionally decreases foot and ankle movement. Exaggerated pelvic tilt and rotation and increased knee flexion are compensatory motions to offset this loss of foot movement.

Contractures of the hip, knee, and ankle joints lead to characteristic gait patterns that may be noted on physical examination of gait. When range of motion of the hip is limited, the affected leg will tend to be held in an externally rotated position to maximize pelvic rotation. Increased motion will be seen in the lumbar spine and the unaffected hip joint. Knee flexion contractures produce a functionally shorter leg with the subsequent gait abnormality most apparent if the contracture is greater than 30 degrees. On the other hand, a knee extension contracture (e.g., fusion) produces a functionally longer extremity. Compensatory strategies include circumduction and hip hiking of the affected "longer" side, or toe walking of the unaffected, "shorter" side. Plantar flexion contractures result in an equinus foot deformity. The limb becomes functionally longer and a steppage gait, with increased hip and knee flexion, is needed to clear the toes.

Painful or antalgic joints generally cause a shortened stance time on the affected side in an effort to minimize painful weight bearing. The altered gait pattern in hip pain resembles a compensated Trendelenburg gait where the shoulder of the affected side is dipped laterally during stance. This moves the center of gravity over the painful side. Knee pain associated with effusion may improve if the joint is held in a small amount of flexion. As with hip pain, heel strike can exacerbate discomfort and is avoided. Arthritis and other painful conditions of the feet can cause a shuffling, flat-footed gait, with decreased heel strike and little or no roll-over.

Do Particular Examination Findings Suggest Serious or Life-Threatening Conditions?

Human locomotion is dependent on the complex interplay of multiple body systems. Gait dysfunction can occur at several levels. Serious or life-threatening disease can have both a chronic or acute presentation. A precipitating event, such as a fall, can unmask an otherwise indolent disease course. Cervical spondylosis exemplifies this concept. Narrowing of the cervical spinal canal may go unnoticed until a fall or other accident causes hyperextension of the neck and contusion of the spinal cord. The patient can present acutely with a central cord syndrome having disproportionately greater upper extremity versus lower extremity weakness and sacral sensory sparing.

Acute changes in cognitive or functional status demand more urgent diagnostic evaluation because they often signal a neurologic emergency. Cerebrovascular accidents, and other intracranial processes, and toxic and metabolic encephalopathies and myelopathies can cause rapid deterioration in function. An accurate diagnosis is based on the combination of relevant history, detailed physical examination, and directed laboratory studies.

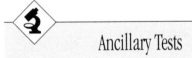

Ancillary Tests

Laboratory and other testing should be based on a patient's history and physical examination. Table 14-11 shows the commonly ordered tests and the underlying disorders to consider.

When a central neurologic process is suspected, diagnostic imaging with computerized tomography scanning or magnetic resonance imaging is warranted. Plain films and CT of the cervical spine are useful to diagnose the cause of a cervical myelopathy.

Electrodiagnostic testing with electromyography and nerve conduction studies can help identify and characterize peripheral neuropathies and distinguish a myopathic process from a neuropathic one. Electrodiagnostic testing can help differentiate a focal neuropathy, such as femoral nerve palsy with quadriceps weakness, from diffuse motor neuron disease such as amyotrophic lateral sclerosis.

Direct observation of gait provides important information regarding gait. The Tinneti Gait and Balance measure (Table 14-12) is a valid and reliable measure of balance and gait abnormalities and can be easily done in the office setting. Figure 14-2 is an alternative office-based mobility screen that includes seven basic functional activities, and can be quickly administered. A formal gait analysis can be performed to quantify movement through the gait cycle. Likewise, vestibular and balance laboratories can measure postural sway and righting reflexes.

Falls, which can be the consequence of a gait and balance abnormality, should also be evaluated to determine the actual cause of the fall. Table 14-13 provides a quick guide for the evaluation of falls in the office setting. This can help differentiate if the fall is due to gait or balance disorders or another underlying disorder (see Table 14-14).

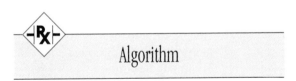

Algorithm

Figure 14-3 shows a general approach to gait disorders. The first decision point is the determination of whether an acute neurologic process exists. This, obviously, must be promptly evaluated and treatment initiated. For a subacute or chronic process, a determination of whether the etiology is primarily a central or peripheral nervous system disorder. The type of central nervous system process is suggested by the gait pattern (see Tables 14-2 and 14-4). The main causes of a peripheral nervous system process resulting in

Table 14-11

Laboratory and Additional Testing for Gait and Balance Disorders

TEST	UNDERLYING PATHOLOGY CONSIDERED
Blood test	
Thyroid-stimulating hormone	Hypothyroidism
Vitamin B_{12}	Deficiency and myelopathy
Schilling's test	Deficiency and myelopathy
Folate	Distal neuropathies
Complete blood count	Megaloblastic anemia
Electrolytes and liver function tests	Encephalopathic disorders
Calcium, phosphorous, alkaline phosphatase	Osteomalacia
Drug levels	Toxicities (anticonvulsants, lithium, diazepam, and antidepressants)
Radiologic evaluation	
Plain films of the spine	Spondylosis and cervical spondylotic myelopathy
Plain films of a joint	Degenerative joint disease and fractures
Chest	Infection and pneumonia
Computed tomography of head	Normal pressure hydrocephalus
	Cerebrovascular accident
	Tumor
	Cerebellar ataxia
Myelography	Cervical spondylotic myelopathy
	Cervical tumors
Lumbar puncture	Amyotrophic lateral sclerosis
	Normal pressure hydrocephalus
	Infection
Electrophysiological studies (EMG)	Peripheral neuropathy
Electrocardiogram	Cardiac event
	Arrhythmia

gait abnormalities are listed in the algorithm. If these conditions are excluded, then muscular, orthopedic, cardiac, and other disorders should be considered.

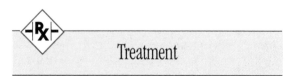

Treatment

If a cause for the gait abnormality is found, the specific treatment should be instituted. For example, ventriculoperitoneal shunting of cerebrospinal fluid can reverse the gait apraxia of normal pressure hydrocephalus. Thyroid replacement therapy can reverse the myopathy associated with hypothyroidism.

Unfortunately, the cause of most gait disorders in elderly individuals is multifactorial and not amenable to a single, specific treatment. Although the underlying etiology of the gait abnormality may not be directly treatable, many interventions can be helpful in improving the patient's mobility. For example, physical therapy to strengthen the unaffected side of a patient with hemiparesis can

Figure 14-2

1. **Sit and rise from a chair**

Watch for ability to sit and rise in a smooth, controlled movement without balance loss or use of armrests. Poor performance signifies lower extremity dysfunction

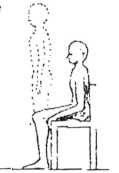

2. **Stand in place for 10 to 15 seconds after rising from chair**

Watch for ability to stand steady unassisted without balance loss or dizziness. Poor performance signifies postural hypotension or vestibular dysfunction

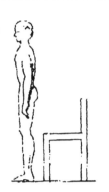

3. **Stand, with eyes closed, arms at sides, and feet about 3 inches apart**

Watch for ability to stand without support and without sway or balance loss. Poor performance signifies proprioceptive loss

4. **Maintain balance when receiving a light nudge on sternum (sternal nudge maneuver)**

Normal reaction is to stretch out arms forward and away from body and to take a step or two backward to regain balance. Poor performance signifies postural instability

5. **Bend down and reach, as if to pick up an object**

Watch for ability to maintain balance. Poor performance signifies altered balance, indicating that retrieving hard-to-reach objects may increase fall risk

6. **Walk in a straight line (about 15 feet), turn around, and walk back**

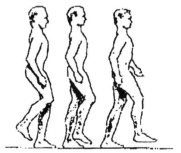

Watch for ability to walk and turn around without hesitation, excessive deviation from side to side, or feet scraping the floor. Poor performance signifies gait/balance dysfunction

7. **Get up from floor**

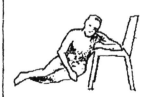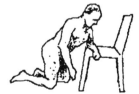

Watch for ability to get up either unassisted or with the help of a chair for support. Poor performance signifies lower extremity dysfunction, indicating risk for long lies

Office-based mobility screen: Seven basic steps.

Table 14-12

Tinetti Balance and Gait Evaluation

BALANCE
Instructions: Participant is seated in a hard, armless chair. The following maneuvers are tested:

Sitting balance

        0 = leans or slides in chair

        1 = steady, safe

Arise

        0 = unable without help

        1 = able but uses arm to help

        2 = able without use of arms

Attempts to arise

        0 = unable without help

        1 = able but requires more than one attempt

        2 = able to arise with one attempt

Immediate standing balance (first 5 seconds)

        0 = unsteady (stagger, moves feet, marked trunk sway)

        1 = steady but uses walker/cane or grabs other object for support

        2 = steady without walker or cane or other support

Standing balance

        0 = unsteady

        1 = steady, but wide stance (medial heels > 4 inches apart) or uses cane/walker or other support

        2 = narrow stance without support

Nudge   (subject at maximum position with feet as close together as possible. Examiner pushes lightly)

        0 = begins to fall

        1 = stagger, grabs, but catches self

        2 = steady

Eyes closed at maximum position

        0 = unsteady

        1 = steady

Turn 360 degrees

        0 = discontinous steps

        1 = continous steps

        0 = unsteady (grabs, staggers)

        1 = steady

Sit down

        0 = unsafe (misjudged distance, falls into chair)

        1 = uses arm or not a smooth motion

        2 = safe, smooth motion

_____/16 BALANCE SCORE

Table 14-12

Tinetti Balance and Gait Evaluation (*continued*)

GAIT
Instructions: Participant stands with examiner, walks down hallway or across room, first at his or her usual pace, then back at a "rapid but safe" pace (using usual walking aid such as cane/walker).
1. Initiation of gait (immediately after told to go)
0 = any hesitancy or multiple attempts to start
1 = no hesitancy
2. Step length and height (right (R) foot swing)
0 = does not pass left (L) stance foot with step
1 = passes L stance foot
0 = R foot does not clear floor completely with step
1 = R foot completely clears floor
3. Step length and height (left foot swing)
0 = does not pass R stance foot with step
1 = passes R stance foot
0 = L foot does not clear foot completely with step
1 = L foot completely clears floor
4. Step symmetry
0 = R and L step length not equal (estimate)
1 = R and L step length appear equal
5. Step continuity
0 = stopping or discontinuity between steps
1 = steps appear continuous
6. Path (estimated in relation to floor tiles, 12 in. wide. Observe excursion of one foot over about 10 feet of course).
0 = marked deviation
1 = mild/moderate deviation or uses a walking aid
2 = straight without walking aid
7. Trunk
0 = marked sway or uses walking aid
1 = no sway but flexion of knees or back or spreads arms out while walking
2 = no sway, no flexion, no use of arms and no walking aid
8. Walk stance
0 = heels apart
1 = heels almost touching while walking
____/12 GAIT SCORE
____/28 TOTAL MOBILITY SCORE (BALANCE AND GAIT)

improve his or her ability to ambulate. Treating spasticity and pain can improve gait, but not cure the underlying disorder.

A team approach to the treatment of gait abnormalities and falls should be employed. Physical therapists and occupational therapists should be integral members of this team. Goals of treatment include providing appropriate pharmacologic intervention, improving functional mobility, improving strength and endurance, preventing deformity, and

Table 14-13

Office Evaluation of Falls

Patient Name _____ Age_____ Gender _____ Date _____

Risk factors for subsequent falls

1. History of previous falls
    a. yes
    b. no
2. Medications
    a. four or more prescriptions
    b. new prescription in the last 2 weeks
    c. use of any of the following medications: tranquilizers, sleeping pills, antidepressants, cardiac medications, antidiabetic agents
3. Known gait problem or muscular weakness
    a. yes
    b. no
4. Dizziness, vertigo, or loss of consciousness at time of fall
    a. yes
    b. no
5. Visual changes
    a. yes
    b. no
6. Environmental problems
    a. clutter
    b. lighting
    c. uneven flooring
    d. footwear or lack of footwear
    e. inappropriate assistive device
7. Major illnesses
    a. neurologic: Parkinson's disease, stroke, dementia
    b. musculoskeletal: arthritis, contracture, fracture
    c. cardiac: hypotension, arrhythmia, acute infarct
    d. new acute illness: infection
    e. other
8. Additional questions
    a. What happened at the time of the fall, i.e., what was the patient doing? _____
    _____
    _____

    b. Were there any injuries associated with the fall?
        1) laceration
        2) sprain/strain
        3) fracture
        4) persistent pain
        5) head trauma
        6) other
    c. How have you been since the fall?
        1) associated fear of falling
        2) change in function
        3) change in cognition
    d. Is the patient able to carry on usual activities, and if not who is available to help with usual activities?_____
    _____
    _____

Table 14-14

Assessment for Fall Risk

Intrinsic	Sensory changes: vision, hearing, touch, and proprioception
	Cardiovasclar: orthostatic hypotension, arrhythmias
	Foot disorders: pain, deformities, and footwear
	Musculoskeletal: mobility, strength, and pain
	Neurologic: gait and balance, tremor, and bradykinesia
	Urologic: incontinence, urgency
	Nutritional: dehydration, malnutrition, anemia, and electrolyte imbalance
	Acute illness: infection
Psychosocial factors	Cognitive changes
	Depression
	Apathy
	Activity level and patterns
	Living situation
Drug use	Number of drugs
	Alcohol use
	Sedative hypnotics
Environmental factors	Outside the home: level surfaces, handrails, no clutter, and no wet surfaces
	Inside the home: marked stairs, handrails, no wet or dusty surfaces, nonskid rugs, covered or hidden cords, and no clutter
	Bathroom: grab bars for tub and toilet, raised toilet seats, shower chair, and nonskid mats
	Kitchen: frequently used objects within reach
	Furniture: proper height to facilitate safe transfers, not easily movable
	Lighting: adequate and nonglare, adequate lighting on stairways, light switches near doorways and beds, and nightlights for bathrooms and bedrooms

developing a safe, energy-efficient gait pattern. Some gait abnormalities can be substantially improved with medications, physical therapy, occupational therapy, or a combination of all three. This section addresses two areas of treatment: assistive devices and medications for spasticity.

Assistive Devices

ORTHOTIC DEVICES

Many gait abnormalities can be improved with the use of an appropriate orthotic device. An orthosis is an externally applied commercially or custom-made device that can support and stabilize a weak joint, optimize limb movements, and promote a safer gait pattern. It can be used to prevent or correct a deformity, relieve pain, and reduce weight bearing on injured structures.

One of the most commonly prescribed orthosis is the plastic molded ankle foot orthosis (AFO). Metal AFOs, while still used today, are less common. AFOs can be manufactured to support both subtalar and ankle joint motion, controlling ankle inversion, eversion, dorsiflexion, and plantar flexion. Knee stability can also be affected by an AFO's design. Stability can be improved by setting the AFO in several degrees of plantar flexion to create an extension force at the knee during stance. Conversely, increasing the rigidity of the AFO or setting it in a small amount of dorsiflexion will

Figure 14-3

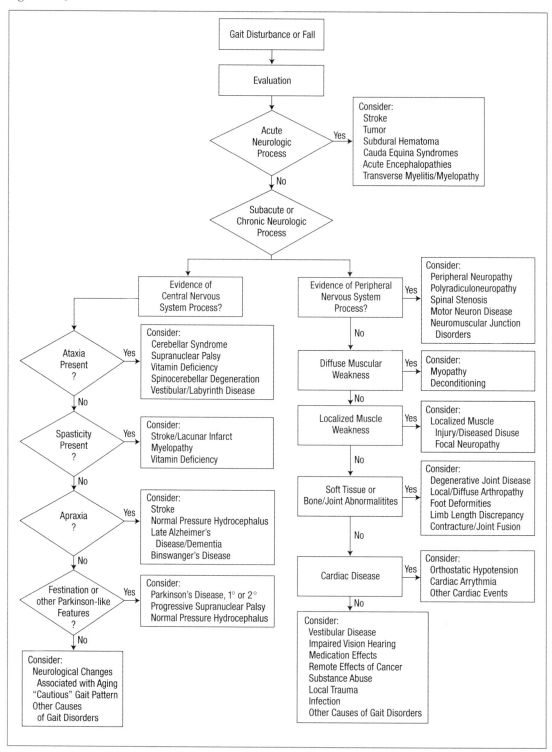

General approach to gait disorders.

increase the flexion force at the knee to reduce genu recuvatum.

AFOs are frequently prescribed for patients with lower limb weakness secondary to stroke. Patients with weak ankle dorsiflexors without spasticity can function well with a plastic leaf spring orthosis. Other patients, particularly those with spasticity, require the additional support of a customized orthosis.

Shoe modifications and foot orthosis can also improve gait abnormalities associated with pain and structural abnormalities. Leg length discrepancies between ½ and ¾ inches can be partially corrected with a heel edge inside the shoe. Corrections greater than this are best made to the outside of the shoe with a heel or heel and sole lift. Leg length discrepancies less than ½ inches are usually not corrected.

WEDGES

Knee pain secondary to degenerative changes in the medial knee compartment can improve with the addition of a lateral heel wedge. Foot pain related to metatarsalgia can be treated by placing a metatarsal pad inside the shoe or by adding a metatarsal bar to the sole of the shoe. Both relieve pressure on the metatarsal heads. Likewise, heel pain can be treated by cushioning the heel area and/or by supporting the medial longitudinal arch.

AMBULATORY ASSISTIVE DEVICES

Ambulatory assistive devices, or gait aids, are often prescribed for patients with gait and balance disorders. Canes, crutches, and walkers increase stability by providing a wider base of support. Gait aids provide additional sensory input and can supplement muscle activity by assisting with both propulsion and deceleration during ambulation. They are often used to reduce compressive forces on an arthritic joint to allow for a less antalgic gait pattern. They are necessary to maintain postoperative weight-bearing restrictions of nonweight bearing (NWB), foot-flat weight bearing (FFWB), touch down weight bearing (TDWB), and partial weight bearing (PWB) common after hip and knee joint replacement surgery.

CANES Canes are the least restrictive of the gait aids. They can be used to improve stability by increasing sensory input and widening the base of support, augment propulsion and deceleration, and reduce forces on painful joints. They are not indicated for ambulation when weight-bearing restrictions must be maintained (e.g., postoperatively). Proper fit is necessary to optimize cane function and safety. The handle of the cane should be near the level of the greater trochanter so that when it is grasped, the elbow rests in 20° to 30° of flexion. A cane is typically held on the side opposite the affected lower extremity and the cane and affected leg are advanced simultaneously. During the stance phase of the gait cycle, weight is distributed between the cane and affected leg. Ipsilateral cane use, where the cane is held on the same side as the affected leg, can be recommended in patients with hip and knee instability or marked hand dominance. The upper extremity functionally becomes a weight-bearing joint when a cane or other gait aid is employed, so pathology in these joints may be exacerbated and preclude contralateral cane use as well.

CRUTCHES Crutches are often prescribed for temporary use to transition a patient through a period of lower extremity nonweight bearing or partial weight bearing. They can also be used as a permanent gait aid in patients with more severe pathology. Crutch use requires good upper extremity strength, adequate upper body range of motion, and an ability to sequence properly. The most stable crutch gait is the four-point gait because three points are always in contact with the ground. The sequence is as follows: one crutch, opposite foot, second crutch, other foot. A two-point crutch gait is faster than the four-point crutch gait because a crutch and opposite extremity move forward in an alternating pattern.

Another advantage of the two-point gait is that it allows for partial weight bearing status in both lower extremities. The three-point crutch gait is useful for the patient who must maintain partial or nonweight bearing status in a lower extremity. The two crutches and the affected leg move forward together, followed by a step with the unaffected leg. This gait pattern is less stable but more energy efficient.

Several types of crutches are available but axillary crutches are the most common. A properly fit axillary crutch should not put pressure on the axilla during weight bearing because this can lead to a radial nerve compression neuropathy. Weight bearing on the axillary pads should be avoided for the same reason. The hand piece is positioned so that there is approximately 30° of elbow flexion.

WALKERS   Walkers provide the most stable base of support and are indicated for those patients requiring maximal mechanical assistance for ambulation, such as following hip and knee arthroplasty procedures. Walkers are often used for elderly patients with lower extremity amputations and other gait disorders resulting in impaired balance and coordination. Rolling walkers can be more energy efficient but requires additional instruction for safe use and are difficult to use on carpeted surfaces. Even standard walkers can tip over, so patients are advised to keep the walker out in front of them and avoid the tendency to "overstep" into the walker.

Medications for Spasticity

The patient with spastic hemiparesis following stroke can benefit from a number of interventions. Treatment of spasticity begins with physical therapy. A daily stretching program can transiently reduce tone and help prevent contractures. Resting splints serve a similar purpose. Various neurofacilitory techniques can also be employed to optimize movement. Transfer and gait training with ambulatory aids optimize functional mobility.

Several oral medications can also be used to treat spasticity associated with stroke. These include baclofen, dantrolene sodium, and tizanidine. Baclofen is often used in this context but is more the drug of choice for spasticity of spinal cord etiology. Baclofen is supplied as 10 mg and 20 mg scored tablets. The suggested dosage titration schedule is 5 mg tid for 3 days, 10 mg tid for 3 days, 15 mg tid for 3 days, and 20 mg tid. The recommended maximal dosage is 80 mg daily; however, the medication is generally well tolerated and higher dosages are not uncommon. Transient drowsiness is the most common side effect. Abrupt discontinuation of the drug can precipitate seizures and hallucinations.

Dantrolene sodium (Dantrium) is a useful medication for spasticity. Dantrium is supplied as 25 mg, 50 mg, and 100 mg capsules. The recommended starting dose is 25 mg once daily, increasing the dose by 25 mg every 4 to 7 days. Dosages above 400 mg per day are rare. Dantrium has a potential to cause hepatotoxicity and cases of fatal and non-fatal hepatitis have been reported. The lowest possible effective dose should be prescribed and liver function studies should be monitored. The drug is discontinued if these become abnormal or if there is no response to treatment after 45 days.

The newest oral medication for the treatment of spasticity is tizanidine (Zanaflex), which has been found to be useful in both spinal and cerebral forms of spasticity. Tizanidine is available as a 4 mg cross-scored tablet. The suggested starting dose is 4 mg at bedtime. A 2 mg morning dose is added after 3 days then a 2 mg mid-day dose is added after another 3 days. Dosages can be increased by 2 mg every 3 days to a maximum daily dose of 24 to 36 mg. Common side effects include dry mouth, somnolence, asthenia, and dizziness. Tizanidine, an α_2-adrenergic agonist, can lower blood pressure producing clinically significant orthostatic hypotension. Additionally, liver function studies should be monitored because of the potential for hepatotoxicity.

Focal spasticity can be treated with chemical neurolysis, with either motor point or nerve block techniques. Tibial nerve blocks, for example, can be used to help correct a spastic, equinovarus foot. More recently, botulinum toxin is being used for the treatment of this type of spasticity. Its effect is to weaken spastic muscles by inhibiting the release of acetylcholine at the neuromuscular junction.

Errors

Clinicians make three common errors in the evaluation of gait disorders. First, they commonly search for a single cause of the gait disorder when abnormalities in gait are commonly multifactorial, having both central and peripheral components. Second, clinicians fail to evaluate a patient's gait in a systematic fashion. The clinician must directly observe the patient's gait, including arising from a seated position, ambulating, and returning to a seated position. Third, physicians fail to recognize that gait abnormalities can be transient and related to cardiovascular effects. Orthostatic hypotension is common, particularly in elderly patients on antihypertensive medications.

Family Approach and Patient Education

There is clearly a relationship between mobility impairment from gait and balance changes and a greater risk of falling for the older adult. Specifically, older adults who had limitations in walking and balance were 10 times more likely to report multiple falling episodes when compared with those elderly without limitations. Lower extremity dysfunction has been reported to especially increase risk. A fall or fall-related injury is a major threat to the loss of independence in this older age group. It has been estimated that about 10 to 15 percent of falls for those over the age of 65 years, result in serious injury. For those older adults who present with a history of recurrent falls, the threat to loss of independence and increased morbidity and mortality is even greater.

In addition to an actual fall, a major effect of gait and balance changes for older adults is a fear of falling. It has been reported that up to 50 percent of those who have fallen report some reduction in activities of daily living to avoid another fall or incurring injury. When risks can be identified and modified to decrease falling, fear of falling can be reduced.

Family members need to be educated regarding the risk of falls when their older family member has an abnormal gait or impaired balance. The goals of fall prevention are to maximize mobility, reduce threat of falls and complications, and maintain autonomy. Family involvement for preventing falls in the community-dwelling elderly should focus on assessing the risk factors for falls, and implementing interventions to decrease those risks.

Assessing for the risk of falls includes consideration of intrinsic factors, psychosocial consideration, drug use and side effects, environmental issues, and there have been prior falls (Table 14-15). Families should be instructed to make sure their older family member has regular physical examinations that can help identify potential problems and changes that may put them at risk for falling. Special consideration should be given

Table 14-15

Resources for Fall Prevention Teaching Guides

National Safety Council
  444 North Michigan Avenue
  Chicago, IL 60611
  (800) 621-7619, Ext. 6900.

Pamphlets: Preventing Falls—A Safety Program
                for Older Adults
                Falling—The Unexpected Trip
                Your Home Safety Checklist
                Ladder Safety
American Association of Retired Persons
  1909 K Street, NW
  Washington, DC 20049

Booklet: Dangerous Products,
         Dangerous Places

to the use of appropriate eyewear, and vision tests to be sure vision is optimal. Hearing aids and periodic removal of impacted cerumen can also improve hearing acuity and allow the older adult to use auditory cues for fall prevention. Adequate nutritional status, particularly adequate fluid intake, is important for the family to consider, as well as assuring that their older family member is eating a balanced diet and taking in 6 to 8, 8-oz. glasses of fluid daily. This can prevent dehydration and other nutritional problems that could result in a fall.

Families are in a key position to make sure that their older family member has appropriate foot care and foot wear. All foot deformities, such as calluses and painful bunions, should be treated. Toenails should be kept short, and shoes should be low heeled, nonskid, and have good support (preferably a tie shoe).

Evaluating the older family members' psychological state, particularly with regard to mood and cognition, can also help decrease the risk of falling. Depression, anxiety, memory loss, and decreased ability to problem solve can result in the older adult putting himself or herself in unsafe situations (such as climbing on a chair to reach something), and result in a fall. Families should be encouraged to report evidence of changes in mood or memory to the older adult's health care provider.

Medications are a well-documented cause of falls, and families should be aware that an older adult taking three or more medications is particularly at risk. Families should encourage their older family member to bring all medications with them to any follow-up medical appointment so that the appropriate use of these medications on an ongoing basis can be evaluated.

Families should also be particularly aware of their family member's use of alcohol or any other medication that can affect judgement and coordination such as sleeping pills or nerve pills. If the older adult uses any of these drugs, families should encourage moderation (e.g., 1 drink daily), and remind their older family member to take special precautions following use of these drugs to prevent falls.

Families have a particularly important role in the evaluation of the environment and helping their family members to make sure the environment is safe. There are a number of important areas to check both inside and outside the home (see Table 14-14). Families should be encouraged to check outside the home for uneven surfaces, objects in the way, broken handrails, and adequate lighting. When areas of concerned are identified, interventions should be taken to decrease these risks.

The inside of the home should be evaluated to be sure areas are free of clutter, that cords are covered and out of the way, that nonskid rugs are tacked down, and that there is adequate nonglare lighting. If there are stairs inside, they should be in good condition with the edges marked in an alternative color to improve visibility, and handrails should be present and sturdy. Bathrooms should be evaluated for the presence of grab bars, raised toilet seats if necessary, a shower chair, and nonskid mats for the tub. All furniture, including beds, should be the proper height for the older adult to transfer. This means that his or her feet reach the floor comfortably when sitting. Kitchens should be evaluated for safety, and cabinets and placement of frequently used materials should be such that the older adult does not have to climb on stools or chairs to reach them.

Families need to be aware of particularly high-risk times for falls. These include: episodes of acute illness, after getting new eyeglasses or eye surgery, after starting on a new medication, in periods of stress or anxiety, following a prior fall, and when in an unfamiliar environment. Families also need to be aware of the even greater importance of making sure their own homes are safe for their older family members when they visit.

The family is an important source of support and encouragement for older adults to engage activities that decrease their risk of falling. Specifically, families need to encourage their older family member to participate in regular exercise, which is an important source of fall prevention. Families can provide the needed verbal encouragement for their older family member to exercise and reinforce the important benefit that exercise will have for them.

Specifically, families should know that regular exercise, particularly muscle strengthening and stretching exercises, improves balance and decreases the incidence of falling.

Handouts for Patient and Families Regarding Fall Prevention

The National Safety Council and the Department of Aging offer programs and literature on home safety and fall prevention (see Table 14-15). Some senior centers have their own programs or literature as well.

Bibliography

Alexander N: Gait disorders in older adults. *J Am Geriatr Soc* 44:434, 1996.

Baloh R, Fife T, Zwerling L: Comparison of static and dynamic posturography in young and older normal people. *J Am Geriatr Soc* 42;405, 1994.

Basmajian JV, Wolf SL: Therapeutic Exercise. In: Basmajian J (ed). Baltimore: Williams & Wilkins; 1990:chap. 6.

Berg WP, Alessio H, Mills EM, et al: Circumstances and consequences of falls in independent community-dwelling older adults. *Age Aging* 26:261, 1997.

Cuncha V: Differential diagnosis of gait disorders in the elderly. *Geriatrics* 43:33, 1988.

Close J, Ellis M, Hooper R, et al: Prevention of falls in the elderly trial (PROFET): a randomized trial. *Lancet* 353:93, 1999.

Dayhoff N, Suhrheinrich J, Wigglesworth J, et al: Balance and muscle strength as predictors of frailty among older adults. *J Gerontol Nurs* 24:18, 1998.

Deathe AB, Hayes KC, Winter DA: The biomechanics of cane, crutches and walkers. *Crit Rev Phys Med Rehabil* 5:15, 1993.

Dobbs R, Chalett A, Bowes S: Is this walk normal? *Age Aging* 22:27, 1993.

Fuh J, Lin K, Wang S: Neurologic diseases presenting with gait impairment in the elderly. *J Geriatr Psychiatr Neurol* 7:89, 1994.

Hageman P, Blanke D: Comparison of gait of young women and elderly women. *Phys Ther* 66:1382, 1986.

Lange M: The challenge of fall prevention in home care: a review of the literature. *Home Healthcare Nurse* 14:198, 1996.

Maki B: Gait changes in older adults: predictors of falls or indicators of fear? *J Am Geriatr Soc* 45:313, 1997.

Mathias S, Nayak V, Isaac B: Balance in elderly patients: the Get-up and Go test. *Arch Phys Med Rehabil* 67:387, 1986.

Ryan JW, Spellbring AM: Implementing strategies to decrease risk of falls in older women. *J Gerontol Nurs* 22:25, 1996.

Sixt E, Landahl S: Postural disturbances in a 75 year old population. *Age Aging* 16:393, 1987.

Steinway K: The changing approach to falls in the elderly. *Am Fam Physician* 56: 1815, 1997.

Sudorsky L: Gait disorders in the elderly. *N Engl J Med* 322:1441, 1990.

Sudorsky L, Ronthal M: Gait disorders among elderly patients: a survey study of 50 patients. *Arch Neurol* 40:740, 1983.

Tideiksaar R: *Falling in Old Age: Prevention and Management*, 2nd ed. New York: Springer Publishing; 1997:6.

Tideiksaar R: Preventing falls: how to identify risk factors and reduce complications. *Geriatrics* 51:43, 1996.

Tinetti M, Baker D, McAvay G, et al: A multifactorial intervention to reduce the risk of falling among elderly people living in the community. *N Engl J Med* 331:821, 1994.

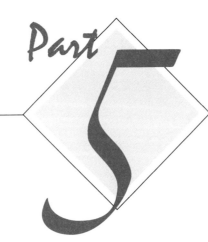

Part

5

Other Common Problems

Barbara Resnick

Constipation

Overview: How Common Is Constipation in the Office Practice?

Constipation is one of the most common digestive complaints in the older adult and accounts for 2.5 million physician visits annually. Annually, more than 4 million people in the United States complain of constipation, with a corresponding prevalence rate of 2 percent. The prevalence of constipation increases with age, is more common in women than in men, in nonwhites than in whites, and in those with lower family income and education. The steepest rise in reported prevalence rates of constipation occurs above the age of 60 years and ranges from 4 to 30 percent.

Constipation can have dangerous complications in older adults including acute changes in cognition, urinary retention, urinary incontinence, and fecal impaction. Chronic constipation, if left untreated, can lead to significant morbidity and, rarely, mortality in the older adult. Fecal impaction from constipation can result in intestinal obstruction, ulceration, and urinary problems. Chronic straining to defecate can cause adverse effects on cerebral, coronary, and peripheral vascular circulations. Constipation must be considered a serious problem for the older adult, and one that is deserving of a comprehensive evaluation and management plan.

Principal Diagnoses

Physiology

Part of the challenge in the diagnosis and management of constipation is the number of body systems involved in the normal defecation process. Defecation is the culmination of strong muscular contractions and colonic peristalsis that propel the feces into the rectum for expulsion. Stool enters and distends the rectal ampulla, causing autonomically mediated reflex relaxation of the internal anal sphincter. To avoid spontaneous evacuation, reflex contraction of the external anal sphincter and pelvic floor muscles, which are innervated by the pudendal nerve, occurs. The brain registers a desire to defecate, the external sphincter is voluntarily relaxed, and the rectum is evacuated, with assistance from abdominal wall muscle contraction. Contractions of the abdominal wall increase abdominal pressure and relax the anal sphincters and levator ani. Both sympathetic and parasympathetic innervation is necessary for defecation to occur. Impairment in any of these functions can cause constipation.

Definition and Prevalence

Studies of constipation, and the understanding of the actual prevalence of this problem in the older adult, are hampered by the subjective nature of the problem and the lack of a universal definition. Constipation was defined as insufficient frequency of defecation, deficient quantity of stool, or abnormally hard and dry stools. This is a qualitative definition, and healthy older adults can pass up to three stools a day or have a comfortable bowel movement once every 3 to 5 days.

In a population-based study of persons older than 65 years of age, 26 percent of the men and 34 percent of the women reported that they suffered from constipation. Fewer older adults who believed themselves to be constipated report that they had three or fewer bowel movements per week. These individuals were more likely to describe themselves as constipated if they had to strain, had incomplete evacuations, difficulty or pain with defecation, or hard stools. Among 200 older adults interviewed about their bowel function, approximately 30 percent described themselves as having problems with constipation at least once a month. Only 3 percent of this group, however, reported that their average stool frequency was less than three per week, the commonly accepted definition of constipation.

Similarly, in a study of 1375 older adults, self-report of constipation poorly correlated with symptoms considered to identify this problem. The patients' subjective report of constipation often was not consistent with the classic definition of constipation.

The International Workshop on Constipation attempted to more clearly define constipation. This group classified constipation on the basis of stool frequency, consistency, and difficulty of defecation. Based on these recommendations, constipation was categorized into two syndromes: functional constipation and rectosigmoid outlet delay (Table 15-1). Functional constipation refers to the slow transit of stool. Rectosigmoid outlet delay refers to anorectal dysfunction. The latter type of constipation is characterized by prolonged defecation, more than 10 mins to complete a bowel movement, or having the feeling of anal blockage. These individuals report a need to press in or around the anus to aid defecation. These definitions of constipation were more consistent with patient symptoms, and based on the definitions, 40 percent of older adults in the community were noted to have constipation, and 21 percent reported a rectosigmoid outlet delay.

CAUSES OF CONSTIPATION

PHYSIOLOGIC CHANGES WITH AGE   Constipation, while normal, is not a normal consequence of the aging process. Normal aging does not result in the slowing of gastrointestinal transit time or in a reduced frequency of bowel movements. Total gastrointestinal transit time is determined by measuring the passage of opaque markers from mouth to anus. In healthy older adults, there was no effect on colonic activity observed before or after meals. Studies of older adults with constipation, however, demonstrated a prolonged total gut transit time ranging from 4 to 9 days (normal is less than 3 days). Markers were noted to pass especially slowly through the left colon, with a striking delay in evacuation from the rectum. The passage of markers in individuals with constipation was slow before and after rectosigmoid disimpaction. This suggests that total transit times in elderly individuals with constipation are prolonged because of segmental dysmotility in the left colon and rectum.

ELECTROPHYSIOLOGY   Direct electrophysiologic measurement of colonic motor activity in elderly subjects has shown that the sigmoid motor response to intraluminal bisacodyl, which directly stimulates the myenteric plexus, is diminished in older adults who are constipated. This implies a deficit in intrinsic innervation. An age-related deficit in the density of inhibitory nerves or in the binding sites for inhibitory neuropeptides on smooth muscle has been reported. This was based on studies of receptor and hormonal function in vitro preparations of colons from healthy older adults. There was a decrease with age in the amplitude of inhibitory junction potentials, but no decline in the levels of

Table 15-1

Definitions of Constipation Established by International Workshop on Constipation

TYPE	CRITERIA
Functional constipation	Two or more of the following complaints present for at least 12 months:
	Straining 25% of the time
	Hard stools 25% of the time
	Incomplete evacuation 25% of the time
	≤2 Bowel movements in a week
Rectal outlet delay	Anal blockage more than 25% of the time
	Prolonged defecation
	Manual disimpaction

inhibitory gut neuropeptides. A decrease in the inhibitory nerve input to circular smooth muscle could result in segmental motor incoordination and functional partial obstruction.

ENDORPHINS   Individuals over 60 years of age are reported to have higher plasma concentrations of beta-endorphins that mediate binding to endogenous opiate receptors in the lower gastrointestinal tract. This can potentially inhibit colonic motility and increase resting anal tone.

SPHINCTER TONE   There is a tendency toward age-related decline in internal sphincter tone. External anal sphincter strength and pelvic muscle strength decline with age, which is more marked in women, especially those with multiple children. Elderly patients with constipation have greater difficulty evacuating a small stool. The subsequent increased straining required can compress the pudendal nerve, further exacerbating any pre-existing weakness.

RECTAL SENSATION AND TONE   Rectal sensation depends on the integrity of the sacral spinal cord, which is not altered with normal aging. Older adults with constipation, however, can have two types of rectal pathology: (1) increased rectal tone and reduced compliance; and (2) rectal dyschezia, which is characterized by reduced rectal tone, variable degree of rectal dilatation, impaired rectal sensory threshold, and a higher volume of rectal distention required to induce reflex relaxation of the internal anal sphincter. Individuals with rectal dyschezia are more likely to have a rectal impaction. The neuropathophysiology of rectal dyschezia is compatible with diminished parasympathetic outflow from the sacral cord, and can occur in older adults with ischemia to the sacral cord, and spinal stenosis. Changes have been observed in older adults with constipation including colorectal dysmotility, increased colorectal diameter, and impaired rectal sensation.

PSYCHOLOGICAL PROBLEMS   Psychological factors, such as depression and cognitive impairment, predispose the older adult to constipation and rectal

impaction, independent of other associated factors such as immobility, dehydration, or medications. Constipation in these individuals may be due to a loss of the awareness of the urge to defecate. This lack of awareness of the urge to defecate is referred to as the "terminal reservoir syndrome." These individuals loose their responsiveness to the gastrocolic reflex and rectosigmoid response to food. It is also possible that psychological distress and depression result in a subjective complaint of constipation and can be a somatic manifestation of the psychological illness.

MEDICATION   Drugs, both prescription and nonprescription, can cause constipation (Table 15-2). Drugs that inhibit neurologic or muscular function of the gastrointestinal tract, particularly the

Table 15-2

Drugs That Commonly Cause Constipation

Analgesics
Inhibitors of prostaglandin synthesis (NSAIDs)
Opiates
Anticholinergics
Antihistamines
Antiparkinsonian agents
Phenothiazines
Tricyclic antidepressants
Antacids
Calcium carbonate
Aluminum hydroxide
Antihypertensives
Diuretics (particularly nonpotassium sparing)
Calcium channel blockers
Clonidine
Vitamins
Iron preparations
Other
Laxative overuse
Bismuth salts
Sedatives
Sympathomimetics
Muscle blockers

colon, can result in constipation. Most commonly implicated are opiates, medications with anticholinergic properties, antacids containing aluminum or calcium, and calcium channel blockers, which slow intestinal transit by affecting autonomic nervous system function or smooth muscle contractility. Diuretics can cause dehydration, resulting in increased absorption of water and decreased stool water content, causing or exacerbating constipation.

Opiates inhibit gastrointestinal motility, particularly in the colon. The major mechanism of opiate action has been proposed to be prolongation of intestinal transit time by causing spastic, nonpropulsive contractions and an increase in electrolyte absorption. All opiate derivatives are associated with constipation, but the degree of intestinal inhibitory effects differs between agents, with codeine having the most potent antimotility effect. Moreover, orally administered opiates appear to have greater inhibitory effect than parenterally administered drugs.

Medications with anticholinergic properties inhibit bowel function by parasympatholytic actions on innervation to many regions of the gastrointestinal tract, particularly the colon and rectum. Many groups of drugs, commonly prescribed for the elderly, such as antihistamines, antiparkinsonian agents, phenothiazines, and tricyclic antidepressants, possess anticholinergic action.

DIET AND EXERCISE The amount of fiber in the diet has been shown to influence bowel function, and increasing fiber intake decreases the incidence of constipation. Increased dietary fiber results in increased stool weight and frequency. Fluid intake of more than 1500 mL per day is important in maintaining bowel function. Increased physical activity reduces both self-reported and objectively measured constipation in older adults.

What Other Diagnoses Should Be Considered as Part of the Cause?

In addition to pathophysiologic causes, there are a number of physical diseases that have been reported to contribute to the incidence of constipation (Table 15-3). Physical diseases that can cause, and/or are associated with, constipation include gastrointestinal disorders, metabolic conditions, muscular or neurologic disease, depression, degenerative joint disease, cognitive impairment, or cardiac disease.

Table 15-3

Common Problems Associated with Constipation

Gastrointestinal disorders
  Colon cancer
  Mechanical obstruction (external lesion)
  Strictures from diverticula or ischemia
  Rectocele
  Megacolon
  Fissures, hemorrhoids
  Irritable bowel disease
  Hernia
  Volvulus
  Helminthic infections
Metabolic and endocrine disease
  Diabetes mellitus
  Hypothyroidism
  Hyperparathyroidism
  Hypercalcemia
  Hypokalemia
  Hypomagnesemia
  Uremia
  Heavy metal poisoning
  Porphyria
Neurologic disease
  Parkinson's disease
  Spinal cord compression (tumor or injury)
  Cerebrovascular disease
Psychogenic and environmental
  Depression
  Cognitive impairment
  Exercise
  Immobility
  Diet and hydration
  Medications
  Terminal reservoir syndrome

GASTROINTESTINAL DISORDERS

Gastrointestinal disorders are a common cause of constipation and generally involve the large bowel. Diseases of the upper gastrointestinal tract, such as gastroduodenal obstruction, can also be responsible. The most common colonic diseases causing constipation are irritable bowel disease and diverticulitis.

IRRITABLE BOWEL DISEASE   Irritable bowel disease (IBD) can be associated with constipation or diarrhea. Irritable bowel disease refers to a combination of symptoms including constipation with or without diarrhea, lower left quadrant discomfort, distention, excessive flatus, and incomplete evacuation. Unlike other pathologic conditions that cause constipation, IBD is not associated with blood in the stool, does not awaken the patient at night, and does not cause a change in appetite or weight loss. Although it is unusual for IBD to present for the first time in late life, the patient may not complain of symptoms until the sixth or seventh decade.

DIVERTICULOSIS   Diverticulosis, or the presence of colonic diverticula, occurs in two-thirds of the American population over the age of 60 years. Diverticulosis represents an outpouching in the colon at sites of insertion of the penetrating blood vessels. Diverticula are most common in the descending colon and sigmoid. Generally, older adults will be asymptomatic unless there is perforation, infection, or bleeding. When there is obstruction of the diverticulum by a fecalith and microperforation, diverticulitis occurs. The older adult can present with left lower quadrant pain, low-grade fever, an elevated white count, and blood in the stool.

NEUROLOGIC DISORDERS

Central neurologic disorders can also cause constipation. The central nervous system is an important component in gastrointestinal regulation, either through gastrointestinal reflexes or by modifying gastrointestinal function in response to conscious effort or emotional stimuli. Trauma to the brain or spinal cord can inhibit bowel function, as can tumors, cerebrovascular accidents, multiple sclerosis, or Parkinson's disease.

METABOLIC AND ENDOCRINE DISORDERS

Metabolic and endocrine disorders, such as diabetes mellitus, can alter bowel function and cause constipation. Diabetes can influence sensory and autonomic function and result in an associated neuropathy that can affect multiple segments of the gastrointestinal tract resulting in an atonic colon and the absence of a gastrocolic reflex. Hypothyroidism can cause hypomotility and slow bowel transit. Metabolic disturbances, such as hypercalcemia and hypokalemia, can produce neuronal dysfunction and minimize acetylcholine stimulation of smooth muscle. This can prolong gastrointestinal transit time. Hypercalcemia also causes conduction delay within the extrinsic and intrinsic innervation of the gut.

What Serious or Life-Threatening Diagnoses Must Always Be Considered, Even If Rare?

Constipation can be indicative of an underlying colonic obstruction due to colon cancer, external compression from some other malignant lesion, strictures, rectocele, postsurgical abnormalities, megacolon, hernias, a volvulus of the bowel, or an anal fissure. Colon obstruction is a potentially life-threatening condition, with a mortality rate of 40 percent. Approximately 50 percent of older adults with bowel obstruction will complain of constipation.

Older adults tend to develop colon obstructions more frequently than younger adults, with neoplasm being the most common cause. Colorectal cancer incidence rates increase from 103 cases in men and 77 cases in women per 100,000 for those age 55 to 59, to about 500 cases in men and 400 cases in women per 100,000 for those 60 years of age and older.

Another common cause of large bowel obstruction in the older adult is volvulus, accounting for 15 percent of all large bowel obstructions. Elongation of the sigmoid colon occurs with time, and the "redundant" segment of sigmoid colon predisposes to a rotation of the segment around the axis of its mesentery. Constipation is seen in 50 percent to 75 percent of these cases. In the small intestine, adhesions and hernias are the most common cause of obstruction.

Typical Presentation

Table 15-4

Associated Symptoms of Constipation

Decreased stool frequency
Sense of incomplete evacuation
Rectal incontinence
Fecal soiling
Pain with defecation
Abdominal pain
Rectal pain
Straining on defecation
Frequent laxative use

Constipation is a common clinical complaint, with a variety of associated signs and symptoms. Patient complaints of constipation do not always correlate with objective measures. Most adults report at least one bowel movement in 24 h, so those who do not will often describe themselves as constipated. For others, constipation implies difficult defecation, with common symptoms being straining and incomplete evacuation. Difficult defecation is a more common complaint reported by the older adult with constipation than infrequent stool. There are a number of associated symptoms (Table 15-4) indicative of constipation in the older adult. These include pain on defecation, a sense of incomplete evacuation, fecal soiling, incontinence, and abdominal pain.

The following areas should be explored with the patient and/or caregivers: stool frequency; the necessity to strain during defecation; the feeling of incomplete evacuation; the sense of outlet obstruction; abdominal bloating or pain; rectal pain; the need for digital manipulation to enable defecation; changes in bowel habits, color, size, or consistency; or pain associated with defecation. A description of the stool is essential information to help with management of constipation. Stools that are hard and dry can be indicative of inadequate fluid and fiber intake. Stools that are putty-like in

consistency are more likely due to decreased segmental contraction and propulsion. Patients should also be asked about diseases that predispose them to chronic constipation such as diabetes mellitus or neurologic and psychiatric disorders, previous abdominal or perianal operations, or hemorrhoidal disease.

Information should be elicited regarding the patient's current medications (including all over-the-counter agents), daily activity level, food preferences, and fiber and fluid intake. Atypical presentation of constipation can occur, particularly for those with some underlying cognitive impairment. Changes in mental status (confusion or increased agitation), elevated temperature, incontinence, and a change in functional performance or unexplained falls can be atypical presentations of constipation.

It is also important to elicit the patient's definition of constipation and description of his or her bowel function. Emotional state should also be evaluated to determine whether depression or stress can be causing the constipation. A simple screening tool for depression that correlates strongly with the 15-item Geriatric Depression Scale is the 1-question Yale Depression Screen "Do you often feel sad or depressed?"

How Do Different Symptoms Suggest One Diagnosis Versus Another?

Constipation in the older adults can be a symptom of acute abdominal events including obstruction (volvulus, adhesions, hernia, ileus, and neoplasm) and inflammation (diverticulitis, appendicitis). When obstruction is present, there can also be fever, pain, guarding, nausea and vomiting, and severe abdominal distention. It is also quite common for older adults with these disorders to have no specific symptoms aside from an acute change in functional performance and cognition.

Older adults with appendicitis can present with constipation and the associated symptoms of right lower quadrant pain, decreased appetite, nausea and vomiting, fever, and a change in function and cognition. Fever, left lower quadrant pain, and/or a change in function and cognition are most likely symptoms of diverticulitis.

Constipation, particularly of new onset, is often the only presenting symptom of a neoplasm. Constipation can be associated with a change in the color of the stools (i.e., darkening), abdominal pain, nausea and vomiting, and if there is a rectal neoplasm, tenesmus (a spastic contraction causing rectal pain), urgency, and hematochezia.

Are Any Symptoms Suggestive of a Serious or Life-Threatening Condition?

Acute abdominal disease is a critical problem in older adults. Of all older patients evaluated in the emergency room with abdominal problems, 51 to 63 percent are admitted to the hospital; they undergo surgery at double the rate of their younger counterparts and have a mortality rate of 8 to 14 percent. It is essential to consider the possibility of either gastrointestinal obstruction, acute inflammation, or the possibility of a neoplasm in all older adults who report constipation of new onset. Abdominal pain, fever, vomiting, and rectal bleeding are suggestive of potential serious or life-threatening disorders. Consequently, it is im-

perative to complete a comprehensive physical examination on any older adult who complains of constipation.

Constipation Score

A constipation scoring system (Table 15-5) was developed by Agachan and colleagues to establish an objective measurement of patients' complaints. This scoring system rates both subjective symptomatic complaints and physiologic findings. Scoring is done by computing individual scores. A score of 15 or more is suggestive of the symptom "constipation." This measure was able to correctly identify those with constipation with 96 percent accuracy; however, the scale must be used in totality since single items were not reliable in determining constipation. The overall score corresponded with the severity of constipation. Although further testing of this measure is needed, it can serve as a useful screening tool to help the practitioner in using a systematic approach to diagnosing constipation.

Physical Examination

A complete physical examination is needed to identify potentially serious problems that can influence bowel function in the older adult. Common physical and laboratory findings associated with the causes of constipation are shown in Table 15-6.

Oral Examination

The practitioner should evaluate dentition and examine the mouth for oral lesions or tumors that might interfere with taste and/or swallowing. A bedside swallowing examination should be considered particularly in patients with dementia,

Table 15-5

Constipation Scoring System

ITEM	SCORE
Frequency of bowel movements	
1–2 times per 1–2 days	0
2 times per week	1
Once per week	2
Less than once per week	3
Less than once per month	4
Difficulty: painful evacuation effort	
Never	0
Rarely	1
Sometimes	2
Usually	3
Always	4
Completeness: feeling incomplete evacuation	
Never	0
Rarely	1
Sometimes	2
Usually	3
Always	4
Pain: abdominal pain	
Never	0
Rarely	1
Sometimes	2
Usually	3
Always	4
Time: minutes in lavatory per attempt	
Less than 5	0
5–10	1
10–20	2
20–30	3
More than 30	4
Assistance	
Without assistance	0
Stimulant laxatives	1
Digital assistance or enema	2
Failure: Unsuccessful attempts for evacuation per 24 h	
Never	0
1–2	1
3–6	2
6–9	3
More than 9	4
History: duration of constipation (yr)	
0	0
1–5	1
5–10	2
10–20	3
More than 20	4

Scoring system: A score of greater than 15 is defined as constipation. The greater the score, the more severe the condition.

SOURCE: Reproduced with permission from Agachan F, Chen T, Pfeifer J, et al: A constipation scoring system to simplify evaluation and management of constipated patient. *Dis Col Rectum* 39;681, 1996.

Table 15-6

Common Causes of Acute Abdominal Disease in Older Adults

CONDITION	PHYSICAL AND LABORATORY FINDINGS	FURTHER WORKUP
Obstruction	Nonreducible hernia	Flat plate of the abdomen
Volvulus	Fever	Barium enema
Neoplasm	Tachycardia	Flexible colonoscopy and/or
Adhesions	Pain and guarding	sigmoidoscopy
Hernia	Leukocytosis	
Ileus	Nausea and vomiting	
	Constipation	
	Abdominal distention	
Inflammation		
Diverticulitis	Left lower quadrant (LLQ) pain	CT scan
	Fever	Barium enema and colonoscopy
	Leukocytosis	contraindicated during acute phase
	Mass in the LLQ	
Appendicitis	Right lower quadrant (RLQ) pain	CT scan
	Decreased appetite	
	Nausea and vomiting	
	Leukocytosis	
	Constipation	
Peptic Ulcer Disease	Decreased appetite	Endoscopy
	Epigastric pain and tenderness	
Ischemia/Vascular Disorders	Abdominal/back pain	Kidney, ureter, and bladder
Abdominal aortic	Hypotension	Ultrasound
aneurysm rupture		

Parkinson's disease, or those who have had a cerebrovascular event or have impairments in cranial nerve functioning.

Abdominal Examination

An abdominal examination can differentiate constipation from a significant acute abdominal event. Inspection of the abdomen should focus on evidence of bloating, distention, or bulges. Percussion of the abdomen can help identify excessive gas. Dullness during percussion can suggest organomegaly, ascites, or a fecal mass. Light palpation of the abdomen can detect tenderness and muscular resistance that can be asso-

ciated with chronic constipation. When abdominal pain is produced with light palpation, or rebound tenderness is detected, peritoneal inflammation must be suspected. Involuntary rigidity or spasm of the abdominal muscles will be detected when there is peritoneal inflammation. Deep palpation can detect abdominal masses, such as an abdominal aortic aneurysm, colon cancer, a distended bladder, or a mass of fecal matter in the descending colon.

Auscultation should be done to assess for hyperactive bowel sounds or no bowel sounds. Friction rubs in the abdomen are rare but indicate inflammation of the peritoneal surface of the organ from tumor, infection, or infarction. Increased bowel sounds can be an indication of diarrhea or impending intestinal obstruction. Decreased, then absent, bowel sounds can suggest paralytic ileus and peritonitis.

Anorectal Examination

An anorectal examination provides important information on the size and condition of the rectum and the amount and consistency of stool in the rectum. Muscle weakness, which is more common in the older adult, is characterized by reduced rectal tone, variable rectal dilatation, and impaired rectal sensory threshold. The combined effects of these changes result in a need for a higher volume of rectal distention to induce defecation. Assessment of the rectal area should include examination for other potential contributors to constipation including hemorrhoids, rectal prolapse, fecal impaction, strength of anal sphincter tone, presence of occult blood (guaiac test), rectal fistula, and rectal masses or nodules.

Ancillary Tests

A complete blood cell count, fasting blood glucose, serum chemistry panel, and thyroid-stimulating hormone can be useful in diagnosing anemia, diabetes mellitus, hypercalcemia, hypokalemia, uremia, and hypothyroidism, respectively. An amylase level can be elevated in pancreatitis or ischemic bowel disease. A urinalysis can be ordered to rule out bladder or kidney infection. If weight loss, anemia, rectal passage of blood, or a family history of colon cancer is present, colonoscopy is appropriate to exclude a malignant lesion. A barium enema study is less sensitive than colonoscopy and does not allow for a tissue biopsy at the time of evaluation; however, a flexible sigmoidoscopy and barium enema are useful as alternative examinations to rule out colorectal neoplasms.

Although most cases of constipation can be evaluated and managed without the need for extensive diagnostic testing, other tests can provide additional useful information in patients. Further workup should be undertaken for patients who have persistent symptoms despite treatment for up to 6 months. Cinedefecography (radiographic evaluation of evacuation of barium paste from the rectum) to evaluate colonic transit abnormalities and demonstrate evidence of functional constipation should be done next. This can determine if there is colonic inertia, in which case, a surgical consultation might be appropriate. If colonic transit time is normal, rectal outlet delay should be considered and anal manometry done. Thereafter further neurologic workup should be considered.

Plain Abdominal X-Rays

Plain abdominal radiographs should be performed on older adults with constipation, particularly those with acute constipation. Volvulus is typically manifested by a focal dilation of the sigmoid or cecal colonic segments. Evidence of colon cancer, especially in the sigmoid area, may be indicated by moderate dilation of the proximal air-filled colon, multiple air-fluid levels, and abrupt termination of air at the site of the tumor. Colon perforation occurs in 7 percent of cases of large bowel obstruction. Therefore, upright abdominal radiographs are useful for detecting free intraperitoneal air.

Barium Enema

In older adults suspected of having colonic obstruction, a barium enema can help to determine the level and often the general nature of the obstruction. Abrupt irregular termination of the barium column suggests colon cancer, whereas smooth tapering is seen in sigmoid or cecal volvulus. Colonic narrowing with mucosal preservation and a "sawtooth" appearance suggests diverticulitis.

Sigmoidoscopy

In the primary care setting, a sigmoidoscopy can be useful in patients with a recent onset of constipation or to confirm chronic constipation. Sigmoidoscopy is a screening procedure that assists in the identification of colorectal carcinoma and premalignant lesions. The colon of older adults who are chronically constipated can reveal melanosis coli, a superficial, spotty, or diffuse dark pigmentation. This condition is caused by chronic use of anthraquinone laxatives such as cascara or senna. Colonoscopy should be considered if there is evidence of occult or gross rectal bleeding.

Colonic Transit Time

Colonic transit time is a procedure that measures the amount of time required for intestinal materials to pass. The study is indicated if the patient has fewer than three to five stools per week, and this persists despite treatment with fluid, fiber, activity, and moderate laxative use. Patients who have a normal number of bowel movements and yet still complain of constipation despite adequate intake of dietary fiber and fluid are also candidates for this test. Abdominal radiographs are taken 5 and 7 days after ingestion of solid radiopaque markers (Sitzmarks). The process is followed by daily x-rays of the abdomen. Expulsion of 80 percent of the markers in 5 days is expected in normal individuals. Retention of markers in the colon or rectum for more than 5 days indicates significant constipation. Holdup of markers in the rectum is indicative of failure of expulsion.

Colonic Motility Testing

This test is used to identify different patterns of colonic activity. It involves the recording of pressure activity in the distal colon and rectum using a water-perfused or solid-state catheter introduced into the lumen via the anus. It can detect spasms associated with irritable bowel syndrome or an atonic colon.

Anorectal Manometry

Anorectal manometry is indicated to diagnose such conditions as amyloidosis, megacolon, a long history of constipation, and colonic transit marker suggesting anorectal dysfunction, melanosis coli, and Hirschsprung's disease, rather than as a routine test for constipation. Manometry is used to measure the pressure in the rectum and anal canal at rest and with a variety of stimuli and to measure the patient's anorectal function. An eight-lumen catheter with individual side holes radially arrayed at 0.5-cm intervals and an inflatable balloon at its distal end is used for testing. The catheter is perfused at a rate of 0.1 mL/min by a low compliance perfusion system and intraluminal pressure changes. These pressure changes are monitored by strain gauge transducers and are recorded. The catheter is inserted rectally, and the patient is asked to squeeze (i.e., voluntarily contract the external sphincter) for at least 60 s or until the pressure increment is decreased to the level of basal sphincter pressure. On completion of squeeze measurements, and with the catheter in the same position, the balloon is rapidly inflated with 60 mL of air to elicit the rectoanal inhibitory reflex. Finally, with the balloon in the rectum, step-wise balloon inflation can be performed at 5-mL increments, and the threshold for rectal sensation can be defined.

Electromyography

Electromyography (EMG) measures anal sphincter electromyographic frequency (i.e., internal sphincter pressure). Single-fiber EMG measures single-fiber nerve density as an expression of motor denervation. Pudendal nerve terminal motor latency is the response time of the external sphincter to transrectal stimulation of the pudendal nerve and is a measure of pudendal nerve atrophy.

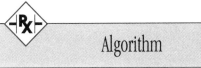

Algorithm

Figure 15-1 provides an algorithm to help differentiate the underlying cause of constipation and/or identify the presence of acute and/or potentially life-threatening associated problems. Once a history and physical examination are done (included within this are a basic serum chemistry panel, CBC, and thyroid function tests), it is essen-tial to rule out the possibility of a colorectal cancer. Flexible sigmoidoscopy and barium enema are suggested as the most practical procedures. Colonoscopy is an alternative choice and is particularly appropriate if a mass and/or polyp is suspected (i.e., if there is blood in the stool and/or a prior history of polyps).

Once a malignancy is ruled out, nonstructural causes of constipation (medications, metabolic problems, endocrine abnormalities, and neuro-logic causes) should be explored. As appropriate, these problems should be treated and/or lifestyle

Figure 15-1

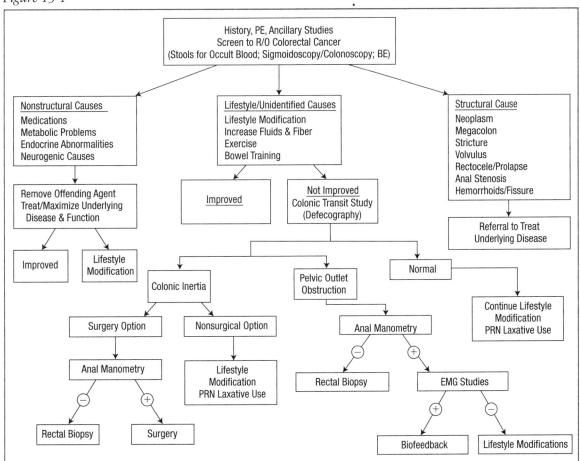

Algorithm.

modifications implemented (as described as fol-lows). Similarly, structural causes of constipation such as megacolon, stricture, volvulus, rectocele, prolapse, anal stenosis, hemorrhoids, or fissures should also be identified and treated. If no known structural or nonstructural causes can be identi-fied, lifestyle modifications should be imple-mented for a period of 6 months.

If there is no improvement in bowel function following adherence to lifestyle modifications such as increased fluids, fiber, and exercise, col-onic transit studies should be recommended. Normal transit studies indicate a need to con-tinue with lifestyle modifications and laxatives as needed. If there is evidence of colonic inertia, a surgical referral should be considered as well as further testing with anal manometry. If there is evidence of pelvic outlet obstruction, anal manometry is indicated, as well as EMG studies. One appropriate treatment plan for abnormal rectal innervation consists of biofeedback. If there is normal nerve innervation, lifestyle mod-ifications are the treatment of choice and should be continued.

Treatment

Treatment of constipation can be nonpharmaco-logic, pharmacologic, or both. The initial man-agement should include nonpharmacologic measures including exercise, fluid and fiber, and environmental interventions. Patients should be educated about the wide variation in bowel habits and that 95 percent of individuals have as many as three bowel movements per day or as few as three bowel movements per week. Patients should also be taught about the gastro-colic reflex and be encouraged to attempt defe-cation 30 min after consumption of a meal. When medications are being used that can cause con-stipation they should be discontinued or replaced by others.

Exercise

Increased levels of activity are recommended for patients with constipation. Physical activity, such as walking for 20 to 30 min, has been suggested as a mechanism to enhance gastrointestinal motility. Alternative exercise programs include riding a stationary bike, doing abdominal and pelvic floor muscle strengthening exercises, and range-of-motion (passive or active) exercises, which can be beneficial for those who are less mobile. Exer-cise, together with abdominal massage, has also been used as an intervention and can result in decreased episodes of fecal incontinence and a significant increase in the number of bowel move-ments with a reduced need for laxatives.

Diet

Dietary fiber is important for the successful long-term management of constipation. Dietary fiber, the portion of vegetable matter not digested in the human gastrointestinal tract, increases stool bulk, retention of stool water, and rate of transit of stool through the intestine. Dietary fiber modifies sev-eral functions of the large bowel including: (1) bac-terial metabolism and fermentation; (2) gas and water concentration; (3) fecal bulk and consis-tency; and (4) intraluminal pressure. It is believed that the therapeutic effect of dietary fiber is due to an interrelationship among all these functions.

Increasing dietary fiber can result in an increased frequency of defecation and a decrease in the intra-luminal pressure in the colon and rectum. A diet that is high in fiber content can be of benefit in managing diverticular disease and irritable bowel syndrome. Bran, a by-product of the milling of wheat, is often added to foods to increase fiber content. Raw bran has generally 40 percent fiber content. Bulk-forming agents, such as psyllium hydrophilic colloids (Metamucil), methylcellulose (Citrucel), or polycarbophil (Fibercon), have prop-erties similar to those of dietary fiber and can be taken as tablets, powders, granules, or wafers (Table 15-7). Many patients object to drinking pow-

Table 15-7

Laxatives Commonly Used in Treatment of Constipation

Type	Dosage	Cost ($)	Side Effects	Action Time (h)	Mechanism of Action
Fiber					
Bran	1 cup	0.50	Bloating, gas, malabsorption	—	Stool bulk
Psyllium (Metamucil)	1 tsp tid	0.10–0.30	Bloating, gas	—	Colonic transit time
Methylcellulose (Citrucel)	1 tsp tid	0.50–1.43	Less bloating	—	GI motility
Calcium polycarbophil (Fibercon)	2–4 tabs	0.44–0.88	Bloating, gas	—	
Stool softener					
Docusate (Colace)	100 mg bid	0.14–0.80	—	12–72	Cyclic adenosine monophosphate stimulated to secrete water, NaCl into lumen
Hyperosmolar agents					
Sorbitol	15–30 mL qd-tid	0.12–0.48	Cramps, gas	24–48	Nonabsorbable sugar metabolized by colonic bacteria
Lactulose (Chronulac)	15–30 mL qd-tid	1.14–4.56	Cramps, gas	24–48	
Stimulants					
Bisacodyl (Dulcolax)	10 mg	0.26–1.50	Cramps, hypokalemia	.25–1	Increase intraluminal fluids; myenteric plexus stimulated
Anthraquinones (Senekot/ Pericolace)	2–4 mg	0.60–2.40	Cramps, dehydration, melanosis coli	8–12	
Phenolphthalein (Correctol/Ex-Lax)	1–2 tabs	0.20–0.60	Rash, malabsorption, dehydration	6–8	
	1–2 tabs				
Saline					
Magnesium (Milk of Magnesia)	15–30 mL	0.11–0.44	Magnesium toxicity, dehydration, cramps	1–3	Fluid osmotically drawn into small bowel
Enemas					
Mineral oil	100–250 mL	1.50	Mechanical trauma, damage to mucosa	6–8	Stool softened
Fleet				.5	Mechanical lavage
Lubricant					
Mineral oil	15–45 mL	1.50	Lipid pneumonia, malabsorption of fat-soluble vitamins, dehydration	6–8	Stool lubricated

dered fiber supplements but are willing to try alternative ways to increase fiber. Many high-fiber breakfast cereals have the advantage of being sugarfree, low fat, and very high in fiber. For example, encouraging a patient to use a half a cup of Fiber-One (General Mills), mixed with other breakfast cereals, can add 13 g of fiber to the patient's daily intake.

The amount of fiber suggested varies and can range between 2.4 g to 40 g, with 14 to 20 g reported to be effective in treatment of chronic nonorganic constipation. Foods high in dietary fiber include whole grain breads and cereals, fresh fruit, root vegetables, and legumes, although cereal fibers seem to have a maximum effect on bowel physiology, There are a variety of natural laxative recipes (Table 15-8) that have been shown to improve bowel function in the older

adult. A mixture of dried fruit was found by Beverley and Travis to be a cost-effective alternative to laxative use for older adults. Power pudding (see Table 15-8) was also effective in improving bowel function. Unprocessed bran can also be mixed into puddings or applesauce to further increase fiber intake.

A trial of dietary modification with high-fiber content should be continued for at least 1 month, although most patients notice effects on bowel function 3 to 5 days after beginning a high-fiber diet. The patient should be cautioned that abdominal distention and flatus may be noticed in the first few weeks of taking a high-fiber diet, particularly if high bran consumption is used. Bulk-forming laxatives have very few side effects and minimal systemic effects. The only major caution for patients is potential obstruction of the esoph-

Table 15-8

Natural Laxative Recipes

Fruit Spread*

2 lb raisins

2 lb currants

2 lb prunes

2 lb figs

2 lb dates

2 28-ounce containers undiluted prune concentrate

Put fruit through a grinder. Mix with prune concentrate in large mixer (mixture will be very thick). Store in large-mouthed plastic container. Refrigerate.

Power Pudding†

1/2 cup prune juice

1/2 cup applesauce

1/2 cup wheat bran flakes

1/2 cup whipped topping

1/2 cup prunes (canned stewed)

Blend ingredients, cover and refrigerate, and keep as long as 1 week. Take 1/4 cup portions of recipe with breakfast. Regulate dose as needed.

SOURCE: *Reproduced with permission from P Ebersole, P Hess: *Toward Healthy Aging.* St Louis: Mosby, 1997. Adapted From L Beverley, I Travis: Constipation: proposed natural laxative mixtures. *J Gerontol Nursing* 18:5, 1992.
†Reproduced with permission from P Ebersole, P Hess: *Toward Healthy Aging.* St Louis: Mosby, 1997. Adapted From J Neal: Power pudding: natural laxative therapy for the elderly who are homebound. *Home Healthcare Nurse* 13:66, 1995.

agus, stomach, small intestine, or colon. Though rare, these obstructions have occurred when the agents were used without fluid. If using powdered agents, patients should add an 8-oz glass of water (or other fluid), and all ingested bulk agents should be followed by an 8-oz glass of water or other fluid.

Environment modification can also be useful in facilitating bowel evacuation. Setting a regular time (preferably after the morning meal) to evacuate is an important first step in improving bowel function. The gastrocolic reflex, the mass propulsion of material through the large intestine that occurs after a meal, is strongest after the morning meal. Adequate time and privacy should also be afforded the patient. In addition, placing the feet on a footstool helps to align the colon in the normal anatomic position for passing stool. This positioning can also help decrease straining.

Pharmacologic Options

For many older adults, a regular regimen of laxatives may be needed. Laxatives are second only to analgesics in sales to elderly persons, but they should be used cautiously. Laxative use over time can result in malabsorption, dehydration, electrolyte imbalances, and fecal incontinence. In general, most agents work by promoting active electrolyte secretion, decreasing water and electrolyte absorption, increasing intraluminal osmolarity, and increasing hydrostatic pressure in the gastrointestinal tract.

LAXATIVES

Laxatives convert the intestine from primarily an organ that absorbs water and electrolytes to an organ that secretes water and electrolytes. Laxatives can be classified as those that: (1) cause softening of the feces in 1 to 3 days (bulk-forming laxatives, docusates, and lactulose); (2) result in soft or semifluid stool in 6 to 12 h (diphenylmethane derivatives and anthraquinone derivatives); or (3) cause water evacuation in 1 to 6 h (saline cathartics, castor oil, and polyethylene glycolelectrolyte lavage solution).

STOOL-SOFTENING AGENTS (EMOLLIENT LAXATIVES)

Emollient laxatives, or surfactant agents, work by facilitating a mixture of aqueous and fatty materials within the intestinal tract. They increase water and electrolyte secretion in the small and large bowel and usually soften the stool in 1 to 3 days. These drugs are mostly effective in preventing constipation. Although they are generally safe, they can increase the intestinal absorption of agents administered concurrently and alter toxic potential. Mineral oil is the only lubricant laxative in routine use. This agent, obtained from petroleum refining, acts by coating stool and allowing easier passage. It inhibits colonic absorption of water, thereby increasing stool weight and decreasing stool transit time. Mineral oil can be given orally or rectally in a dose of 15 to 45 mL. Generally, this will be effective in 2 to 3 days. Similar to the emollient laxatives, mineral oil is effective in preventing constipation. There is, however, a greater risk profile with this drug. Mineral oil can be absorbed systemically and cause a foreign-body reaction in lymphoid tissue, and in debilitated or recumbent patients, mineral oil can be aspirated, causing lipoid pneumonia. Mineral oil has also been reported to decrease the absorption of fat-soluble vitamins (A, D, E, and K) with chronic use and can also result in rectal leakage with subsequent pruritus and soiling of clothes.

Lactulose, a disaccharide, and sorbitol, a monosaccharide, can be used either orally or rectally. These agents are not absorbed by the small intestine and are metabolized by colonic bacteria to low-molecular-weight acids, resulting in an osmotic effect whereby fluid is retained in the colon. The fluid retained in the colon lowers the pH and increases colonic peristalsis. Lactulose use can be expensive for the older adults; can cause flatulence, cramps, diarrhea, and electrolyte imbalances; and can alter the colonic microbial activity. Sorbitol is equally as effective as lactulose for constipation, but costs considerably less. Both agents can be used in dosages starting at 15 mL/d and can increase as needed to 60 mL/d or bid.

CATHARTICS　Cathartics cause a soft or semifluid stool in 6 to 12 h. Diphenylmethane derivatives, such as bisacodyl (Dulcolax) and phenolphthalein (Correctol), work primarily on the colon. Bisacodyl stimulates the mucosal nerve plexus of the colon, and phenolphthalein is believed to inhibit active glucose absorption and sodium absorption resulting in fluid accumulation in the colon by osmotic action. These agents are not recommended for daily use but rather for intermittent acute constipation as they cause severe cramping as well as significant fluid and electrolyte imbalances if used chronically.

Anthraquinone derivatives, such as cascara sagrada, sennosides, and casantrol, are metabolized by gut bacteria to their active compounds, but the exact mechanisms of action are not understood. A major advantage of these drugs is that their effects are limited to the colon, making them physiologically more natural and potentially safer. Recommendations for the use of these agents are similar to those of the diphenylmethane group. In addition, the anthraquinone derivatives can cause melanosis coli, an accumulation of dark pigment, mainly in the cecum and rectum, after chronic use (4 to 13 months). There is no known pathologic effect of melanosis coli, and it is reversible if the drugs are discontinued.

SALINE CATHARTICS　Saline cathartics cause water evacuation in 1 to 6 h. Saline cathartics are composed of relatively poorly absorbed ions such as magnesium, sulfate, phosphate, and citrate, which produce their effects primarily by osmotic action to retain fluid in the gastrointestinal tract. Magnesium stimulates the secretion of cholecystokinin, a hormone that causes stimulation of bowel motility and fluid secretion. These agents can be given orally or rectally. A bowel movement can result within a few hours after oral doses, and in an hour or less following rectal administration. These agents should not be used on a routine basis to treat constipation because fluid and electrolyte depletion can result. Also, magnesium or sodium accumulation can occur with chronic use, particularly in patients with renal dysfunction or heart failure.

ENEMAS

Enemas evacuate the rectal ampulla and sometimes, the descending and sigmoid colon. Enemas should be used very cautiously in older adults. Soapsuds, or large-volume enemas in particular, cause discomfort and can disrupt homeostasis and give rise to shock. Soapsuds and phosphate enemas should also be used with caution because they can cause mucosal injury. When giving an enema to an older adult, a small-volume Fleet Bisacodyl enema (37.4 mL) is preferable. The safest enema, however, is a lukewarm tap-water enema because this will not irritate the colonic mucosa.

RECTAL STIMULANTS

Glycerin suppositories can be used to stimulate the rectum locally and can induce evacuation. These suppositories can be used to augment the gastrocolic reflex as part of a bowel retraining program. Glycerin exerts its effect by osmotic action in the rectum. As with most agents given as suppositories, the onset of action is usually less than 30 min, but can be a little longer in the older adult. Glycerin is considered a very safe laxative, although there have been some reports of rectal irritation.

OTHER AGENTS

Sitz baths and topical ointments, such as pramoxine hydrochloride (Anusol) or Tucks pads, can be beneficial in relieving the discomfort of hemorrhoids and thereby facilitating defecation. Prokinetic agents, such as cisapride, can be used when there is known evidence of a gastrointestinal motility disorder. This drug is more expensive than most laxatives, and has more adverse effects, so should not be used as a first-line treatment.

SURGICAL INTERVENTION

Total abdominal colectomy is recognized as a therapeutic option for patients with intractable constipation due to colonic dysmotility. Total colectomy with ileoproctostomy seems to be more effective than a partial colectomy. The success rate is variable and over time decreases to as low as 50 percent. Redmond and associates differentiated between patients with colonic inertia versus those with generalized intestinal dysmotility. The researchers followed the patients after surgical interventions for constipation. More than 90 percent of the patients with colonic inertia had resolution of constipation, and 100 percent had resolution of pain after total abdominal colectomy. This improvement persisted for 2 years post-surgery. In contrast, patients with generalized intestinal dysmotility showed initial improvement of their constipation; however, there was a recurrence of constipation in 63 percent of these individuals after 2 years, increasingly severe diarrhea in 13 percent, and no relief in pain.

inappropriate based on the underlying cause of the individual's constipation. Mineral oil, for example, can predispose the older adult to inhalation pneumonia, deficiencies of fat-soluble vitamins, fecal incontinence, and colorectal cancer. If the stool is soft, senna or bisacodyl should be the first choice of treatment since they will stimulate the bowel to evacuate the soft stool. If the stool is hard, however, a laxative that increases the water content of the stool, such as lactulose, should be considered. Careful attention needs to be given to the use and appropriateness of each laxative.

Treatment of the immobile older adult with constipation should be considered separately from those who are mobile. Immobile individuals should not be given bulking agents such as Metamucil. Rather, for these individuals, the best treatment and prevention of constipation can be to use enemas or suppositories as needed. It should be stressed, however, that even immobile older adults can demonstrate an improvement in bowel function by doing daily exercise in bed or in the wheelchair.

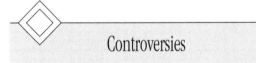

Controversies

Errors

One of the major controversies in the use of fiber supplementation is how much fiber intake should be recommended. The amount of fiber suggested varies and can range between 2.4 g and 40 g, with 14 to 20 g reported to be effective in the treatment of chronic nonorganic constipation. Certainly, there may be individual variations regarding how much fiber is sufficient, and titration of dosing should be done based on effectiveness of the treatment.

Practitioners and patients have a tendency to believe that laxatives, since they are sold over the counter, are all safe and equally effective. Regular use of some laxatives can cause potentially life-threatening complications and may be

The most common error is assuming that constipation is a normal age-related change, and not attempting to do a comprehensive evaluation of the patient. This can result in a missed diagnosis of the underlying cause of the constipation and thus inadequate treatment. If constipation is left untreated, the complications can be life-threatening. These complications include idiopathic megacolon and megarectum.

A second common error relates to laxative abuse. Older adults frequently abuse laxatives. Overuse is due, in part, to misconceptions about the need for a daily bowel movement and the easy availability of laxatives as in chocolates, gums, teas, as well as in traditional pill or powder forms. This error is compounded when clinicians prescribe laxatives, thereby seeming to approve of their use. It has repeatedly been demonstrated that laxative use can be diminished by increasing fluid intake, dietary fiber, increasing exercise, and adhering to a regular bowel schedule. These interventions should be used as the first line of treatment, before instituting laxatives. Chronic laxative abuse can result in serious illnesses such as electrolyte imbalances, protein-losing gastroenteropathy, and hypoalbuminemia.

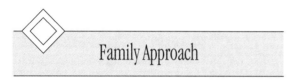

Family Approach

Families need to be educated that constipation, especially new-onset constipation, is a serious problem in older adults and should not be considered a normal age-related change. Families should encourage their older family member to discuss this problem with a health care provider so that a comprehensive evaluation of the problem can be done and an appropriate treatment plan developed. Family members should receive the same guidelines for the lifestyle modifications given to patients so that they can reinforce these guidelines. The lifestyle modifications may not be easy for the older adult to adhere to, and families will need to motivate these individuals not only to initiate the treatment guidelines but adhere to these guidelines over time.

Specifically, families can help motivate their older family member by use of the following guidelines. The family member should be encouraged to increase fluid and fiber intake and to exercise regularly. This can be done by providing verbal encouragement that he or she is capable of adapting to these behaviors. It should also be stressed that these interventions will improve bowel function. Small attainable goals

should be set, and reinforcement given for goal attainment. For example, initially the goal might be to drink four to six 8-oz glasses of fluid daily for 1 week, then increase to six to eight 8-oz glasses daily. Similarly, fiber intake might be increased by adding a new high-fiber food each day. Regular exercise can be initiated by starting a walking program, which initially might mean walking for 5 to 10 min daily and building this to 20 min three times per week. Positive reinforcement should be given by the family and might include using a chart, which demonstrates successes daily. Role modeling can also help to motivate older adults to adhere to health-promoting activities, and family members themselves should consider engaging in the same activities. Moreover, if family members are doing the grocery shopping and/or cooking for their older family member, attempts should be made to include high-fiber foods. Unrefined bran can be added to recipes (muffins, pancakes, cookies, and breads) or sprinkled into yogurt or over salads to further increase fiber intake for the whole family.

The response to treatment of lifestyle modifications can be slow and may require trial and error to determine how much fiber and fluid intake is needed to improve bowel function. Family members should also be instructed that with an increase in fiber intake, there may be an associated increase in gas, but this side effect decreases after a few weeks. Continual verbal encouragement, positive reinforcement, and role modeling will be required by the family to help their older family member adhere to the treatment plan. The consequences of this hard work, however, will mean improved bowel function without dependence on laxatives.

If the lifestyle modifications do not sufficiently improve bowel function, or the older adult is not able or willing to adhere to these modifications, laxative use can be indicated. Families should encourage their older family members to discuss this with a primary health care provider to assure that they are taking appropriate laxatives in the correct dosages.

Table 15-9

Fiber Content of Common Foods

TYPE OF FOOD	AMOUNT OF DIETARY FIBER (GRAMS/AVERAGE SERVINGS)
Cereals	(1/2 cup serving)
Fiber-One	13
Raisin Bran	3.0
All-Bran	8.4
Bran Flakes	7.8
Shredded Wheat	2.3
Vegetables	(1/2 cup serving)
Lettuce	1.0
Carrots	2.0
Celery	1.0
Cabbage	2.0
Broccoli	3.2
Brussels sprouts	2.3
Peas	6.0
Potato	3.0
Corn	2.6
Legumes	(1/2 cup serving)
Beans	8.5–10.0
Sunflower seeds	3.8
Sesame seeds	6.3
Walnuts	2.1
Peanuts	2.7
Almonds	2.6
Pecans	2.3
Fruit	
Banana	1.5
Apple	2.0
Grapefruit	0.6
Orange	2.0
Peach	2.0
Raspberries	4.6
Strawberries	1.6
Breads	(one slice)
English muffins	1.0
White bread	1.0
Whole wheat breads	1.3
Meats/fish/chicken/cheese	0

Patient Education

Education of the patient should include reassurance and a thorough explanation of normal bowel habits. Specifically, it should be stressed to the older adult that a daily bowel movement is not necessary for the maintenance of health and that there is a great deal of individual variations with regard to what is normal bowel function. Patients should be educated about the many common causes of constipation by explaining to them that constipation can be caused by emotional stress, lack of exercise, and medications including diuretics, medications to lower blood pressure, calcium pills, medications that are used to help decrease anxiety, and those that treat Parkinson's disease. They should also be advised to report any changes in their bowel patterns, especially after starting a new medication.

Every effort should be made to have patients reduce the use of laxatives and increase fluid and fiber intake, exercise regularly, and use postprandial increases in colonic motility by trying to defecate after meals. The following guidelines should be given to patients.

1. Diet: Increase fiber intake to at least 15 to 20 g of fiber (Table 15-9). This can be easily done by eating 2 cups of Fiber-One cereal and an apple. If you absolutely can not increase your fiber intake, you may supplement your diet with a store-bought psyllium hyrophilic mucilloid product, such as Metamucil or Perdiem. Mix a tablespoon of this product in 8 oz of water, and then follow it with 8 oz of water.
2. Time: Set up time daily each morning after your first meal to sit on the commode and try to move your bowels. This is the time of the day when your bowel is most active. During the day, make sure that you respond immediately to the need to move your bowels.
3. Fluids: It is essential to drink six to eight 8-oz glasses of fluid daily to make sure that your bowel elimination is the right consistency for easy passage.
4. Exercise: Regular exercise, which includes activities such as walking, swimming, or bike riding, should be done three times a week for at least 20 min. This helps to keep your bowel moving.
5. Laxatives: Laxatives, enemas, and suppositories can be harmful to your body and should only be used after consulting with your health care provider.

Emerging Concepts

Biofeedback

Biofeedback is increasingly recognized as an effective treatment for certain groups of severely constipated patients, such as those with pelvic outlet obstruction defecation. The effectiveness of this technique is variable however, this can be due to patient selection rather than the efficacy of biofeedback. Biofeedback is a behavioral technique of operant conditioning to train the mind to control the activity of somatic function. It is a painless, noninvasive means of cognitively retraining the pelvic floor and the abdominal wall musculature. Patients are guided by electromyographic (EMG) surface electrodes or an anal plug and an abdominal wall surface electrode (Table 15-10). This has helped to better standardize biofeedback techniques for patients with constipation. Continued research is needed to determine how much of the benefit is actually due to biofeedback versus the fact that there is a strong supportive environment of caring people who provide an array of potentially useful interventions to improve constipation. Biofeedback requires a good deal of patient motivation, as well as an extensive workup prior to initiation. Cost and availability must also be considered.

Table 15-10

Biofeedback Technique

1. Patients were instructed to maintain daily logs of dietary intake, water, and bowel movements. The dietician assessed the patient and made appropriate dietary interventions and suggestions.

2. Biofeedback included electromyography with a 12-mm diameter, 45-mm-long PerryMeter anal EMG sensor EPS-21 (PerryMeter Systems, Strafford, PA), connected to an Orion 8600 (Self Regulation Systems, Redmond, WA) biofeedback computer. After insertion of the sensor, the patient remained fully clothed during the session. A full color graphic display was used as the video unit to let both the patient and the therapist visualize the patient's sphincter muscle activity to facilitate teaching. A horizontal blue line on the video display marked the goal that was adjusted as the patient improved.

3. Exercises included Kegel exercises and "constipation exercise" (bearing down maneuver).

4. Biofeedback sessions were conducted weekly until the patient's goal was met.

5. Home training consisted of instructing the patient to use the sensor at home and to practice the exercises with a home trainer aided by a training tape.

Cost Analysis

The cost of evaluating older adults with constipation must be considered and balanced against the yield of the positive findings and the impact that these findings have on the treatment plan. In a study of 51 older adults with a 30- to 40-month history of constipation who were known to be free of colorectal neoplasm, the total cost of a comprehensive evaluation was $140,369, for a mean cost per patient of $2,752. Overall, 31 (61 percent) of the participants had no etiology identified for their constipation. Only 12 patients (24 percent) benefited from the extensive workup. Thus, the cost of successful treatment to benefit one patient by means other than conservative measures was $11,697.

Since the cost of comprehensive testing is high and yield low, careful consideration needs to be given to when referrals for further testing are appropriate. The algorithm in Fig. 15-1 helps to contain costs by suggesting a step-by-step approach to the evaluation of the patient, with referrals made for specific testing/treatment only when indicated. As in all other areas of geriatric care, patients should always be asked if they are: (1) willing to participate in further testing; and (2) willing to use the information obtained from testing for more invasive or involved treatment such as surgery or biofeedback.

An estimated $400 million is spent on laxatives annually in the United States, and there are currently over 700 commercially produced products. Costs will vary by location and generic versus name brand item. Current cost estimates are provided in Table 15-7. Chronic use of these medications can be costly to the patient and/or the health care system. Therefore, all attempts should be made to avoid laxative use by adhering to the lifestyle modifications suggested previously. If laxatives are needed, generic forms should be suggested.

Bibliography

Abdul A, Mourad F: Constipation: common-sense care of the older patient. *Geriatrics* 51:28, 1996.

Agachan F, Chen T, Pfeifer J, et al: A constipation scoring system to simplify evaluation and management of constipated patients. *Dis Colon Rectum* 39:681, 1996.

Badiali D, Corazziari E, Habib FI, et al: Effect of wheat bran in treatment of chronic nonorganic constipation. *Dig Dis Sci* 40:349, 1995.

Barloon, T, Lu C: Diagnostic imaging in the evaluation of constipation in adults. *Am Fam Physician* 56:513, 1996.

Beverley L, Travis I: Constipation: proposed natural laxative mixtures. *J Gerontol Nurs* 18:5, 1992.

Cheskin L, Kamal N, Crowell M, et al: Mechanisms of constipation in older persons and effects of fiber compared with placebo. *J Am Geriatr Soc* 43:666, 1995.

Clausen MR, Mortensen PB: Lactulose, disaccharides and colonic flora. *Drugs* 53:930, 1997.

Dahl J, Lindquist BL, Tysk C, et al: Behavioral medicine treatment in chronic constipation with paradoxical anal sphincter contraction. *Dis Colon Rectum* 34:769, 1991.

Enok P: Biofeedback training in disordered defecation: a critical review. *Dig Dis Sci* 38:1953, 1993.

Gattuso J, Kamm A: Adverse effects of drugs used in the management of constipation and diarrhea. *Drug Saf* 10:47, 1994.

Hale W, Perkins L, May F, et al: Symptom prevalence in the elderly: an evaluation of age, sex, disease and medication use. *J Am Geriatr Soc* 34:333, 1986.

Harari D, Gurwitz J, Minaker K: Constipation in the elderly. *J Am Geriatr Soc* 41:1130, 1993.

Heaton K, Crips H: Straining at stool and laxative taking in an English population. *Dig Dis Sci* 38:1004, 1993.

Hogan T: Geriatric emergencies. In: Cassel C (ed): *Geriatric Medicine.* New York: Spring-Verlag; 1996:131.

Johanson JF: Geographic distribution of constipation in the United States. *Am J Gastroenterol* 93:188, 1998.

Johnson R, Vollner W: Comparing sources of drug data about the elderly. *J Am Geriatr Soc* 39:1079, 1991.

Kinnunen O: Study of constipation in a geriatric hospital, day hospital and old people's home and at home. *Aging* 3:161, 1991.

Kleessen B, Sykura B, Hans-Joachim Z, et al: Effects of inulin and lactose on fecal miroflora, microbial activity, and bowel habit in elderly constipated persons. *Am J Clin Nutr* 65:1397, 1997.

Ko C, Tong J, Lehman R, et al: Biofeedback is effective therapy for fecal incontinence and constipation. *Arch Surg* 132:829, 1997.

Koch A, Voderholzer W, Klauser A, et al: Symptoms in chronic constipation. *Dis Colon Rectum* 40:902, 1997.

Longe R, DiPiro J: Diarrhea and constipation. In: DiPiro J, Talbert R, Yee G, et al (eds): *Pharmacotherapy: a Pathophysiologic Approach,* 3rd ed. Stanford: Appleton & Lange; 1996:767.

Mahoney J, Drinka T, Abler R, et al: Screening for depression: single question versus GDS. *J Am Geriatr Soc* 42:1006, 1994.

Merkel I, Locher J, Burgio K, et al: Physiologic and psychologic characteristics of an elderly population with chronic constipation. *Am J Gastroenterol* 88:1854, 1993.

Messmer J: Abdominal plain film: gas and soft tissue abnormalities. In: Core R, Levin M, Laufer I (eds): *Textbook of Gastrointestinal Radiology.* Philadelphia: Saunders; 1994:169.

Neal L: Power pudding; natural laxative therapy for the elderly who are homebound. *Home Health Nurse* 13:66, 1988.

Patankar S, Ferrara A, Levy J, et al: Biofeedback in colorectal practice. *Dis Colon Rectum* 40:827, 1997.

Rantis PC, Vernava AM, Daniel GL, et al: Chronic constipation—is the work-up worth the cost. *Dis Colon Rectum* 40:280, 1997.

Redmond J, Smith G, Barofsky I, et al: Physiological tests to predict long-term outcome of total abdominal colectomy for intractable constipation. *Am J Gastroenterol* 90:748, 1995.

Resende T, Brocklehurst J, O'Neill P: A pilot study on the effect of exercise and abdominal massage on bowel habit in continuing care patients. *Clin Rehabil* 7:204, 1996.

Resnick B: Functional performance of older adults in a long term care setting. *Clin Nurs Res* 7:230, 1998.

Resnick B: The presentation of acute illness in the older adult with dementia. *Clin Lett Nurse Practitioner* 2:1, 1997.

Resnick B: Constipation: common but preventable. *Geriatr Nurs* 6:213, 1985.

Rieger NA, Wattchow D, Sarre R, et al: Prospective study of biofeedback for treatment of constipation. *Dis Colon Rectum* 40:1143, 1997.

Romero Y, Evans J, Fleming K, et al: Constipation and fecal incontinence in the elderly population. *Mayo Clin Proc* 71:81, 1996.

Sandler R, Jordan M, Sherlton F: Demographic and dietary determinants of constipation in the U.S. population. *Am J Public Health* 80:185, 1990.

Somers S: Constipation, diarrhea and IBS. In: Core R, Levin M, Laufer I (eds): *Textbook of Gastrointestinal Radiology*. Philadelphia: Saunders; 1994:2485.

Sonnenberg A, Koch T: Physician visits in the United States for constipation. *Dig Dis Sci* 34:606, 1989.

Talley NJ, Flemin KC, Evans JM, et al: Constipation in an elderly community: a study of prevalence and potential risk factors. *Am J Gastroenterol* 91:19, 1996.

Towers A, Burgio K, Locher J, et al: Constipation in the elderly: influence of dietary psychological and physiological factors. *J Am Geriatr Soc* 42:701, 1992.

Wexner S, Cheape J, Jorge J, et al: Prospective assessment of biofeedback for the treatment of paradoxical puborectalis contraction. *Dis Colon Rectum* 35:145, 1992.

Whitehead W, Chaussade S, Corazziari E, et al: Report of an international workshop on management of constipation. *Gastroenterol Int* 4:99, 1991.

Whitehead W, Drinkwater W, Cheskin L: Constipation in the elderly living at home: definition, prevalence, and relationship to lifestyle and health status. *J Am Geriatr Soc* 37:423, 1989.

Mel P. Daly
Alan M. Adelman

Nutritional Status
and Involuntary Weight Loss

Although most elderly persons are well nourished, the prevalence of obesity and protein-calorie undernutrition is significantly increased in older persons. Age-related changes in body habitus, and disease, physiologic, and medication-related interactions can affect "normal" nutritional requirements of elderly persons. This can be further compounded by difficulties that older persons experience in accessing grocery stores and in cooking healthy foods. Many older persons rely on the convenience of buying processed foods or ordering "fast foods" that can contribute to both obesity and deficiencies in essential nutritional requirements.

Primary care providers often fail to recognize that patients have nutritional problems and frequently fail to recommend nutritional supplements when they are indicated. Recent initiatives sponsored by the American Academy of Family Physicians, the American Diabetes Foundation, and the National Council on Aging are focusing on identifying older persons at risk for malnutrition and upon providing education for caregivers and health care providers.

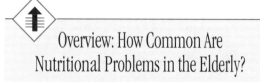

Overview: How Common Are Nutritional Problems in the Elderly?

Among community-dwelling elderly persons, approximately 10 to 15 percent have difficulties in feeding themselves, and up to 50 percent of older persons admitted to an acute care hospital are malnourished at the time of admission. Many more become undernourished during hospitalization. Among hospitalized elderly patients who have evidence of undernutrition at the time of admission or become undernourished during the course of an admission, length of stay is prolonged and rates of readmission are increased. Among patients in long-term care settings, the prevalence of undernutrition or obesity may be in the range of 40 percent.

About 25 to30 percent of older persons are overweight [Body Mass Index (BMI) >28] and 10 percent are severely overweight (BMI >31 for men, and 32 for women). Obesity is a major risk for mortality and morbidity. Obesity is associated with a greater likelihood of developing coronary artery disease, diabetes mellitus, hypertension, and sleep apnea. In very advanced age, however, obesity and hypercholesterolemia can be protective; lower levels of cholesterol can indicate that serious conditions (cancer, dementia, congestive heart failure, etc.) can be causing malnutrition. There is evidence that hypocholesterolemia is associated with increased mortality.

Age-Associated Changes

In normal older persons, weight usually increases through the age of 50. Then, in older men, weight usually declines, with the most rapid declines occurring in the 60s and 70s. These changes are influenced by many factors such as cultural norms, exercise patterns, and comorbid illness. In older women these changes are less dramatic.

In general, total body fat increases with age (up to 30 percent, by age 70). Lean body mass and muscle mass decrease, as does total body water. Thus, while older persons may not change much in weight, their body composition changes dramatically. Truncal obesity is the most usual manifestation of increased fat deposition and is usually accompanied by a reduction in muscle mass and a decline in muscle strength. Many of these changes can be attenuated and reversed by exercise and dietary interventions.

Older persons are more likely to eat foods that are high in saturated fats, cholesterol, and salt (fried and fast foods). In general, older adults have dietary intakes that are low in protein and vitamin content.

Age-Related Physiologic and Anatomic Changes

Many age and disease-associated changes contribute to a greater likelihood of nutritional deficiencies in older persons. These changes in physiologic functioning affect older persons differently (Table 16-1) and variably affect nutritional intake in older persons.

Oral and Esophageal Changes

Older persons may not enjoy food as much as when they were young because of age-associated and disease-associated decreases in olfactory and taste perceptions. Many older persons are edentulous (40 percent of persons over the age of 70)

Table 16-1

Age- and Disease-Associated Changes That Contribute to Nutritional Deficiencies in Older Persons

Oral and esophageal
  Decreased olfactory and/or taste perceptions
  Lack of teeth
  Dentures
  Dry mouth
  Decreased peristalsis
  Dysphagia

Gastrointestinal
  Atrophic gastritis
  Reduced absorption of important nutrients
  Lactose intolerance
  Atrophy of bowel

Other
  Decreased ability to shop and cook
  Cognitive impairment
  Depression
  Medications

or have significant periodontal disease that can affect the ability of an older person to chew. It is estimated that dentures restore 15 percent of the average person's ability to chew when compared to natural dentition. Dentures are also sometimes uncomfortable and embarrassing for older persons and require frequent readjustments and often need to be replaced. Medicare reimburses for neither dental care nor dentures, and, as a result, many older persons elect not to avail themselves of dental care or dentures because of cost.

Salivary glands usually have preserved function over time and years, but many older adults complain of having a "dry mouth." Saliva is important in protecting the tissues of the oral cavity and in facilitating mastication, taste perception, and swallowing. The most common cause of "dry mouth" is medications (anticholinergic drugs, antidepressants, antihistamines, narcotic analgesic agents, etc.). In addition, oral diseases (salivary gland tumors, blocked or infected ducts) and systemic illness (autoimmune disorders, cancer, radiotherapy, diabetes mellitus, and hypothyroidism) can also play a role.

Biopsy and autopsy data suggest that esophageal muscles become thicker with advancing age. As a result of these changes, esophageal motility and peristalsis frequently becomes impaired. Age-associated changes in esophageal function are often compounded by pathologic conditions that can affect esophageal motility (diabetes mellitus, Parkinson's disease, and progressive supranuclear palsy). Cardiac disorders such as congestive heart failure can cause enlargement of heart chambers (left atrium, right ventricle) that can impinge on the esophagus. Neoplasms of the esophagus can also interfere with motility but most often cause pain or a sensation of food becoming "stuck." Gastroesophageal reflux disease (GERD) occurs in about 15 percent of older persons and is caused by an abnormal laxity of the gastroesophageal sphincter that results in reflux of gastric contents (acid, bile, etc.) into the esophagus. Hiatal hernias occur when the stomach encroaches on the chest cavity because of an abnormal laxity of the diaphragm. This condition frequently predisposes to GERD and other long-term sequelae, such as esophagitis or cancer.

Gastrointestinal Changes

Age- and disease-associated changes in gastric functioning are common. Up to 70 percent of older individuals have evidence of atrophic gastritis and a decrease in parietal cell mass, resulting in reduced gastric acid and intrinsic factor production. These changes can result in a reduced ability of older persons to extract vitamin B_{12} from salivary R-binding protein (requires gastric acid) and cause impaired vitamin B_{12}, calcium, and iron absorption (intrinsic factor– and gastric acid– mediated). While stomach motility and emptying are minimally reduced with age, the ability of the stomach to relax and dilate to accept a food bolus is impaired.

Age- and disease-associated changes of the small and large intestines includes a variable amount of villous atrophy and loss of lymphoid tissue. This can cause a reduction in absorption of iron, calcium, vitamin D, and lactose. Many older persons (especially African-Americans) are lactose intolerant. Other changes that occur with aging in the large intestine include atrophy of the mucosa (predisposing to diverticular disease) and slowing of colonic transit time (often resulting in constipation).

Whereas the mass of the liver declines by about 10 percent with aging, liver function, in the absence of disease, remains preserved. Pancreatic function also remains preserved with age.

Other Changes

With advancing years, older persons are more likely to become impaired in their abilities to carry out normal activities of daily living because of an increase in disability. The prevalence of disability increases with each decade after the age of 70 years. These impairments can lead to decreased ability to shop for food and cook. Thus, physical disability resulting from medical conditions, such as Parkinson's disease, arthritis, cerebrovascular disease, and congestive heart failure, often result in impaired nutrition.

Cognitive impairment is also more likely to occur with advancing years and can result in a reduction in energy needs, a reduced appetite, and behavioral problems that can interfere with feeding. Depression, although relatively uncommon in "normal" older adults, is common in hospitalized and institutionalized older persons and is associated with anorexia, reduced metabolism, and decreased activity levels. Patients who are taking medications to treat depression (serotonin reuptake inhibitors, tricyclic antidepressants) often experience anorexia or weight gain as a side effect.

Older persons are more likely to be taking prescription and nonprescription medications that can cause anorexia or interfere with absorption or metabolism of essential nutrients.

Normal
Nutritional Requirements

Energy and Calories

Total energy requirements decrease with age, mostly because of reduced levels of physical activity (60 to 70 percent). The remainder is accounted for by a reduced lean body mass (20 to 25 percent), and a reduced resting metabolic rate (15 to 30 percent), often as a result of reduced levels of physical activity. Total energy intake among older men declines from about 3000 kcal for men aged 30 years, to about 2000 kcal for men aged 60 to 75 years. Energy expenditure depends on activity levels; however, it is estimated that a sedentary elderly person requires approximately 30 kcal/kg per day. This figure is multiplied by factors of 1 to 2, depending on activity levels and illness (e.g., fever, pain, dehydration, etc.).

Protein

Daily protein requirements increase with aging, partly because of an age-associated decline in hepatic production of somatic proteins and a decrease in muscle mass (that may be potentially reversed or attenuated by exercise). Total daily protein requirements for older persons are in the range of 1.0 to 1.5 g/kg per day. Among patients who are malnourished, or who are in catabolic states (illness, fever, burns, hypermetabolic states) because of acute illness or hospitalization, protein intake should be increased to 2 to 3 times normal. When making dietary recommendations to older individuals, catabolic and age-associated states must always be considered.

Fat

Total fat calories should not exceed 30 percent of total calorie intake. Monounsaturated fats (olive oil) are associated with a reduced incidence of coronary artery disease, as are polyunsaturated fats (soybean, fish-oils, canola, etc). By contrast, trans-fatty acid derivatives are associated with higher levels of circulating low-density lipoproteins and lower levels of high-density lipoproteins.

Fiber

Older persons are more likely to ingest less than the recommended amount of dietary fiber. Lower than recommended fiber ingestion is associated with a greater risk of developing cancer (especially colorectal cancer) and coronary artery disease. The typical older American ingests about 10 g of total fiber, which is much less than the 20 to 25 g that is currently recommended.

Micronutrients

VITAMINS

There is considerable controversy about age-appropriate recommendations for micronutrient intake. The recommended daily allowances (RDA) for vitamin and mineral intake developed in the late 1980s are controversial, and older persons are more likely to ingest less than is required. Many older persons consume less than the RDA for vitamins A, B_6, B_{12}, D, E, K, and folic acid. This is further compounded by age- and disease-associated factors. There is uncertainty about appropriate RDAs for many vitamin and minerals in older adults (Table 16-2).

Table 16-2

Required Daily Allowance (RDA) for Common Vitamins and Minerals

VITAMIN OR MINERAL	RDA	FOOD SOURCES HIGH IN VITAMIN OR MINERAL
A	5000 IU	Carrots, squash, sweet potato, cantaloupe, dark leafy greens (kale, greens, and broccoli), apricots, peaches
B_6	2.0 mg	Grains, beans, spinach, broccoli, wheat germ
B_{12}	6.0 μg	Red meat, cottage cheese, milk, eggs, cheese, yogurt
D	400 IU	Fortified milk
E	30 IU	Oils (wheat germ, sunflower, and safflower), nuts and seeds (almonds, filberts, sunflower seeds, and walnuts), spinach, sweet potato, greens, leeks
Thiamin	1.5 mg	Grains, legumes (soy beans, kidney beans)
Folic acid	0.4 mg	Dark green leafy vegetables, sweet potato, beans
Zinc	15 mg	Meat, legumes, grains, peas

Abbreviations: CSF, cerebrospinal fluid; IV, intravenous.

Age-associated changes and diseases that occur more commonly among older persons can result in significant deficiencies in these nutrients. Clinical manifestations of deficiencies of these nutrients can be confused with symptoms (subtle or otherwise) of other comorbid illness, thus potentially delaying the diagnosis. For example, whereas deficiencies of vitamins C and some B vitamins can occur over a period of weeks, fat-soluble vitamin (vitamins A, D, K, and E) deficiency can only occur over a period of months. Thus, nonspecific symptoms of vitamin deficiency such as weakness, aches, skin rashes, bone pain, and weight loss can be considered as manifestations of other conditions or as variations of "normal."

FOLIC ACID Folic acid deficiency is more common in older persons, especially those who abuse alcohol. Folic acid is readily available in fresh vegetables and fruits. Over-cooking vegetables will frequently result in loss of folic acid content. Little folic acid is stored, so deficiencies can quickly occur (months) and can result in serious neurologic and hematologic abnormalities. Older persons taking medications, such as methotrexate, trimethoprim, phenytoin, and sulfasalazine, can become folate deficient because of drug–nutrient interactions.

VITAMIN B_{12} Although dietary deficiency of vitamin B_{12} can rarely occur, older persons most commonly become deficient in vitamin B_{12} because of other factors. These include pernicious anemia or an impaired ability to extract vitamin B_{12} from foods because of an age- or disease-associated change in intrinsic factor and gastric acid production. Rarely, vitamin B_{12} deficiency occurs because of malabsorption at the terminal ileum.

VITAMIN D Vitamin D deficiency states occur more commonly among older adults. This occurs largely because older persons spend less time exposed to sunlight. This relative deficiency of vitamin D, when compounded with age-associated impairments of calcium absorption and age-related impairments in cholecalciferol metabo-

lism, result in a greater likelihood of older persons developing osteoporosis.

VITAMIN K Vitamin K is an important cofactor in the clotting cascade. Low levels of vitamin K result in impaired hemostasis. Vitamin K also plays a role in bone metabolism (probably related to osteoblastosis and calcium absorption), and deficiencies of vitamin K may play an as-yet-undetermined role in osteoporosis.

MINERALS

ZINC Most elderly persons ingest less than the RDA for zinc. In addition, older persons with diabetes mellitus who take diuretic medications are more likely to excrete zinc in the urine. Absorption of zinc can also become impaired in older persons. Zinc deficiency can be associated with many symptoms including anorexia, dysgeusia, visual impairments (macular degeneration), impotence, and impaired wound healing.

IRON Most elderly persons have adequate iron stores. In general, older persons become deficient in iron only if a pathologic condition, such as bleeding, occurs. Dietary deficiency of iron in Western societies is extremely uncommon. Iron absorption remains preserved. Iron absorption is decreased where gastric acid secretion is reduced, (atrophic gastritis, achlorhydria). Iron absorption can be enhanced by concomitant administration of vitamin C. The body's ability to mobilize iron from visceral iron stores and transport iron to the marrow erythroblasts is reduced in chronic diseases. This accounts for the high prevalence of anemia of chronic disease in older adults.

Water and Salt

Water metabolism significantly changes even in "normal" elderly persons. Thirst perception in response to increased serum osmolality and the ability to concentrate urine (ADH-mediated) in response to fluid deprivation (hemoconcentration) is often impaired in older persons.

Older persons are often less able to appreciate the taste of salt, can have impaired thirst appreciation, and frequently add salt as a garnishment to food. In addition, most Americans are accustomed to a high salt intake. This combination of factors may not be of benefit for many older patients with hypertension and congestive heart failure. Older individuals only require 500 mg/d of sodium (~1.5g).

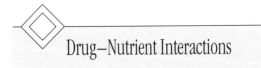

Drug–Nutrient Interactions

For older persons with borderline nutritional status, the addition of a medication can result in anorexia. Many drugs are potentially anorexogenic including digoxin, theophylline, hydrochlorthiazide, nonsteroidal anti-inflammatory agents, and triamterene. Some drugs interfere with taste perception (allopurinol, clindamycin, and antihistamines), whereas others can result in vitamin and trace mineral deficiencies. Isoniazid can result in vitamin B_6 deficiency. Tetracycline reduces the absorption of calcium and iron. Folic acid deficiency often occurs with the use of anticonvulsants, triamterene, and trimethoprim.

Many interactions between drugs and nutrients have been described. Antacids interfere with the absorption of folic acid, iron, phosphorus, and vitamin B_1. Barbiturates reduce absorption of vitamin D and folic acid. Cholestyramine binds with bile salts and interferes with the absorption of vitamins A and K. Colchicine interferes with the absorption of protein, fat, and lactose. This drug can also cause villous damage and impair vitamin B_{12} absorption. Dilantin can cause a loss of structural integrity of the small intestinal lining, resulting in reduced absorption of calcium, fat, and fat-soluble vitamins. Salicylates can interfere with vitamin C absorption and folic acid absorption. Tetracycline reduces the absorption of fat-soluble vitamins (vitamins A, K, E, and D). Many other

drug nutrients have been described and should always be taken into consideration when evaluating an older person's nutritional state.

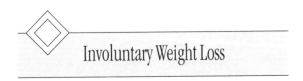

Involuntary Weight Loss

Involuntary weight loss is of concern to both patients and clinicians because it often signifies a serious, life-threatening illness. Older persons with protein-calorie undernutrition are also more prone to infections and are less likely to recover from illness in a timely fashion.

Older persons who consume a normal variety of foods are unlikely to have any dietary deficiency; however, not all older persons consume a "normal" diet. Thus, weight loss occurring in an older person, whether they consume a "normal" diet or not, should be of concern.

How Common Is Involuntary Weight Loss?

Involuntary weight loss is defined as a loss of 1 to 2 percent per week, 5 percent per month, or 10 percent in a 6-month period. Wallace et al reported that involuntary weight loss in ambulatory patients more than doubled their risk of death. Involuntary weight loss should be promptly evaluated and appropriate interventions initiated.

The prevalence of involuntary weight loss in the ambulatory setting is unclear due to differing definitions and the fact that weight loss is not usually coded as the primary diagnosis. Thompson and Morris reported that 45 patients in a population of approximately 10,000 over the age of 63 years were identified with an involuntary weight loss of greater than 7.5 percent. Other data would suggest that up to 20 percent of community-dwelling elderly persons consume less than 1000 kcal/d and that 15 percent have lost more than 5 percent of their body weight in the previous year. Up to 5 percent of community-dwelling elderly may be overtly malnourished. The prevalence of malnutrition significantly increases among hospitalized and institutionalized older persons.

Principal Diagnoses

Several factors can contribute to weight loss including poor oral intake, alterations in metabolism, or increased loss of nutrients through the urine or bowel. Poor oral intake can be due to nausea, early satiety, depressed mood, and alterations in taste. Many other factors including living circumstances, accessibility to grocery stores, ability to cook, and finances are of importance in the nutritional assessment of older persons. Causes of inadequate nutrient intake that can be frequently over-looked include poverty (unable to afford needed foodstuffs), bereavement, ethnic or cultural food restrictions, abuse and neglect, and perceived or real food intolerances. Other contributing causes include impaired vision or hearing, dental or chewing problems, upper extremity dysfunction, diminished sense of taste and smell, outdated "therapeutic diets," drug–drug and drug–food interactions, and food preferences or fads.

A number of medical conditions can present with a chief complaint of weight loss. Table 16-3 lists these conditions. Thompson and Morris reported the following identifiable major causes of weight loss. These included depression (18 percent), cancer (16 percent), gastrointestinal disorders other than cancer (11 percent), hyperthyroidism (9 percent), medications (9 percent), and neurologic disorders that can affect intake of food (7 percent).

Less common causes of weight loss among older persons are chronic infections (tuberculosis, bacterial endocarditis, and pyelonephritis), end-stage chronic disease (emphysema, cirrhosis, uremia, and congestive heart failure), alcoholism, connective tissue disorders, uncontrolled diabetes mellitus, and other endocrine conditions (Addison's disease, Cushing's disease).

Invariably, the cause is multifactorial, frequently the result of a combination of medication effects,

Table 16-3
Causes of Involuntary Weight Loss

Diabetes mellitus
Depression
Drugs
Selective serotonin reuptake inhibitors (SSRIs)
Digoxin
Anticholinergic agents
Theophylline
Malignancy
Hyperthyroidism
Hypothyroidism
Infection
Tuberculosis
Bacterial endocarditis
Systemic fungal infections
Gastrointestinal disease
Malabsorption
Hepatitis
Peptic ulcer disease
Chronic diseases
Congestive heart failure
Chronic lung disease
Chronic renal failure
Connective tissue disease
Oral disorders
Poor dentition
Ill-fitting dentures
Neurologic conditions
Dementia
Stroke
Swallowing disorders
Parkinson's disease
Social factors
Poverty
Isolation
Inability to shop, prepare food
Other
Alcoholism

social factors, psychiatric conditions (a variant of anorexia nervosa), and physical disorders resulting in disability. In about one fourth of cases, no cause can be found. In these persons it is postulated that weight loss occurs because of age-associated factors (reduced metabolic rate, reduced activity levels) together with higher than normal circulating levels of anorexogenic hormones (cachectin, tumor necrosis factor) that are associated with chronic conditions. A syndrome of "failure to thrive" has been described in which weight loss is associated with a slow and progressive withdrawal (physical, social, and emotional) from society. Persons with this "syndrome" become depressed and apathetic and, over time, slowly deteriorate and continue to lose weight.

Key History

Patients may or may not complain of weight loss. Thompson and Morris reported that weight loss was the chief complaint in only 42 percent of patients with weight loss. When patients complain of weight loss, it is important to document the amount. Because many patients will not complain of weight loss, weight should be assessed regularly.

Associated symptoms will depend on the underlying cause of the weight loss. Common nonspecific symptoms are listed in Table 16-4. Functional impairment due to the fatigue and malaise of malnutrition may be reported. Patients may state that their clothing is loose. Depending on the degree of weight loss, they may even change clothing size. Other symptoms can include nausea, vomiting, diarrhea, constipation, problems with chewing or dentures, dysphagia, and symptoms that are specific to disease states (congestive heart failure, Parkinson's disease, cancer, cerebrovascular disease, etc.).

Table 16-4

Common Nonspecific Symptoms in Patients With Weight Loss

| Anorexia |
| Fatigue, malaise |
| Nausea |
| Vomiting |
| Loose-fitting clothing |

There are a number of ways to assess the caloric intake of elderly individuals including diet recall, food records, diet history, and food frequency questionnaires. Twenty-hour and 3-day calorie recall can help quantify intake. These approaches are time-consuming and often not practical for the practicing clinician. A quick way to assess the nutritional status of a patient is to question the individual regarding recent changes in the appetite and food intake. Clinicians must ask the patient to compare his or her current calorie intake and exercise level with the intake 1, 6, or 12 months ago.

Clinicians should inquire about medications, especially drugs that can potentially interfere with nutritional intake. A careful review of social circumstances is always indicated. Income, food accessibility, cooking facilities, home circumstances, and availability of help should always be asked about.

SCREENING FOR MALNUTRITION

There are several instruments available to screen for malnutrition in the elderly including the Nutrition Screening Initiative (NSI) Checklist and the Nutritional Risk Index (NRI). The NSI is the result of a joint effort between the American Academy of Family Physicians, the American Dietetic Association, and the National Council on Aging. The NRI was derived from the National Health and Nutrition Examination Survey (NHANES). Both were developed for use in ambulatory populations, but have not been widely tested and validated.

Detsky and associates developed a Subjective Global Assessment scale for the evaluation of malnutrition in hospitalized patients. Although it has not been tested on ambulatory patients, it forms a good framework to evaluate patients for malnutrition. The three key elements in their examination were (1) the amount of weight loss; (2) dietary intake; and (3) evidence of fat loss or muscle wasting. The rating scale and criteria are shown in Table 16-5. It is simple and can be readily used by a clinician.

Table 16-5

Subjective Global Assessment

> Well nourished
>   Weight loss of less than 5% or
>   Weight loss of more than 5%, but recent gain
>   or improved appetite
> Moderately malnourished
>   5%–10% weight loss without recent gain
>   Poor dietary intake
>   Mild loss of subcutaneous tissue
> Severely malnourished
>   Weight loss of more than 10%
>   Severe subcutaneous tissue loss and
>   muscle wasting
>   Edema often present

Physical Examination

A complete physical examination, including the patient's weight, should be performed. At each visit, weight should be measured and compared to previous measures and normative data for age and gender. Height should be measured periodically. Nonspecific signs of weight loss include loss of subcutaneous fat and muscle wasting. Other signs of undernutrition can include alopecia, confusion, dependent edema, dry and depigmented hair, skin desquamation, glossitis, and generalized muscle wasting and weakness. An oropharyngeal examination should also be done to exclude cancer, glossitis, severe gingivitis, or other oral or dental pathology.

A useful measure of nutritional state that incorporates both height and weight is the BMI (weight in kg divided by height in meters squared). BMI is quantifiable and can be followed over time. This measure of body habitus and nutritional state had been shown in prospective studies to be strongly associated with significant outcomes, such as mortality, cardiovascular events, and diabetes control. A normal BMI is defined as 18 to 25 kg/m^2, overweight is defined as BMI of 25 to 30 kg/m^2, and obesity is defined as a BMI of 30 to 40 kg/m^2. Morbid obesity is defined as BMI levels of over 40 kg/m^2. By contrast, protein-energy undernutrition can also be classified as mild (BMI = 18 to $17/m^2$), moderate (BMI = 17 to 16 kg/m^2), and severe (BMI < 16 kg/m^2). This measure of nutritional status is widely used in research studies and is useful as a general guide for predicting risk for serious long-term adverse outcomes among older persons.

Measuring mid-arm muscle circumference (triceps) or subscapular skinfold thickness can approximate adipose mass, and these measures can be useful if done serially and consistently. These are indirect measurements of body fat and muscle protein, respectively. Whereas these measures can be useful in younger persons and normal standards have been established, these measurements are not as accurate in older persons and may not add sufficient additional information to warrant their regular measurement.

Rapid increases in weight are usually due to fluid retention and rarely due to increases in muscle mass or lean body mass. This type of rapid weight gain is usually suggestive of pathologic processes such as worsening congestive heart failure, cancer, hepatic failure, or kidney failure.

The appearance of edema or ascites can be an indication of severe malnutrition. Examination in the area of the 5th metacarpal is a convenient place to search for loss of subcutaneous tissue. The best locations to examine for muscle wasting are the shoulders (deltoid muscles) and thighs (quadriceps muscle).

Ancillary Tests

ASSESSMENT OF MALNUTRITION

Hypoalbuminemia is a useful biochemical measure of nutritional status. A serum albumin level of less than 3.5 g/dL is suggestive of malnutrition. Low serum cholesterol (< 160 mg/dL) and transferrin levels (< 200 mg/dL) are also found in persons with malnutrition, but they are not considered as useful an indicator as the serum albumin. Transferrin has a half-life of 9 days and thus may be more sensitive than albumin (half-life of 21 days) as a measure of short-term undernutrition. An even more sensitive measure of nutritional status may be serum levels of prealbumin, which has a half-life of 2 days. Prealbumin levels of less than 11 mg/dL suggest significant undernutrition. Other measures such as C-reactive protein, insulin-like growth factor, thyroxin-binding protein, and tumor necrosis factor are research tools and have no current clinical role.

Biochemical measures, such as total lymphocyte count, serum ferritin level, and hemoglobin count, have been suggested as measures of nutrition status. In general, they are inaccurate and can be affected by factors other than nutritional status. Persons with protein-calorie undernutrition are often anergic to common antigens such as mumps or *Candida*. Testing for responsiveness to these antigens has also been suggested as a measure of malnutrition.

ASSESSMENT OF MEDICAL CAUSES OF WEIGHT LOSS

Initial laboratory testing for documented weight loss is shown in Table 16-6. Further testing should be guided by the history and physical examination and initial laboratory testing. If the cause is still undiagnosed, endoscopic studies, computerized tomographic (CT) studies of the abdomen or chest, and measuring serum tumor markers (CEA, CA-125) should be considered. The diagnostic yield of extensive testing in patients with unexplained weight loss and a normal history, physical examination, and initial laboratory testing is low.

If a trial of supervised nutritional supplementation is unsuccessful and weight loss persists, the cause of the patient's weight loss should be reevaluated and more extensive testing may be required.

Treatment

The treatment of involuntary weight loss should be directed at the underlying cause. Because the cause of weight loss is usually multifactorial, the treatment must be highly individualized and frequently involves addressing many issues simultaneously. Functional (impaired ability to perform activities of daily living [ADLs] and instrumental activities of daily living [IADLs]), cognitive (depression, dementia), psychological (anorexia nervosa, alcoholism), social (poverty, isolation, and bereavement), and economic (fixed income) factors can all play significant roles in contributing to poor nutrition. Each must be addressed appropriately. The approach to each person's situation must be individualized and take into consideration factors such as cost and available support. When instituting a nutritional intervention, baseline measures should be obtained (e.g., weight, albumin, and prealbumin) and frequently reassessed to evaluate progress. Calorie, protein, fat, and micronutrient intake should also be monitored at regular intervals.

Consultation with a registered dietician can be helpful. A registered dietician can advise patients how to increase their caloric intake. Among patients who are homebound and who have poor caloric intake, referral to community services such as meals-on-wheels can be helpful. Meals-on-wheels can provide nutritionally complete meals that are delivered to a person's home on a daily basis. Usually, one meal is provided for a nominal fee. Arrangements can be made for supplemental food (sandwiches, cookies, milk, etc.) to be provided, if a need exists. Some senior centers have group lunch programs that can be helpful for isolated elderly persons.

Table 16-6

Initial Laboratory Testing in the Patient With Documented Weight Loss

Complete blood count
Thyroid stimulating hormone (TSH)
Urinalysis
Serum chemistries (including liver and renal function, albumin, total protein, and calcium)
Hemoccult testing
Chest x-ray

APPETITE STIMULANTS

In general, appetite stimulants are not effective in stimulating weight gain. The most commonly used agent is megestrol acetate, a progesterone preparation that has been used with some variable success to stimulate appetite in patients with cancer. Other agents that have been tried in patients with anorexia associated with AIDS and cancer include anabolic steroids (dronabinol, medroxyprogesterone) and psychostimulants. These drugs have thus far not been shown to be effective in helping frail older persons gain weight or improve their appetites. Human growth hormone has been recently shown to be potentially helpful in treating undernutrition in older persons. Further study is required before this expensive therapeutic modality becomes readily available for this indication.

Other drugs that can help stimulate appetite are cyproheptadine (serotonin inhibition) and chlorpromazine. There are no good studies of their effectiveness. Small amounts of alcohol are felt by some to stimulate the appetite.

Patient Education

In general, educational efforts should be targeted at individuals who are at an increased risk for protein-calorie undernutrition. All older persons should be counseled about foods that are high in nutritional value (lean meats, chicken, fish, fruits, and vegetables) and how best to cook and prepare them.

It can be important to feed older persons with anything that they prefer simply to stimulate their appetite and desire to eat. Most persons who are undernourished respond well to feeding at scheduled intervals. Liquid protein supplements are most often used. Instant breakfast drinks mixed with whole milk are high in calories and protein (e.g., Carnation Instant Breakfast) and are excellent nutri-

tional supplements. Many commercial supplements are now available including liquids, puddings, shakes, and powders (e.g., Ensure, Sustacal). These preparations can be selected to provide adequate supplementation of calories, protein, and micronutrients. For patients who are lactose-intolerant, many of these products are lactose-free and nutritionally complete (Sustacal, Isocal, and Ensure).

Bibliography

Corti M, Guralnik JM, Salive ME, et al: Serum albumin level and physical disability as predictors of mortality in older persons. *JAMA* 272:1036, 1994.

Detsky AS, Smalley PS, Chang J: The rational clinical examination: is this patient malnourished? *JAMA* 271:54, 1994.

Hoffman N: Diet in the elderly. Needs and risks. *Med Clin North Am* 77:745, 1993.

Klonoff-Cohen H, Barrett-Connor EL, Edelstein SL: Albumin levels as a predictor of mortality in the healthy elderly. *J Clin Epidemiol* 45:207, 1992.

Lipshitz DA, Ham RJ, White JV: An approach to nutrition screening for older Americans. *Am Fam Physician* 45:601, 1992.

Reife CM: Involuntary weight loss. Common Medical Problems in Ambulatory Care. *Med Clin North Am* 79:299, 1995.

Reuben DB, Greendale GA, Harrison GG: Nutrition screening in older persons. *J Am Geriatr Soc* 43:415, 1995.

Rush D: Evaluating the Nutrition Screening Initiative. *Am J Public Health* 83:944, 1993.

Sullivan DH, Martin W, Flaxman N, et al: Oral health problems and involuntary weight loss in a population of frail elderly. *J Am Geriatr Soc* 41:725, 1993.

Thompson MP, Morris LK: Unexplained weight loss in the ambulatory elderly. *J Am Geriatr Soc* 39:497, 1991.

Wallace JI, Schwartz RS, LaCroix AZ, et al: Involuntary weight loss in older outpatients: incidence and clinical significance. *J Am Geriatr Soc* 43:329, 1995.

Whitehead C, Finucane P: Malnutrition in elderly people. *Aust NZ J Med* 27:68, 1997.

Wilson MG, Vaswani S, Liu D, et al: Prevalence and causes of undernutrition in medical outpatients. *Am J Med* 104:56, 1998.

James P. Richardson

Infections

The elderly are prone to variety of infectious diseases. The accumulation of years of environmental insults, the development of chronic diseases, generalized changes of aging, and changes of aging in the immune system itself are all factors in the increased incidence of infections in the elderly. For important geriatric infectious diseases, the mortality rate is 3 to 10 times higher than in younger individuals (Table 17-1). Although antibiotic regimens are discussed in this chapter, readers are cautioned that dosages for some antibiotics vary by the patient's weight, renal and liver function, and whether comorbidities are present.

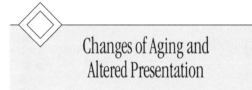

Changes of Aging and Altered Presentation

Many changes in host defenses, as well as dysfunction of the immune system itself, affect elderly persons' susceptibility to infection. For example, incomplete emptying of the bladder and the production of less acid urine contribute to the increased incidence of urinary tract infection (UTI). Reduced mucociliary function and diminished cough reflex lead to a greater incidence of pneumonia. The thinning of the epidermis and decreased vascularity of the dermis can increase the risk of cellulitis and infected pressure ulcers in the elderly.

Diminished cell-mediated immunity, as evidenced by the increased prevalence of anergy, is the major alteration of the immune system in the elderly. T-lymphocyte proliferation in response to mitogens and antigens is less in the elderly. Helper T-cell and cytotoxic T-cell activity also decline with age. Cytokine synthesis or receptors can be reduced in older adults, mediated through errors in mRNA expression or signal transduction. Cytokine antagonists can be increased in older adults, which result in decreased T-cell proliferation and immune suppression.

Less is known about the effects of aging on neutrophil and macrophage function. Although changes in the functions of these cells have been found in aging animals, whether these changes are clinically important is not clear. B-lymphocyte function, primarily the production of antibodies, is not significantly impaired in the aged, but studies

Table 17-1

Important Geriatric Infectious Diseases and Their Relative Mortality Rates

INFECTIONS	RELATIVE MORTALITY RATES COMPARED WITH YOUNG ADULTS*
Pneumonia	3
Urinary tract infection	5–10 (for renal infection)
Infective endocarditis	2–3
Bacterial meningitis	3
Tuberculosis	10[†]
Sepsis	3
Cholecystitis	2–8
Appendicitis	15–20

*Number equals multiplier factor compared with young adults.
[†]Excluding HIV-infected younger adults.
SOURCE: Modified with permission from TT Yoshikawa. Perspective: aging and infectious diseases: past, present, and future. *J Infect Dis* 176:1053, 1997.

have produced conflicting results because B-cell function is dependent on T lymphocytes.

Despite these changes, the presence of chronic illness, so common in older adults, is more important to evaluation, outcome, and treatment than are immunologic changes of aging. Elderly persons suffering from infectious diseases often present atypically, either because of changes in aging or comorbid conditions. Changes in function, such as falls, delirium, poor appetite, and incontinence, can be the only clues to early infection. Indeed, infections are a common cause of delirium in older adults. Ill elderly often underreport symptoms and complaints arising from chronic disease can mask other symptoms. Even those with serious infections, such as sepsis syndrome, can be afebrile, possibly because of a reduced temperature response to pyrogenic cytokines such as interleukin 1 (IL-1) and tumor necrosis factor (TNF). When fever is present, however, elderly patients are more likely than younger patients to have a serious or life-threatening infection.

The patient's environment is a critical component of the assessment of patients with infections. In general, community-acquired illnesses are less severe and are less likely to be caused by antibiotic-resistant organisms than are those infectious diseases contracted by patients residing in nursing homes or hospitals.

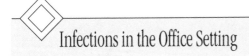

Infections in the Office Setting

Older adults experience fewer trivial infectious illnesses ("colds") than younger adults and children. Whether this is the result of decreased exposure or acquired immunity is not clear. Nevertheless, seniors can be more likely than younger persons to suffer significant complications of upper respiratory infection, such as pneumonia. Because older adults are especially prone to complications from antibiotic therapy,

such as antibiotic-associated colitis and drug-drug interactions, it is important that antibiotic therapy be reserved for illnesses that require such interventions.

Pharyngitis

As in younger adults and children, viruses (usually rhinoviruses, coronaviruses, influenza, parainfluenza, and adenovirus) cause most episodes of sore throat. When pharyngitis has a viral etiology, nasal congestion and a clear or mucoid discharge usually accompany the sore throat. Complaints of malaise and fatigue are common. Findings on examination are minimal, limited primarily to pharyngeal erythema and nasal turbinate swelling and redness.

The sudden development of severe odynophagia without nasal symptoms suggests the diagnosis of streptococcal pharyngitis. Although uncommon, older adults who care for grandchildren or great-grandchildren may be exposed to streptococcus. On examination, a beefy red pharynx, significant tonsillar exudate, and tender anterior cervical nodes significantly increase the probability that group A streptococcus is the cause of the pharyngitis. Clinicians can elect to treat a patient with a typical presentation without further testing, but even in these cases, the likelihood of streptococcal infection is only about 50 percent, as adenovirus can cause pharyngeal exudate as well. Most authorities recommend throat culture or a swab for rapid group A streptococcal antigen before treating with antibiotics. This is because of the benefits of withholding antibiotics from patients with viral illnesses and because delays of a few days prior to treatment for streptococcal pharyngitis have not resulted in a higher incidence of first attacks of rheumatic fever or a reduction in the severity of symptoms. Immediate treatment, however, is recommended for patients with known rheumatic heart disease.

Very rare causes of pharyngitis in older adults include infectious mononucleosis, caused by Epstein-Barr virus, and herpangina, caused by coxsackievirus. These viral infections can be treated symptomatically. Mouth pain or pharyngitis can also be the initial presentation of granulocytopenia, especially in patients on chemotherapy or other hematotoxic drugs such as clozapine, carbamazepine, phenytoin, or propylthiouracil (PTU). Multiple painful ulcers are usually seen on examination in these patients.

Symptomatic relief is one of the primary goals in the treatment of pharyngitis. Patients should be asked which symptoms are most bothersome, and treatment recommendations are aimed at these symptoms. For example, cough usually responds to dextromethorphan. Severe coughs, especially those that interfere with sleep, can require a codeine-containing cough syrup. Nasal congestion can be relieved by decongestants such as pseudoephedrine, although caution is advised in men with benign prostatic hypertrophy (BPH), who may experience urinary hesitancy due to stimulation of alpha-adrenergic receptors in the bladder neck. Throat pain can be resistant to any one therapy, but combining acetaminophen or ibuprofen with topical agents, such as phenol sprays, almost always results in significant improvement in symptoms. Severe pain can require the short-term use of oral opioids like codeine.

Appropriate treatment for group A streptococcal pharyngitis is penicillin V 500 mg qid or 1.0 g bid for 10 days. If oral therapy cannot be assured, 1.2 million units of benzathine penicillin G is given intramuscularly. Erythromycin 250 mg qid for 10 days is a suitable alternative for patients allergic to penicillin.

Epiglottitis is a rare cause of pharyngitis in older adults that is life-threatening and requires immediate recognition and treatment. Cellulitis at the base of the tongue can spread to the epiglottis, which may become swollen. This threatens the airway. The usual cause is *Haemophilus influenzae*. In addition to severe throat pain and a toxic appearance, adults can present with shortness of breath or drooling. Stridor can be present. Clinicians should not attempt to view the throat directly; instead immediate referral to an otolaryngologist for direct viewing by endoscopy in an operating room where the airway can be protected is recommended. Appropriate antibiotic coverage for adults includes cefuroxime, ceftriaxone, and ampicillin/sulbactam.

Influenza

Older adults, just as do individuals of younger ages, often complain of "the flu," especially during the winter season. The flu syndrome presents as the sudden onset of fever, headache, myalgias, and pharyngitis. In common usage, "the flu" has become synonymous with a severe upper respiratory infection of any etiology, but clinicians should attempt to distinguish true influenza from "the flu" because of the implications for treatment and prevention. Infection can spread to the lower respiratory tract, resulting in a secondary pneumonia, especially in the elderly. Older adults are especially susceptible in institutional settings, such as nursing homes, where epidemics have occurred.

Influenza syndromes can be caused by parainfluenza, adenovirus, and respiratory syncytial virus (RSV), but most cases are caused by the influenza viruses, especially during an epidemic. Influenza viruses are classified into three types: A, B, and C. Influenza C is nonvirulent. Influenza B attacks children and is antigenically stable; thus adults are often immune. Influenza A attacks persons of all ages. Influenza A viruses also show antigenic shift among the hemagglutinin (H) and neuraminidase (N) antigens. Therefore vaccination with one strain of influenza A will not necessarily confer protection against others.

Influenza is an acute respiratory illness. Constitutional symptoms, especially fever, myalgias, and headache often predominate. Fever can be severe and usually lasts about 3 days, although it can last longer. Myalgias usually involve the eyes, extremities, and torso. As the constitutional symptoms resolve, respiratory symptoms such as a nonproductive cough, sore throat, and nasal discharge can begin or worsen. Examination will show a somewhat toxic appearing person, often with conjunctival erythema, tender cervical nodes, and a clear nasal discharge.

Treatment with amantadine or rimantadine usually results in shorter duration of fever and the length of the overall illness, but only if treatment is begun within 1 to 2 days. Both drugs are dosed at 100 mg twice a day in the healthy elderly. This dosage, however, can cause significant central nervous system effects (e.g., delirium, insomnia, and anxiety) in the frail elderly or in those with reduced creatinine clearance. For these patients, a dose of 100 mg a day should be used. Acetaminophen, ibuprofen, or aspirin should be given to control fever and myalgias, and adequate fluid intake should be advised. Cough and cold symptoms can be treated as discussed elsewhere in this chapter.

Pulmonary complications of influenza include airway hyperreactivity, secondary bacterial pneumonia, and, rarely, primary influenza pneumonia. Airway hyperreactivity can be manifested as a continual or worsening cough, dyspnea on exertion, or wheezing. An aerosolized bronchodilator, such as albuterol or ipratropium dosed as two inhalations four times a day, can be helpful. Severe coughs can require the addition of codeine. Patients with an improving flu illness who then develop shortness of breath, fever, and a productive cough can have a secondary bacterial pneumonia caused by pneumococcus, *H. influenzae*, or *Staphylococcus aureus*, or primary influenza pneumonia. These patients should be managed as noted in the section on pneumonia.

Otitis Media

Otitis media is not as common in adults as children, but can occur after severe viral respiratory infections. In addition to symptoms resulting from the preceding viral upper respiratory infection (URI), symptoms include ear pain, hearing loss, and purulent discharge (when the tympanic membrane ruptures). The value of antihistamines is still a subject of debate, but they can be helpful if there is an allergic component. Antibiotics effective for sinusitis are usually effective for episodes of otitis media.

Sinusitis

Viral upper respiratory infections sometimes lead to bacterial infection in the sinuses, or sinusitis. Additionally, mucosal thickening and increased mucus production in the sinuses from allergic rhinitis can set the stage for bacterial infections. The diagnosis of sinusitis is difficult to make no matter what age of the patient. Suggestive symptoms are facial pain, purulent nasal discharge, tooth pain, fever, and headache. Nasal congestion is often severe, but without the presence of the previously mentioned symptoms, sinusitis is unlikely. Most patients with sinusitis do not have significant physical findings, but they can have swelling over the sinuses, tenderness to palpation of the sinuses, and pus in the ostia or on the turbinates. The value of transillumination remains debatable. Sinusitis rarely can be the presenting symptom of Wegener's granulomatosis or cancer of the head or neck.

Treatment with antibiotics usually results in rapid improvement when patients truly have infection in the sinuses, but the importance of shrinking the mucous membranes to allow drainage of infected debris from the sinuses is often overlooked. The latter can be provided by oral decongestants (if the patient's blood pressure is controlled and urinary retention is not a concern) or by limited use (3 to 4 days) of a topical decongestant such as oxymetazoline. If there is an allergic component, antihistamine therapy, preferably with a nonsedating antihistamine, can be helpful. Alternately, some experts recommend topical nasal steroids.

Antibiotic therapy is aimed at the usual etiologic factors (*Streptococcus pneumoniae, Streptococcus pyogenes, H. influenzae, Moraxella catarrhalis*, and, rarely, *S. aureus*). A recent meta-analysis showed that amoxicillin or trimethoprim/sulfamethoxazole (TMP/SMZ) was as effective as newer, more expensive antibiotics, such as amoxicillin/clavulanate, clarithromycin, azithromycin, or cefuroxime. The cost of these newer antibiotics is often prohibitive. In this study, two thirds of patients with sinusitis improved without antibiotics. The recommended duration of treatment is 10 days, but one study that compared a 3-day course with a 10-day course of TMP/SMZ showed equal efficacy. Chronic infections can be caused by anaerobic infections, which can require the addition of metronidazole or clindamycin to clear. Patients with infections resistant to appropriate antibiotic treatment should be referred to an otolaryngologist for possible drainage.

Acute Bronchitis and Exacerbation of Chronic Bronchitis

Viral URIs often involve the lower respiratory tract as well. When cough becomes severe or productive, bronchitis is diagnosed. Despite the common practice of treating bronchitis with antibiotic therapy, most episodes will resolve with symptomatic treatment only. Antihistamines should be avoided because they cause thickening of mucus. A subset of patients who do not have a diagnosis of asthma or chronic obstructive pulmonary disease (COPD) will manifest wheezing or cough. In these patients, treatment of bronchospasm with an aerosolized bronchodilator such as albuterol, if present, will reduce coughing and shortness of breath. For patients who worsen despite these measures and in whom incipient pneumonia is suspected, amoxicillin 500 mg three times a day, TMP/SMZ (1 double-strength tablet twice a day), erythromycin 1 g a day in divided doses, or a newer macrolide or a second-generation cephalosporin is usually effective.

On the other hand, patients with acute bacterial exacerbation of chronic bronchitis usually improve with antibiotic therapy. The thickened mucus found in patients with COPD promotes the growth of bacteria, and these patients often have a difficult time clearing these secretions. In addition to antibiotic therapy, bronchodilation, usually by inhaler, is helpful. Patients can require a short course of steroids as well. Prophylactic antibiotic therapy during the winter months is controversial and can lead to exacerbation caused by resistant organisms. Patients with COPD should be immu-

nized with influenza and pneumococcal vaccines (see Chap. 3).

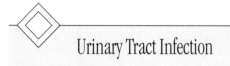

Urinary Tract Infection

Urinary tract infections (UTIs) are the most common bacterial infections in the elderly. Compared with younger patients, however, proportionately more men develop UTIs. Functionally impaired elderly, such as those living in a nursing home, and those elderly with indwelling or condom catheters, also are at increased risk of UTIs.

Community-Acquired Urinary Tract Infections

The presentation of urinary tract infection can range from minor suprapubic discomfort to the classical symptoms of dysuria, urinary frequency, and urgency, to fever and hypotension from sepsis syndrome. Older adults with dementia can present with new-onset incontinence, poor appetite, lethargy, agitation, or a change in functional status, such as a loss of an ADL (activity of daily living, e.g., the ability to feed oneself). Elderly patients with pyelonephritis can have gastrointestinal or respiratory symptoms. Most authorities do not treat patients with asymptomatic bacteriuria.

Escherichia coli accounts for the vast majority of UTIs in both elderly men and women. UTIs in institutionalized elderly, however, are often caused by other gram-negative bacilli. These include *Klebsiella* species, *Proteus* species, *Enterobacter*, or other Enterobacteriaceae.

As in younger patients, laboratory assessment consists of urinalysis and urine culture. Pyuria is a sensitive test for UTI, but its absence does not exclude infection. A urine culture that grows 10^5 pathogenic bacteria/mL remains diagnostic of UTI in a symptomatic elderly patient, but lesser counts can also indicate infection and may merit treatment. Multiple blood cultures are indicated in those with pyelonephritis or sepsis syndrome. Imaging studies, such as ultrasonography, should be considered for patients who remain febrile for more than 96 h, who have obstruction, who are bacteremic, or who have persistent bacteriuria.

Antibiotic treatment for UTI depends on the severity of infection and the presumed site of infection (kidney or bladder). Patients with minor or no systemic signs or symptoms are treated with oral antibiotic therapy, whereas those with sepsis syndrome or pyelonephritis are hospitalized for parenteral antibiotics, intravenous fluids, and other supportive treatment. Antibiotics usually appropriate for outpatients include amoxicillin 250 mg or 500 mg three times a day, TMP/SMZ (1 double-strength tablet twice a day), norfloxacin 400 mg twice a day, and first- or second-generation cephalosporins. Culture results should dictate therapy when available. Duration of treatment can be as short as 3 days in minimally ill patients for which follow-up can be assured. If patients do not improve after 3 days, a culture should be obtained (if not yet done), and treatment continued for 2 weeks. Moderately ill patients should receive 2 weeks of therapy.

Broad-spectrum antibiotic treatment is usually given for seriously ill elderly patients, such as those with sepsis syndrome or with difficult to eradicate infections (e.g., those with indwelling bladder catheters). Appropriate parenteral antibiotic regimens are as follows: ampicillin or a first-generation cephalosporin combined with an aminoglycoside; a third-generation cephalosporin, ampicillin/sulbactam, imipenem/cilastatin, piperacillin/tazobactam; or a fluoroquinolone. Aztreonam can be substituted for an aminoglycoside in those patients in whom aminoglycosides are relatively contraindicated (dehydration, chronic renal failure). Elderly patients with less serious systemic illness and who do not have a history of an indwelling catheter can be treated with intravenous trimethoprim/sulfamethoxazole, first- or second-generation cephalosporin, or ciprofloxacin. The duration of therapy should be guided by the severity of illness but should be a minimum of 2 weeks.

Catheter-Associated Urinary Tract Infections

Older adults are the most common population in which chronic indwelling urinary catheters are used. A substantial proportion of hospitalized patients will have a bladder catheter at some time during their stay. An estimated 100,000 nursing home residents have urethral catheters at any one point.

Bacteria can enter the bladder of a catheterized patient during insertion, by ascending the lumen of the catheter or the space between the outside of the catheter and the urethral mucosa, or after removal of the catheter. Once in the bladder, bacteria multiply significantly within 3 days. Almost all patients are colonized within 30 days of catheter placement. In patients recently catheterized, *E. coli* is most commonly found. Other frequent isolates are *Pseudomonas aeruginosa, Klebsiella pneumoniae, Proteus mirabilis,* and enterococci. In addition to these pathogens, long-term catheterized patients can have less common bacteria such as *Providencia stuartii* and *Morganella morganii.*

Most episodes of bacteriuria are asymptomatic in patients with short-term catheterization, but fever occurs in 10 to 30 percent. Progression to pyelonephritis and sepsis syndrome can occur. At least one study demonstrated that routine administration of antibiotics to catheterized patients with bacteriuria does not lower the incidence of symptomatic UTI and, instead, leads to resistant organisms. Both routine irrigation with antibacterial solutions or sterile saline and routine replacement of catheters have also been ineffective in reducing the incidence of UTIs in these patients because the risk of a symptomatic UTI is related to the frequency of manipulation of the catheter.

UTI should be suspected in a catheterized patient with a fever, elevated white blood cell count, or a change in functional status. In these patients, urine and blood cultures should be obtained. Some authorities recommend changing the catheter prior to obtaining a urine specimen for culture (to avoid culturing a colonizing organism instead of an invasive one). Because many of these infections are caused by enterococci, appropriate regimens include ampicillin with gentamicin, imipenem/cilastatin, piperacillin/tazobactam, or meropenem. An intravenous fluoroquinolone, such as levofloxacin, is an alternative. Once patients improve and the organism is known, patients can often be switched to an oral antibiotic to complete 2 weeks of therapy. Catheterized patients with symptoms of UTI but without fever or signs of systemic illness can be treated with oral antibiotics directed at the organisms previously mentioned.

Prostatitis

The diagnosis of acute prostatitis is suggested by the symptoms of dysuria, low back pain, and fever. On examination, the prostate is painful and enlarged. A urine culture should be obtained but prostatic massage is not recommended because this increases the risk of bacteremia. Empiric therapy should be started before urine culture results are available. A sexually transmitted agent such as *Chlamydia* or *Neiserria gonorrhoeae* rarely causes prostatitis in this age group. Rather, Enterobacteriaceae are usually the offending organism. Appropriate regimens are oral fluoroquinolones or TMP/SMZ 160 mg/800 mg twice daily for 14 days.

Chronic low back pain with perineal or low back discomfort together with dysuria, frequency, or nocturia suggests the presence of chronic prostatitis. To confirm the prostate as the source of bacteriuria, a urethral urine sample (first 10 mL), a midstream sample, and expressed prostatic secretions (EPS) should be cultured. Bacterial counts in the EPS exceeding those in the other samples confirm the diagnosis of bacterial prostatitis. The same antibiotics can be used for chronic prostatitis as for the acute disease, but the course of treatment should be for at least 4 weeks (ofloxacin should be given for 6 weeks).

Prostatosis is suggested when the patient has symptoms of prostatitis but cultures are negative. Although the etiology is unknown, suggested causes include *Chlamydia* and *Ureaplasma*. Doxycycline at 100 mg twice a day for 14 days can be helpful.

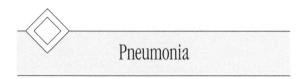

Pneumonia

Together, pneumonia and influenza rank as the fifth leading cause of death in the elderly in the United States. Increasing age, confusion, admission from a nursing home, dehydration, hypotension, and leukocytosis have been associated with increased mortality from pneumonia in the elderly. Recognition of pneumonia can be problematic: a significant proportion of older adults with pneumonia will not have a fever greater than 101°F or a cough productive of sputum. Instead, delirium can be the major manifestation. An increased respiratory rate is a sensitive sign of pneumonia in the elderly.

Some types of pneumonia, such as tuberculosis and influenza, can be acquired by direct contact with infected individuals, and infection can spread through the bloodstream from a distant source (e.g., endocarditis). Most frequently, however, pneumonia results from aspiration of oropharyngeal secretions that contain respiratory pathogens. As a result, although *S. pneumoniae* remains an important pathogen in the elderly, other pathogens occur more commonly in the elderly than they do in younger age groups (Table 17-2). This change can be due to the alteration of the usual respiratory flora to a predominance of gram-negative rods in older adults who are admitted to the hospital or nursing home. In addition, *S. aureus* and anaerobes are much more common in the elderly and are frequent nosocomial causes of pneumonia. Atypical pneumonia is uncommon in older adults. So-called atypical pneumonia is said to have a more gradual onset than the usual pneumonia syndrome, with a predominance of extrapulmonary symptoms including headache, myalgias, sore throat, vomiting, and diarrhea. *Legionella pneumophila* is the most frequent

Table 17-2

Most Common Bacterial Agents That Cause Community-, Nursing Home–, and Hospital-Acquired Pneumonia in Elderly Patients*

Community-Acquired
  Streptococcus pneumoniae
  Staphylococcus aureus
  Haemophilus influenzae
  Aerobic gram-negative bacilli
  Aspiration (aerobes and anaerobes)
  Moraxella catarrhalis
  Legionella pneumophila
  Streptococcus agalactiae
  Polymicrobial†
Nursing Home–Acquired
  Streptococcus pneumoniae
  Aspiration (aerobes and anaerobes)
  Klebsiella pneumoniae
  Staphylococcus aureus (both methicillin-sensitive and methicillin-resistant)
  Haemophilus influenzae
  Escherichia coli
  Moraxella catarrhalis
  Mycobacterium tuberculosis
  Polymicrobial†
Hospital-Acquired
  Aerobic gram-negative bacilli (including *Pseudomonas aeruginosa*)
  Aspiration (aerobes and anaerobes)
  Streptococcus pneumoniae
  Staphylococcus aureus
  Haemophilus influenzae
  Legionella sp.
  Polymicrobial†

*In approximate order of frequency.
†Increase in frequency in institutional settings.
Source: Reprinted with permission from TJ Marrie: Pneumonia. *Clin Geriatr Med* 8:721, 1992.

cause of atypical pneumonia in the elderly. Other causes include *Mycoplasma pneumoniae, Chlamydia pneumoniae,* and *Pneumocystis carinii.* Community-acquired pneumonia is considered first. Because of the importance of the patient's location in selecting therapy for pneumonia, nursing home–acquired pneumonia will be considered separately.

Community-Acquired Pneumonia

A community-dwelling patient with a typical presentation of acute pneumonia has fever, chills, and cough productive of purulent sputum; leukocytosis; and infiltrates on a chest radiograph. Some patients, especially those with chronic illnesses, can present with altered mental status, or changes in function, such as a fall or loss of appetite. Neither fever nor leukocytosis may be present.

After the history and physical examination, evaluation of the elderly patient with suspected pneumonia should include a chest radiograph, although a classic lobar pattern of involvement often is not present. This study can help eliminate other causes of dyspnea and fever. All hospitalized patients should also have at least two blood cultures drawn. All patients with pneumonia should have routine hematologic and chemistry studies.

The value of sputum smears has been debated. Traditionally, it has been taught that if the sputum specimen shows more than 25 white blood cells and less than 5 epithelial cells under low-power microscopic examination, then it probably represents true respiratory secretions, and a Gram stain and culture should represent the actual pathogen. The sensitivity and specificity of these tests have varied widely, however, and there are no studies that correlate results of these tests with tests of alveolar material in large numbers of patients. Direct staining can be helpful for some pulmonary pathogens, including *Mycobacterium* species, fungi, *Pneumophilia Legionella* (by direct fluorescent antibody staining) and *P. carinii.* In severely ill patients who are unable to produce sputum, sputum can be obtained by nebulization, transtracheal aspiration, or by bronchoscopy with a protected brush catheter or bronchoalveolar lavage. Of these methods, the latter two procedures have the best sensitivity and specificity.

Treatment of older adults with pneumonia is guided by the severity of the illness (i.e., the patient's ability to oxygenate his or her blood) and comorbid conditions such as hydration status. The patient, any advance directives (because of the high mortality of pneumonia in this population), or his or her family should be consulted for guidance regarding the extent of support the patient desires.

The sputum Gram stain guides antibiotic therapy, if one is available, with the aforementioned caveats. In the absence of reliable sputum smears, empiric therapy should be started that covers the pathogens in Table 17-2, considering the patient's residence. Mildly ill older adults can be treated with an oral agent such as azithromycin, clarithromycin, or if penicillin resistance is suspected, levofloxacin. An alternative is amoxicillin/clavulanate. Still another choice is second-generation cephalosporins such as cefuroxime. These drugs are usually well tolerated and will treat most pathogens likely to cause community-acquired pneumonias, but they do not cover "atypicals" such as *Legionella*.

The decision to hospitalize an older adult with pneumonia is a clinical one, as no hard and fast rules apply. Many risk factors have been recognized that increase mortality or the risk of complications from pneumonia. The American Thoracic Society (ATS) guidelines list age greater than 65 years as one such factor, so all older adults are at slightly increased risk. Additionally, the ATS guidelines list several other risk factors including physical findings, laboratory results, and the presence of chronic diseases (Table 17-3). Fine and colleagues devised a prediction rule to identify low-risk patients with community-acquired pneumonia. Most adults older than 74 years with a chronic illness and any significant physical or laboratory findings would fall into the highest risk categories and, thus, would warrant hospitalization. In practice therefore, it is probable that all but the healthiest and youngest elderly patients with pneumonia will need hospitalization.

Hospitalized patients with pneumonia should receive a second- (e.g., cefuroxime) or third-generation (e.g., ceftriaxone) cephalosporin or a β-lactam/β-lactamase inhibitor (e.g., ampicillin/clavulanic acid). Some authorities would add either erythromycin or a newer macrolide (azithromycin) to cover "atypicals" such as *Legionella* or *Mycoplasma*. Severely ill patients with pneumonia, such as those requiring treatment in an intensive care unit, should be given a third-generation cephalosporin and erythromycin, and the addition of vancomycin should be considered to cover staphylococcus. Levofloxacin is an alternative to these. Seriously ill patients with hospital-acquired pneumonias should be treated with a third-generation cephalosporin and an antipseudomonal aminoglycoside, or imipenem, or an antipseudomonal penicillin (e.g., ticarcillin/clavulanate) and an antipseudomonal aminoglycoside. Erythromycin or azithromycin are added if *Legionella* is suspected.

Patients with aspiration pneumonias require treatment with clindamycin in addition to a third-generation cephalosporin. If *Legionella* has been found in the institution's water supply, then erythromycin may also need to be a part of the regimen. All patients with progressive pneumonias should be considered for the addition of erythromycin and an aminoglycoside. With proper monitoring (i.e., drug levels, BUN, and creatinine), aminoglycosides can be used even in elderly patients with reduced renal function.

Nursing Home–Acquired Pneumonia

Although accepted as a distinct clinical entity in geriatric medicine, whether patients with nursing home–acquired pneumonia (NHAP) require a distinct approach clinically has been debated. The ATS guidelines do not recognize NHAP as a separate clinical entity because residence was considered to be of less importance than the presence of comorbidities and increased age in the evaluation and treatment of adults with pneumonia. Although nursing home (NH) residents tend to have oropharyngeal colonization with gram-negative bacteria, their heterogeneity with respect to function and the presence of chronic illnesses lends support to this view. In a prospective study

Table 17-3

Risk Factors for Mortality or Complications from Pneumonia

Chronic diseases
    Chronic obstructive pulmonary disease
    Diabetes mellitus
    Chronic renal failure
    Congestive heart failure
    Chronic liver disease
Physical findings
    Respiratory rate > 30/min
    Diastolic blood pressure ≤ 60 mmHg or systolic blood pressure ≤ 90 mmHg
    Temperature < 101°F (38.3°C)
    Evidence of extrapulmonary sites of disease (arthritis, meningitis, etc.)
    Confusion or decreased level of consciousness
Laboratory findings
    White blood cell count < 4×10^9/L or > 30×10^9/L or an absolute neutrophil count below 1×10^9/L
    Pa_{O_2} < 60 mmHg or Pa_{CO_2} of > 50 mmHg while breathing room air
Need for mechanical ventilation
    Evidence of abnormal renal function (serum creatinine > 1.2 mg/dL or a blood urea nitrogen
        > 20 mg/dL > (7 mmol/L)
    Presence of unfavorable chest radiographic findings, (e.g., more than one lobe involved, presence
        of a cavity, rapid radiographic spreading, and a pleural effusion)
Hematocrit < 30% or hemoglobin < 9 g/dL
Other evidence of sepsis or organ dysfunction as manifested by metabolic acidosis, an increased
    prothrombin time, an increased partial thromboplastin time, decreased platelets, or the presence of fibrin
    split products > 1:40

SOURCE: Adapted with permission from American Thoracic Society. Guidelines for the initial management of adults with community-acquired pneumonia: diagnosis, assessment of severity, and initial antimicrobial therapy. *Am Rev Respir Dis* 148:1418, 1993.

comparing patients with NHAP, CAP, and NH patients without pneumonia admitted to the hospital, Marrie and Blanchard found that mortality at 1 year was predicted not by residence. It was, however, predicted by complications during the initial hospitalization and by functional status at the time of admission.

Much attention has focused on the issue of whether patients with NHAP have better outcomes when treated in the nursing home rather than in the hospital. In a retrospective study in an academic nursing home, Fried and colleagues compared function and mortality in NH residents treated for pneumonia in the hospital and the NH.

Although both groups had similar mortality rates (13 percent in NH vs. 12 percent in hospital), those patients treated in the nursing home had better functional outcomes at 2 months. After adjusting for differences in the groups, the improved functional outcomes remained only in those patients with lower initial respiratory rates, suggesting that treatment for pneumonia in an appropriately staffed NH can be better for patients with milder pneumonias. Suggested requirements for NH treatment of patients with NHAP include daily physician rounds and availability of intravenous therapy. Selection of antibiotic therapy has already been discussed. Patients with NHAP should be treated according to the severity of their illness, as noted previously.

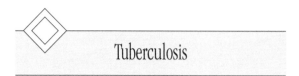

Tuberculosis

Excluding those individuals infected with HIV, older adults are the age group at greatest risk both for contracting and dying from tuberculosis (TB). TB is particularly common in minority elderly populations, who have higher mortality rates. The diagnosis and treatment of tuberculosis is a broad subject that is constantly changing. Readers are advised to consult current recommendations prior to treatment. The following discussion highlights areas of interest to those who treat older adults.

The majority of the current cohort of the "oldest old" with tuberculosis contracted the disease when they were younger. Most survived the initial infection but retained live *Mycobacterium tuberculosis* in caseous lesions in the lungs. Endogenous reactivation accounts for most cases of tuberculosis occurring in older adults today. Others can become infected with primary TB, especially in the nursing home setting. Predisposing factors for reactivation include the presence of diabetes, poor nutrition, alcoholism, and waning T-lymphocyte activity.

Diagnosis

TB can be more difficult to diagnose in older adults. This is because of a higher incidence of false-negative purified protein derivative (PPD) skin tests and because pulmonary TB can occur in middle or lower lobes on chest radiography rather than in the apices. Nevertheless, older adults suspected of have TB should have skin testing with 5 tuberculin units of PPD. A positive test is defined by the Centers for Disease Control and Prevention according to the probability that a positive test represents a true infection and determines which patients without active infection

should be considered for chemoprophylaxis (Table 17-4). Thus, a cutoff of 5 mm or more is used for those with close contact with an active TB patient, previously untreated persons with a chest radiograph consistent with healed tuberculosis, and those persons with HIV infections. Persons with a high-risk medical condition, such as diabetes mellitus, prolonged therapy with systemic glucocorticoids, immunosuppressive therapy, or end-stage renal disease, have a cutoff of 10 mm or more. Those with positive tests but without evidence of active tuberculosis should be considered for prophylaxis from active TB with 6 to 12 months of isoniazid (INH). Older adults treated with INH have a higher risk of hepatitis than do younger adults, but most tolerate chemoprophylaxis well. Those who complain of nausea or other gastrointestinal side effects should have liver function tests (LFTs) drawn. If LFTs remain elevated, chemoprophylaxis should be stopped.

Although prophylactic therapy is not always tolerated by older adults, the risk/benefit ratio is favorable for recent convertors at any age. Those with negative reactions should have a repeat test within 2 weeks to elicit the booster effect. The two-step test helps to distinguish true conversion in initial nonreactors in the event exposure to TB necessitates another test. Those with positive tests should have chest radiography to determine the presence of active or old disease. Careful note should be made of patients with radiographs negative for active disease since they are still at risk of developing active TB in the future. About 20 to 30 percent of persons with active TB will have a negative tuberculin test. Thus, patients with negative tests in whom TB is highly suspected should have further evaluation. Two or three sputa should be sent for smear and culture if possible. Occasionally, bronchoscopy can be necessary to obtain bronchial washes or biopsies for smear and culture.

Extrapulmonary TB is diagnosed by examination of tissue specimens, such as liver biopsy, which is especially useful in disseminated TB. Examination of early morning urine specimens can help detect genitourinary TB. In addition to the usual studies (cell count, glucose, protein, and

Table 17-4

Criteria for Positive Tuberculin Reaction

SKIN TEST CRITERIA (mm INDURATION)	POPULATION AT RISK
≥5 mm	Persons with known or suspected HIV infection*
	Close contacts of person(s) with infectious tuberculosis*
	Person with chest radiographs consistent with tuberculosis (e.g., fibrotic changes)*
≥ 10	Recent converters ≥ 10 mm with ≥ 6 mm increase within 2 years; ≥ 15 mm for those age ≥ 35 years*
	Intravenous drug users known to be HIV seronegative*
	Persons with certain risk factors: silicosis; gastrectomy; jejunoileal bypass; ≥ 10% below ideal body weight; chronic renal failure; diabetes mellitus; corticosteroid and other immunosuppressive therapy; hematologic and other malignancies*
	Foreign born from country with high tuberculosis prevalence[†]
	Medically underserved low-income populations (homeless, blacks, Hispanics, Native Americans)[†]
	Residents of long-term care facilities (nursing homes, correctional facilities)[†]
≥ 15 mm	None of the above factors[†]

*Chemoprophylaxis recommended for all persons regardless of age.
[†]Chemoprophylaxis recommended for persons less than 35 years.
ABBREVIATION: HIV, human immunodeficiency virus.
SOURCE: Reproduced with permission from Centers for Disease Control. The use of preventive therapy for tuberculosis infection in the United States; recommendations of the Advisory Committee for Elimination of Tuberculosis. *MMWR* 39:9, 1990.

staining), cerebrospinal fluid should be sent for culture when TB meningitis is suspected.

Treatment

Standard treatment for TB has been antimycobacterial treatment with at least two active drugs to prevent the emergence of resistant organisms. Because of the emergence of multiresistant TB, however, the Centers for Disease Control and Prevention currently recommends treatment with at least four drugs for the first 2 months. This is because the drug susceptibility of patients' organisms usually is not known at the beginning of therapy (Table 17-5). Once susceptibility testing has been completed (usually after 2 months of therapy), the regimen can be altered accordingly, and drug treatment is continued for a total of at least 6 months. Patients with HIV infection should be treated for at least 9 months. Based on the

current prevalence of drug-resistant organisms, at least 95 percent of patients will receive adequate treatment using this regimen. Because drug-resistant TB is less common in older adults, some authorities recommend that older adults with a new infection be treated with isoniazid and rifampin for 9 months rather than with the four-drug regimen.

Drug susceptibility testing should be performed on isolates from patients whose cultures are still positive after 3 months of treatment. Therapy should be based on the likelihood of drug resistance if the results of drug-susceptibility tests are not available. If the prevalence of isoniazid resistance is 4 percent or higher, then pyrazinamide should be stopped after 8 weeks, but either ethambutol or streptomycin should be continued, along with isoniazid and rifampin, for a total of 6 months. Primary care physicians should consult a physician experienced in the treatment of patients with multidrug-resistant tuberculosis

Table 17-5

Regimen Options for the Initial Treatment of Tuberculosis (TB) in Children and Adults

	TB WITHOUT HIV INFECTION		TB WITH HIV INFECTION
OPTION 1	OPTION 2	OPTION 3	
Daily isoniazid, rifampin, and pyrazinamide for 8 weeks followed by 16 weeks of isoniazid and rifampin daily or 2–3 times weekly.* Ethambutol or streptomycin should be added to the initial regimen until sensitivity to isoniazid and rifampin is demonstrated. Continue treatment for at least 6 months total and 3 months beyond culture conversion. Consult TB medical expert if patient remains smear or culture positive after 3 months.	Daily isoniazid, rifampin, pyrazinamide, and streptomycin or ethambutol for 2 weeks followed by twice weekly* administration of the same drugs for 6 weeks, and subsequently, twice weekly isoniazid and rifampin for 16 weeks. Consult TB medical expert if patient remains smear or culture positive after 3 months.	Treat with directly observed therapy 3 times weekly,* with isoniazid, rifampin, pyrazinamide, and ethambutol or streptomycin for 6 months. Consult TB medical expert if patient remains smear or culture positive after 3 months.	Options 1, 2, or 3 can be utilized, but treatment regimens must continue for a total of 9 months and at least 6 months beyond culture conversion.

*All regimens administered twice weekly or three times a week should be monitored by directly observed therapy.
SOURCE: Reproduced with permission from *MMWR* 42:1, 1993.

for patients who remain symptomatic or whose cultures remain positive after 3 months.

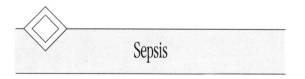

Sepsis

Both bacteremia and sepsis are more common in the elderly. The presentation of elderly patients with these syndromes can be subtle, and their treatment is often very difficult. Mortality in the elderly ranges from 20 to 50 percent.

Probable risk factors for sepsis syndrome and bacteremia in geriatric patients are similar to those for other infections discussed earlier. The decline in the aging immune system makes some contribution, but more likely serious comorbidities, such as pulmonary and renal disease, and changes of aging in other systems (impaired cough reflex, increased post-void bladder residuals) are more important. Catheterization of the urinary bladder was a strong predictor of bacteremia in one study. A case-control study of NH residents with bacteremia found significant associations between bacteremia and the presence of a urinary catheter and urinary incontinence. Hypocholesterolemia on admission to the facility was associated with death from bacteremia. A recent prospective study of 242 consecutive adults with bacteremia in a community hospital found that hypotension, impaired function, nosocomial infection, absence of fever, and immunocompromised status were significantly associated with increased mortality. Age greater than 65 years was not associated with increased mortality after adjustment by logistic regression.

Diagnosis

Bacteremia is defined as the presence of bacteria in the blood, as detected by standard blood cultures. The term sepsis denotes the clinical response to an invasive infection (often bacteremia) and is usually manifested by fever, chills, and malaise or collapse. The nomenclature of sepsis has been expanded and clarified recently. A new entity has been described called systemic inflammatory response syndrome (SIRS) in recognition of the occurrence of a clinical picture of sepsis in patients with noninfectious etiologies, such as burns or trauma. To diagnose SIRS, patients must have two of the following: (1) temperature greater than 38°C or less than 36°C; (2) heart rate faster than 90 beats/min; (3) respiratory rate of more than > 20/min; or (4) white blood cell count higher than 12,000/μL or more than 10 percent bands. Sepsis is diagnosed when SIRS is present and there is an infection documented with a positive culture. Severe sepsis is present when there is evidence of organ dysfunction, such as hypotension or hypoperfusion, as indicated by lactic acidosis, oliguria, or altered mental status. Finally, septic shock is present when there is sepsis-induced hypotension (systolic blood pressure < 90 mmHg) not responsive to a 500-mL intravenous fluid challenge.

As with other serious infections in the elderly, a nonspecific presentation is common (Table 17-6).

Most elderly patients have temperatures in excess of 100°F, but normal temperatures are not uncommon. Hypothermia can also occur. Delirium is also frequently noted, exceeding 50 percent in some series. Signs of altered function, such as falls or incontinence, are also frequent.

Gram-negative organisms are the most common cause of sepsis syndrome in the elderly, accounting for about two-thirds of blood culture isolates in most studies. *S. aureus* and group A beta-hemolytic streptococci are the most common gram-positive organisms isolated. Sources of sepsis are, in approximate descending order: the genitourinary tract, lungs, skin, and the biliary tract. Sources of gram-negative infections are usually the genitourinary tract, intraabdominal sites, and the lungs, whereas gram-positive infections usually start in the lungs, skin, or genitourinary tract (enterococci). Mortality is highest in elderly patients with a nongenitourinary source of infection and in patients with hospital-acquired bacteremias.

Table 17-6

Presenting Signs and Symptoms of Sepsis in the Elderly*

Fever
Lethargy
Confusion
Incontinence
Tachycardia
Rigors and chills
Falls
Nausea and vomiting
Hypotension
Abdominal pain
Dysuria
Diarrhea

*Listed in descending order of approximate frequency.
SOURCE: From JP Richardson: Bacteremia in the elderly. *J Gen Intern Med* 8:89, 1993. Reprinted by permission of Blackwell Science, Inc.

Treatment

Treatment of sepsis and bacteremia includes appropriate antibiotic therapy and supportive therapy. Antibiotic regimens should be chosen according to organisms most likely to be isolated from the presumed site of infection, but because the range of organisms is great, broad spectrum coverage is recommended initially. Possible regimens are imipenem/cilastatin, meropenem, or ticarcillin/clavulanate. Another alternative is a third-generation cephalosporin or ampicillin and an aminoglycoside. The combination of ampicillin, clindamycin, and an aminoglycoside is an appropriate regimen when anaerobic infection is a possibility. Vancomycin should be added only if methicillin-resistant *S. aureus* (MRSA) is a concern. Treatment of septic shock includes volume replacement to reverse hypotension (with a vasoactive agent such as dopamine if necessary) and monitoring of central venous or pulmonary wedge pressure. Antiendotoxin antibodies have not been effective.

Bibliography

American College of Chest Physicians—Society of Critical Care Medicine Consensus Conference. Definitions for sepsis and organ failure and guidelines for the use of innovative therapies in sepsis. *Crit Care Med* 20:864, 1992.

American Thoracic Society. Guidelines for the initial management of adults with community-acquired pneumonia: diagnosis, assessment of severity, and initial antimicrobial therapy. *Am Rev Respir Dis* 148:1418, 1993.

Bender BS: Sepsis. In: Yoshikawa TT (ed): Infectious Diseases. *Clin Geriatr Med* 8:913, 1992.

Ben-Yehuda A, Weksler ME: Host resistance and the immune system. In: Yoshikawa TT (ed): Infectious Diseases. *Clin Geriatr Med* 8:701, 1992.

Catania A, Airaghi L, Motta P, et al: Cytokine antagonists in aged subjects and their relation with cellular immunity. *J Gerontol* 52A:B93, 1997.

Centers for Disease Control and Prevention. Initial therapy for tuberculosis in the era of multidrug resistance—recommendations of the Advisory Council for the Elimination of Tuberculosis. *MMWR* 42:1, 1993.

Centers for Disease Control and Prevention. The use of preventive therapy for tuberculosis infection in the United States: recommendations of the Advisory Committee for Elimination of Tuberculosis. *MMWR* 39:9, 1990.

De Ferranti SD, Ioannidis JP, Lau J, et al: Are amoxycillin and folate inhibitors as effective as other antibiotics for acute sinusitis? A meta-analysis. *BMJ* 317:632, 1998.

Deulofeu F, Cervello B, Capell S, et al: Predictors of mortality in patients with bacteremia: the importance of functional status. *J Am Geriatr Soc* 46:14, 1998.

Dutt AK, Stead WW: Tuberculosis. In: Yoshikawa TT (ed): Infectious Diseases. *Clin Geriatr Med* 8:761, 1992.

Falsey AR, McCann RM, Hall WJ, et al: The "common cold" in frail older persons: impact of rhinovirus and coronavirus in a senior daycare center. *J Am Geriatr Soc* 146:706, 1997.

Fine MJ, Auble TE, Yealy DM, et al: A prediction rule to identify low-risk patients with community-acquired pneumonia. *N Engl J Med* 336:243, 1997.

Fried TR, Gillick MR, Lipsitz LA: Short-term functional outcomes of long-term care residents with pneumonia treated with and without hospital transfer. *J Am Geriatr Soc* 45:302, 1997.

Funnye AS, Ganesan K, Yoshikawa TT: Tuberculosis in African Americans: clinical characteristics and outcome. *J Nat Med Assoc* 90:73, 1998.

Gilbert DN, Moellering RC Jr, Sande MA: *The Sanford Guide to Antimicrobial Therapy.* Vienna, VA: Antimicrobial Therapy, Inc; 1998.

Gleckman RA: Urinary tract infection. In: Yoshikawa TT (ed): Infectious Diseases. *Clin Geriatr Med* 8:793, 1992.

Gonzales R, Sande M: What will it take to stop physicians from prescribing antibiotics in acute bronchitis? *Lancet* 345:665, 1995.

Kennedy DJ: Pneumonia in the elderly. In: Powers DC, Morley JE, Coe RM (eds): *Aging, Immunity, and Infection.* New York: Springer Publishing Company; 1994:191.

Mahmoudi A, Iseman MD: Pitfalls in the care of patients with tuberculosis: common errors and their association with the acquisition of drug resistance. *JAMA* 270:65, 1993.

Marrie TJ: Pneumonia. In: Yoshikawa TT (ed): Infectious Diseases. *Clin Geriatr Med* 8:721, 1992.

Marrie TJ, Blanchard W: A comparison of nursing home–acquired pneumonia patients with patients with community-acquired pneumonia and nursing home patients without pneumonia. *J Am Geriatr Soc* 45:50, 1997.

McFadden JP, Price RC, Eastwood HD, et al: Raised respiratory rate in the patients: a valuable physical sign. *BMJ* 284:626, 1982.

Norman DC, Castle SC, Cantrell M: Infections in the nursing home. In: Yoshikawa TT (ed): *J Am Geriatr Soc* 35:796, 1987.

Norman DC, Toledo SD: Infections in elderly persons. In: Yoshikawa TT (ed): Infectious Diseases. *Clin Geriatr Med* 8:713, 1992.

Richardson JP: Bacteremia in the elderly. *J Gen Intern Med* 8:89, 1993.

Richardson JP, Hricz L: Risk factors for the development of bacteremia in nursing home patients. *Arch Fam Med* 4:785, 1995.

Rudman D, Hontanasas A, Cohen Z, et al: Clinical correlates of bacteremia in a Veterans Administration extended care facility. *J Am Geriatr Soc* 36:726, 1988.

Stead WW, To TT, Harrison RW, et al: Benefit-risk considerations in preventive treatment for tuberculo-sis in elderly persons. *Ann Intern Med* 107:843, 1987.

The Expert Committee on the Diagnosis and Classification of Diabetes Mellitus. Report of the Expert Committee on the Diagnosis and Classification of Diabetes Mellitus. *Diabetes* 20:1183, 1997.

Warren J: Catheter-associated bacteriuria. In: Yoshikawa TT (ed): Infectious Diseases. *Clin Geriatr Med* 8:805, 1992.

Warren JW, Anthony WC, Hoopes JM, et al: Cephalexin for susceptible bacteriuria in afebrile, long-term catheterized patients. *JAMA* 248:454, 1982.

Williams JW, Holleman DR, Samsa GP, et al: Randomized controlled trial of 3 vs 10 days of trimethoprim/sulfamethoxazole for acute maxillary sinusitis. *JAMA* 273:1015, 1995.

Yoshikawa TT: Perspective: aging and infectious diseases: past, present, and future. *J Infect Dis* 176:1053, 1997.

Yoshikawa TT: The challenge and unique aspects of tuberculosis in older patients. *Infect Dis Clin Pract* 3:62, 1994.

Zimmer JG, Hall WJ: Nursing home–acquired pneumonia: avoiding the hospital. *J Am Geriatr Soc* 45:380, 1997.

Alan M. Adelman

Chapter 18

Common Dermatologic Problems

Dermatologic conditions are commonly seen in the primary care setting. In a national survey, approximately 5 percent of all visits to general internists were for dermatologic conditions. In addition, the majority of dermatologic conditions are diagnosed by clinicians other than dermatologists. Many of the skin conditions that occur in older patients can be easily diagnosed and managed by the primary care clinician. This chapter reviews the most common dermatologic problems seen in the geriatric age group.

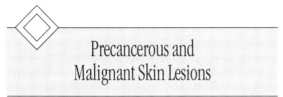

Precancerous and Malignant Skin Lesions

Actinic Keratosis

Actinic keratoses are also known as solar keratoses because they are caused by sun exposure. They are considered precancerous. Because of their relation to sun exposure, individuals who worked or spent time outdoors have a higher prevalence of the lesions.

PHYSICAL EXAMINATION

Actinic keratoses appear as dry, rough, hyperkeratotic lesions (Figs. 18-1 and 18-2). They may or may not have an erythematous base. Usually round or oval, actinic keratoses appear most often in sun-exposed areas such as the face, neck, and forearms. The borders are sharp and well demarcated. As opposed to seborrheic keratoses, actinic keratoses adhere tightly to the skin and are not easily picked off.

TREATMENT

Prevention is the best treatment. Patients should always be advised to avoid prolonged sun exposure and to use sun block appropriately.

Figure 18-1   (Plate 1)

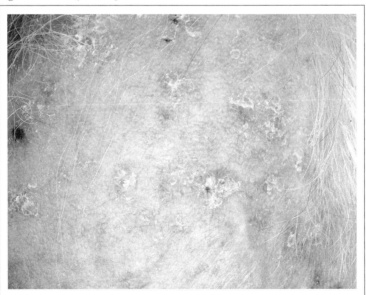

Solar keratosis. Erythematous macules and papules with coarse, adherent scale becoming confluent on the forehead, arising in a background of dermatoheliosis. Gently abrading lesions with a fingernail usually induces pain, even in early subtle lesions, a helpful diagnostic finding.

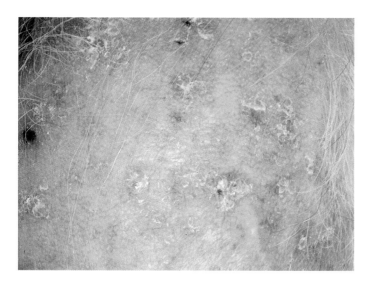

Plate 1 (Figure 18–1) Solar keratosis Erythematous macules and papules with coarse, adherent scale becoming confluent on the forehead, arising in a background of dermatoheliosis. Gently abrading lesions with a fingernail usually induces pain, even in early subtle lesions, a helpful diagnostic finding.

Plate 2 (Figure 18–2) Spreading pigmented actinic keratosis (SPAK) This is a rather uncommon variant of actinic keratosis. The distinctive features of SPAK include size (1.5 cm or larger), pigmentation (brown to black and variegated), and history of lateral spreading, especially the verrucous surface. The lesion is important because it can mimic lentigo maligna (LM). It is, however, easily distinguished from LM because LM is completely flat without evidence of verrucous change. The epidermal change in SPAK may appear as a slightly verrucous surface perceptible only with a hand lens and oblique lighting. Biopsy is necessary to confirm the clinical diagnosis. The lesion responds to a combination of cryosurgery (a very light freeze) followed by application of 5% 5-fluorouracil ointment for 10 to 12 days; the application of the ointment is begun 3 days after the cryosurgey, after the scale falls off.

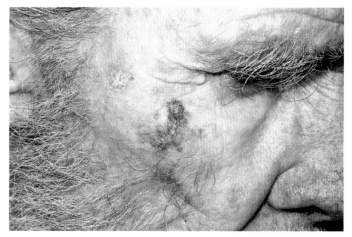

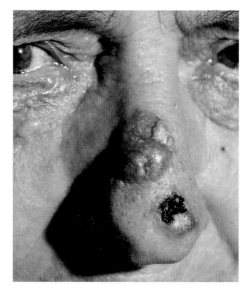

Plate 3 (Figure 18–4) Basal cell carcinoma: nodular and ulcerative types Two lesions are seen on the nose: a large, shiny, red nodule with a cobblestoned surface and an ulcerated nodule near the tip, arising in the setting of dermatoheliosis.

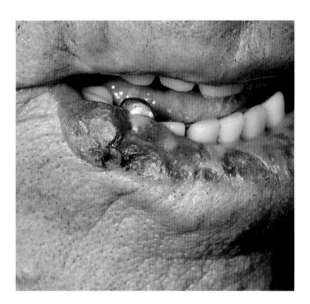

Plate 4 (Figure 18–5) Squamous cell carcinoma A large but subtle nodule, which is better felt than seen, on the vermilion border of the lower lip with areas of hyperkeratosis and erosion, arising in the setting of dermatoheliosis.

Plate 5 (Figure 18–6) Squamous cell carcinoma A large notch on the superior aspect of the helix, a nodule of SCC with hyperkeratosis and ulceration.

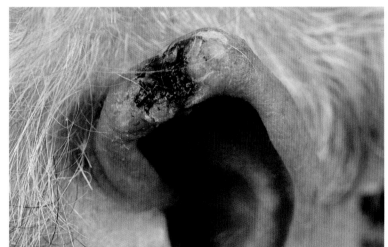

Plate 6 (Figure 18–7) Varicella zoster virus infection: herpes zoster in a single dermatome Dermatomal, grouped and confluent vesicles and pustules arising in the third sacral dermatome; note extension of lesions 1–2 cm across the midline.

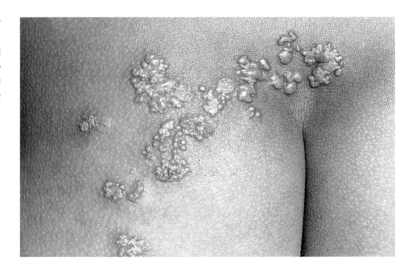

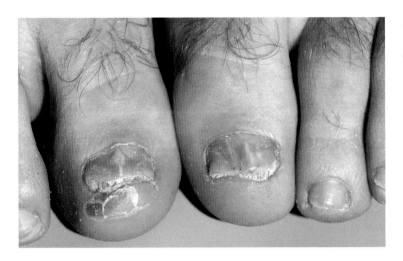

Plate 7 (Figure 18–8) ***Onychomycosis of toenails: distal and lateral subungual type*** Distal subungual hyperkeratosis and onycholysis involving most of the nail bed of the great toenails; these findings are usually associated with tinea pedis.

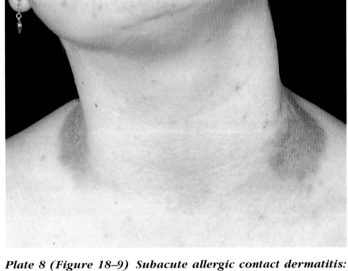

Plate 8 (Figure 18–9) ***Subacute allergic contact dermatitis: nickel*** Red/tan plaques consisting of tiny confluent papules with indistinct borders on the lateral base of the neck recurred whenever a necklace containing nickel was worn. The reaction also commonly occurs when nickel-containing jewelry is worn on the earlobes, wrists, and/or fingers of nickel-sensitized individuals.

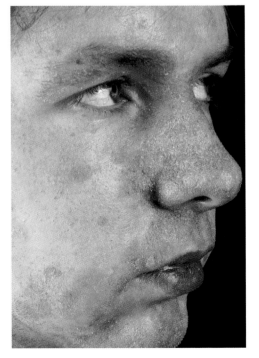

Plate 9 (Figure 18–10) ***Seborrheic dermatitis*** with involvement of nasolabial folds, cheeks, eyebrows, and nose.

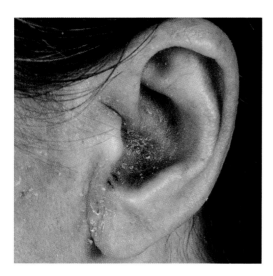

Plate 10 (Figure 18–11) Seborrheic dermatitis of the earlobe The ear canal is also involved.

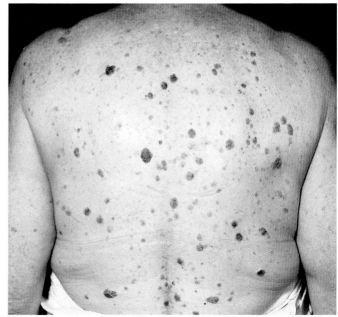

Plate 11 (Figure 18–12) Seborrheic keratoses, multiple Multiple brown, warty papules and nodules on the back, having a "stuck on" appearance.

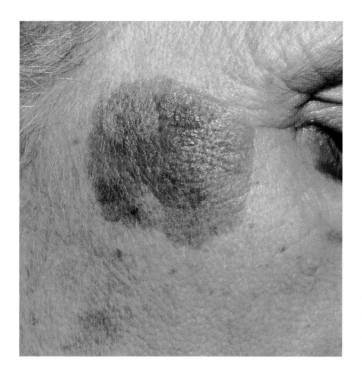

Plate 12 (Figure 18–13) Seborrheic keratosis, solitary A very large, slightly raised, keratotic, brown, flat plaque on the temple in an older female. The differential diagnosis includes lentigo maligna and lentigo maligna melanoma.

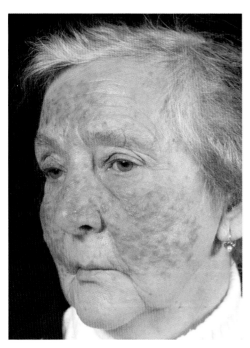

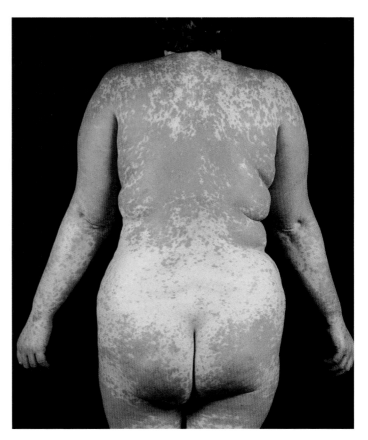

Plate 13 (Figure 18–14) Rosacea Typical moderately severe involvement with confluent erythematous papules and pustules on the forehead, cheeks, and nose. Note the absence of comedones that are typically seen with acne vulgaris.

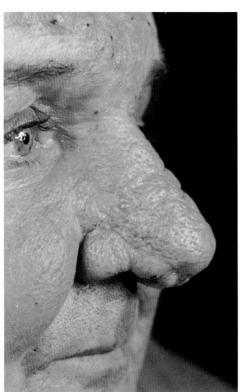

Plate 15 (Figure 18–17) Exanthematous drug eruption: ampicillin Symmetrically arranged, brightly erythematous macules and papules, discrete in some areas and confluent in others, on the back and extremities.

Plate 14 (Figure 18–16) Rosacea Long-standing disease with edema and hyperplasia of the tissues of the nose (rhinophyma), cheeks, and forehead.

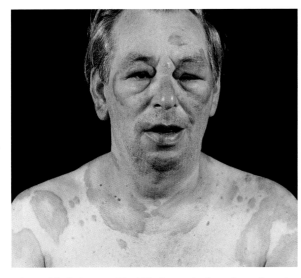

Plate 16 (Figure 18–18) Drug-induced urticaria: penicillin Large, urticarial wheals on the face, neck, and trunk, with angioedema in the periorbital region.

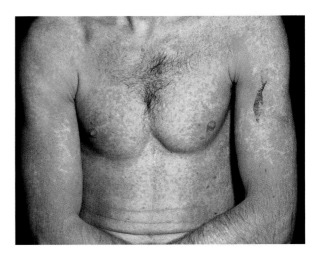

Plate 17 (Figure 18–19) Drug hypersensitivity syndrome: phenytoin Symmetrical, bright-red, exanthematous eruption, confluent in some sites; the patient had associated lymphadenopathy.

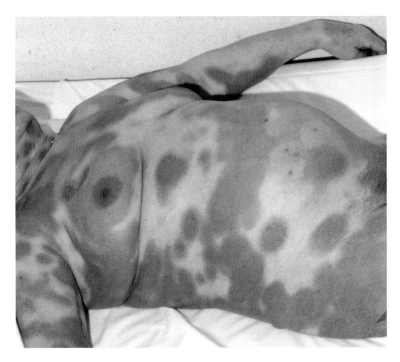

Plate 18 (Figure 18–20) Generalized fixed drug eruption: tetracycline Multiple, confluent, violaceous-red, oval erythematous areas, some of which later became bullous. The eruption may be difficult to distinguish from toxic epidermal necrolysis.

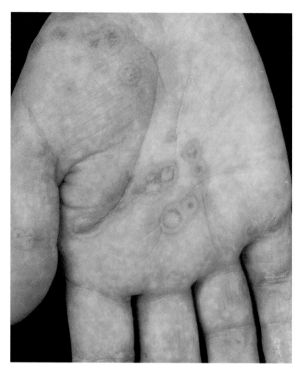

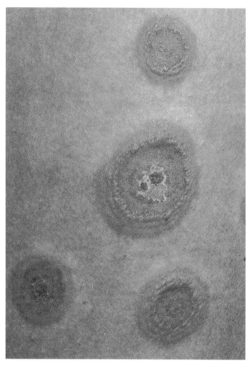

Plate 19 (Figure 18–21A) Erythema multiforme minor Papular, urticarial, and vesicular target lesions in acral distribution. *(Courtesy of Dr. K. Wolff)*

Plate 20 (Figure 18–21B) Erythema multiforme minor Herpes iris of Bateman. *(Courtesy of Dr. K. Wolff)*

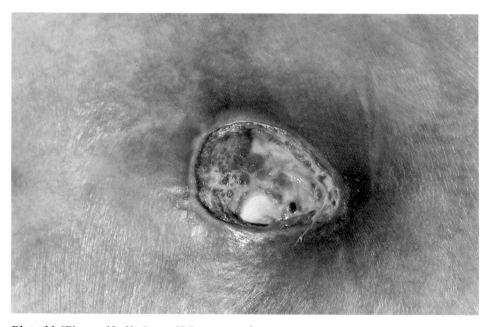

Plate 21 (Figure 19–1) Stage II Pressure ulcer

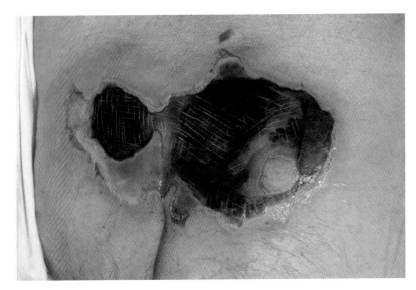

Plate 22 (Figure 19–2) Stage IV Pressure ulcer

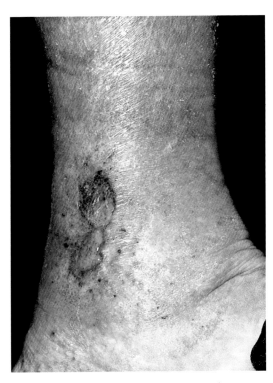

Plate 23 (Figure 19–3) Venous Statis ulcer

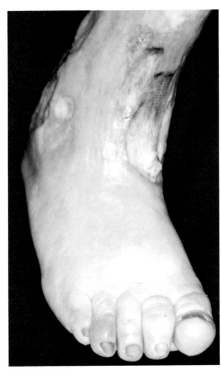

Plate 24 (Figure 19–4) Arterial ulcer

Figure 18-2   (Plate 2)

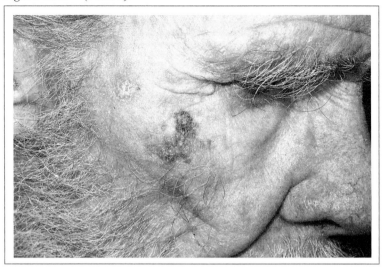

Spreading pigmented actinic keratosis (SPAK). This is a rather uncommon variant of actinic keratosis. The distinctive features of SPAK include size (1.5 cm or larger), pigmentation (brown to black and variegated), and history of lateral spreading, especially the verrucous surface. The lesion is important because it can mimic lentigo maligna (LM). It is, however, easily distinguished from LM because LM is completely flat without evidence of verrucous change. The epidermal change in SPAK may appear as a slightly verrucous surface perceptible only with a hand lens and oblique lighting. Biopsy is necessary to confirm the clinical diagnosis. The lesion responds to a combination of cryosurgery (a very light freeze) followed by application of 5% 5-fluorouracil ointment for 10 to 12 days; the application of the ointment is begun 3 days after the cryosurgery, after the scales fall off.

The most common treatment of established lesions is freezing with liquid nitrogen. Small lesions can be frozen for about 20 s and then allowed to thaw. Larger lesions can warrant a second freeze at the same session. Patients should be advised that the lesions usually turn black and fall off in a few days. A blister can form, but it will heal. If the first treatment is inadequate, a second treatment can be required.

5-Fluorouracil cream (5%) can also be used to treat actinic keratoses. The cream is applied once daily to the lesions for several weeks.

Basal Cell Carcinoma

The most common skin cancer is basal cell carcinoma (BCC), accounting for 75 percent of all skin cancers diagnosed in the United States. Its etiology is sun exposure and thus commonly occurs on sun-exposed areas such as the face, ears, neck, and forearms. It rarely metastasizes.

PHYSICAL EXAMINATION

BCC has a pearly or translucent appearance (Figs. 18-3 and 18-4). It is usually round or oval in shape with sharply demarcated borders. As the carcinoma grows, it develops a rolled edge and a central ulceration can appear. If allowed to continue to expand, it can cause disfigurement and destruction of underlying structures, particularly when located in the nasolabial area, around the eyes, or on the ears.

TREATMENT

Treatment of BCC is surgical excision, although small lesions can be treated with electrodesicca-

Figure 18-3

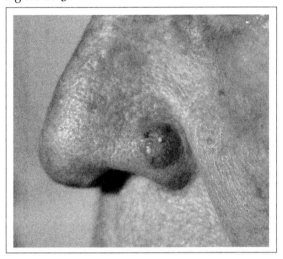

Basal cell carcinoma: nodular type. A solitary, shiny, red nodule with large telangiectatic vessels on the ala nasi, arising on skin with dermatoheliosis (solar elastosis).

Figure 18-4   (Plate 3)

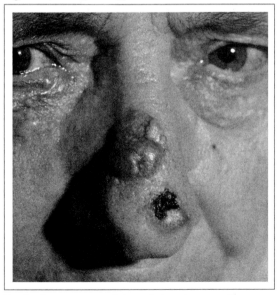

Basal cell carcinoma: nodular and ulcerative types. Two lesions are seen on the nose: a large, shiny, red nodule with a cobblestoned surface and an ulcerated nodule near the tip, arising in the setting of dermatoheliosis.

tion and curettage. In areas where the cancer can be potentially disfiguring, Mohs' surgery can be performed to minimize the extent of the surgical excision, yet still remove the carcinoma. Mohs' surgery is an office procedure, but should be performed by a dermatologist with special training in the procedure. The procedure involves taking microscopic slices and then examining each specimen for cancerous cells. If cancerous cells are present, another slice is taken, until the specimen is cancer-free.

Squamous Cell Carcinoma

Squamous cell carcinoma (SCC) is also related to sun exposure. It can also develop in old scars or chronic ulcers. Men are more frequently affected than women. As with other sun-related skin disorders, outdoor workers or individuals who spent more time outdoors are at greater risk for developing SCC. Lesions caused by sun-damage are less likely to metastasize than those associated with other causes.

SCC accounts for over 90 percent of lip cancers. The risk of recurrence can be as high as 10 percent in sun-related SCC and is greatest during the first few years after the cancer is excised.

PHYSICAL EXAMINATION

SCC is a slow growing tumor. In its early stages, the surface of the lesion can be erythematous. As SCC develops, it can have the appearance of an indurated papule, plaque, or nodule with well-demarcated borders (Fig. 18-5). As the lesion continues to grow, it can ulcerate and develop an elevated margin (Fig. 18-6). A keratotic, "horny" material (called a cutaneous horn) can also develop. Any persistent ulcerated lesion should be suspected.

TREATMENT

The same techniques used to treat BCC are used to treat SCC.

Figure 18-5   (Plate 4)

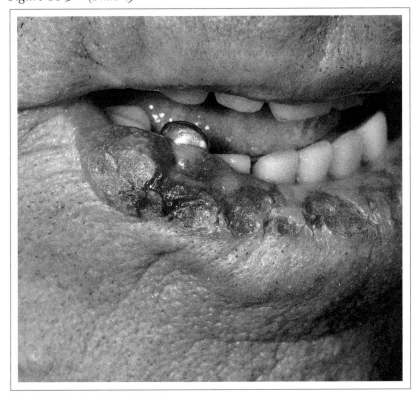

Squamous cell carcinoma. A large but subtle nodule, which is better felt than seen, on the vermilion border of the lower lip with areas of hyperkeratosis and erosion, arising in the setting of dermatoheliosis.

Infectious

Herpes Zoster

Herpes zoster (HZ), commonly known as "shingles," is caused by the reactivation of the varicella zoster virus. After an episode of chickenpox, the zoster virus lies dormant in one or more dorsal sensory ganglia. The exact mechanism of virus reactivation is uncertain. Immunosuppression

associated with malignancy, HIV infection, lymphoproliferative disorders, and chemotherapy are risk factors. The incidence of HZ increases with age. There is no difference in the incidence by gender or race.

PATIENT SYMPTOMS

Pain is a common initial complaint and can precede the appearance of the rash by several days. Patients can also complain of difficulty sleeping because of nocturnal pain. Other symptoms can include malaise, fever, headache, and pruritis.

Figure 18-6   *(Plate 5)*

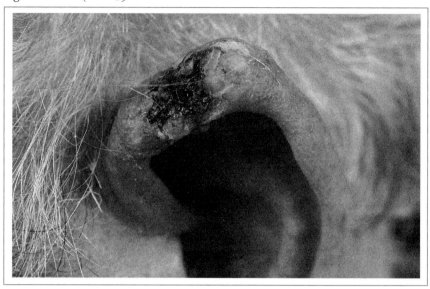

Squamous cell carcinoma (SCC). A large notch on the superior aspect of the helix, a nodule of SCC with hyperkeratosis and ulceration.

PHYSICAL EXAMINATION

The rash of HZ presents as a clustered, vesicular eruption on an erythematous base, distributed along a unilateral or multiple contiguous dermatome(s) of the affected dorsal root ganglion (Fig. 18-7). The most commonly affected dermatomes are the trunk (> 50 percent) and trigeminal nerve (10 to 20 percent). Involvement of the ophthalmic division of cranial nerve V (herpes zoster ophthalmicus) can be a serious condition since it can spread to the globe itself.

LABORATORY TESTING

No further work-up is usually required, as the presentation is classical. A Tzanck stain, looking for giant and/or multinucleated cells, or a skin biopsy can be used to confirm the diagnosis, if the diagnosis is uncertain. Direct fluorescent antibody testing and viral cultures are also available.

TREATMENT

Treatment with antiviral agents is most effective if started within 72 h of the appearance of the rash. Acyclovir 800 mg 5 times per day for 7 to 10 days has been shown to decrease pain, improve sleep, and decrease time to resume normal activities. Famciclovir 500 mg 3 times daily or valacyclovir 1000 mg 3 times daily are also effective and more convenient because of the reduced dosing schedule. The recommended duration of treatment for both agents is 7 days. Topical antiviral agents are not effective.

Local treatments with moist dressings can often provide pain relief. Pain management is important, as the pain from HZ can be very disabling. If there is ophthalmic involvement, an ophthalmologist should be consulted.

Postherpetic neuralgia (PHN) is a common complication of herpes zoster. This neuropathic pain is continued pain in the distribution of the affected nerve after the rash has resolved. The incidence of this complication of HZ increases

Figure 18-7   (Plate 6)

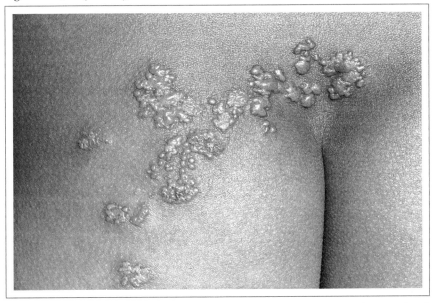

Varicella zoster virus infection: herpes zoster in a single dermatome. Dermatomal, grouped and confluent vesicles and pustules arising in the third sacral dermatome; note extension of lesions 1-2 cm across the midline.

with age and affects as many as 50 percent of affected individuals over the age of 60 years. PHN can last for years.

A recent meta-analysis reported that patients treated within 72 h of the onset of rash with acyclovir 800 mg 5 times per day for 7 to 21 days had a 46 percent reduction in the incidence of pain. The number needed to treat (NNT) was 6.3 to prevent one case of postherpetic neuralgia. Although there are no good studies demonstrating effectiveness of corticosteroids, a 2- to 3-week course of prednisone, starting at the time of diagnosis, with an initial dose of 30 to 60 mg, with a subsequent taper, is often recommended to prevent postherpetic neuralgia.

Several treatments have been tried to relieve the pain of postherpetic neuralgia including tricyclic antidepressants (TCAs), antianxiety agents, anticonvulsants, capsaicin, acupuncture, and transcutaneous electrical nerve stimulation. A meta-analysis by Volmink and associates reported that TCAs

seemed to be of benefit, although it helps only about half the patients treated. Recently, Rowbotham and colleagues showed that gabapentin (neurontin) was effective in improving the pain and reducing the sleep disturbance of postherpetic neuralgia. A TCA should be the initial drug of choice because of its cost, but gabapentin is an effective alternative for elderly patients who cannot tolerate the side effects of TCAs. Pain management including the use of narcotic analgesics can be necessary for relief of the pain of PHN.

Onychomycosis

Onychomycosis is a fungal infection of the nails that affects 2 to 14 percent of the general population and can affect almost half the elderly population by the age of 70 years. The most common causative agent is a dermatophyte *(Trichophyton, Microsporum, Epidermophyton). Candida albi-*

cans causes less than 5 percent of infections. Since the vast majority of infections affect the toenails (tinea unguium), the remaining discussion focuses only on disease of the toenails.

PATIENT SYMPTOMS

Patients usually complain of the abnormal appearance of the nails, but can also complain of pain. Onychomycosis can also affect a patient's psychological well-being and his or her performance of daily activities of living.

PHYSICAL EXAMINATION

Tinea unguium starts at the distal or lateral margin of the nail and then spreads centrally and can eventually affect the entire nail. The toenails of the first and fifth toes are most commonly affected. The appearance of the nail is opaque and whitish (Fig. 18-8). As the infection progresses, the nail can become brownish, thickened, and can easily crack. The distal portion of the nail can rise from the nail bed because of hyperkeratotic debris.

LABORATORY TESTING

The diagnosis can be confirmed prior to initiating therapy. The simplest method that can be performed in the office setting is the examination of abnormal nail samples. The keratinaceous material is mixed with potassium hydroxide (KOH), heated, and then examined under the microscope. Hyphae can be visualized. If hyphae are not present, a culture should be performed. Some insurance companies and health maintenance organizations (HMOs) require a confirmatory culture before authorizing antifungal treatment. If the culture is negative and onychomycosis is still suspected, clippings of the abnormal nail can be sent for histologic analysis.

TREATMENT

The decision to treat is based on several factors. If an abnormal appearance of the nail is the only symptom, treatment can often be withheld. If the patient complains of pain or that the infected nail(s) are affecting the performance of his or her daily activities, there are several treatment options.

Figure 18-8   (Plate 7)

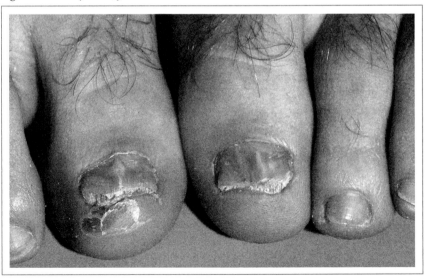

Onychomycosis of toenails: distal and lateral subungual type. Distal subungual hyperkeratosis and onycholysis involving most of the nail bed of the great toenails; these findings are usually associated with tinea pedis.

Table 18-1

Topical Agents for the Treatment of Onychomycosis

TOPICAL AGENT	BRAND NAME
Butenafine	Mentax
Naftifine	Naftin
Terbinafine	Lamisil AT
Clotrimazole	Lotrimin, Mycelex
Nystatin	Mycostatin
Ciclopirox	Loprox

One option is surgical debridement or nail avulsion. This can be an effective form of therapy especially when combined with oral/topical therapy. Total removal of the nail should be considered only as a last resort.

Another option is the use of one of several topical antifungal agents available for the treatment of onychomycosis (Table 18-1). Topical agents are usually not sufficient therapy, and should be combined with surgical debridement or nail avulsion.

There are several options for oral therapy including fluconazole, terbinafine, or itraconazole (continuous or pulse) (Table 18-2). All three oral medications are hepatotoxic, and liver function

tests need to be monitored on a regular basis. Pulse therapy for itraconazole can be less toxic than continuous therapy.

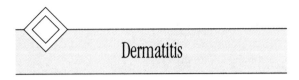

Dermatitis

Dermatitis is a general term used to describe acute or chronic inflammatory conditions of the skin. In a national survey, it was the most common skin condition diagnosed by internists. Dermatitis represents a cluster of different conditions. Table 18-3 lists the different types of dermatitides.

Dermatitis can be divided into two types: exogenous (contact dermatitis) and endogenous (the remaining types). The terms dermatitis and eczema are often used interchangeably.

Contact Dermatitis

Contact dermatitis is the most common form of dermatitis. Contact with almost any substance with the skin can cause contact dermatitis. Table 18-4 lists the common causes of contact dermatitis.

Table 18-2

Oral Agents for the Treatment of Onychomycosis of the Toenails

AGENT	BRAND NAME	DOSE	COMMENTS
Fluconazole	Diflucan	150–300 mg once weekly for 6 months	Cure rate of 60% at 9 months with a 25% relapse rate; Dose needs to be adjusted for renal failure
Terbinafine	Lamisil	250 mg once daily for 12 weeks	Cure rate of 80%; Not recommended if with renal failure
Itraconazole	Sporanox	Pulse: 200 mg twice daily for 1 week then without therapy for 3 weeks (for 3 months) Continuous: 200 mg once daily for 12 weeks	Cure rate of 60% at 9 months with a 20% relapse rate

Common Types of Dermatitis

Contact dermatitis
Atopic dermatitis
Seborrheic dermatitis
Xerotic eczema
Nummular eczema
Dyshidrotic eczema

PATIENT SYMPTOMS

The main complaint of patients with contact dermatitis is pruritis, which can range from mild to severe. Other complaints include the cosmetic appearance of the rash or drainage from the rash.

PHYSICAL EXAMINATION

The diagnosis is usually made by the visual appearance of the rash. Acute reactions consist of plaques of erythema and edema (Fig. 18-9). The lesions can be punctate or cover larger areas, depending on the exposure. The rash associated with poison ivy and poison oak is most often linear in configuration. The skin can be intact, macerated,

Table 18-4

Common Causes of Contact Dermatitis

Cosmetics
Perfumes
Sunscreen
Nickel (jewelry)
Hygienic products
Skin care preparations
Fragrances
Formaldehyde resins (sometimes found in new
   clothing)
Plants (poison ivy, poison oak, and poison
   sumac)

cracked, fissured, or crusted. The lesions can also be erosive and weeping. Vesicles can also be part of the presentation. More chronic lesions become thickened (lichenification). Finally, there can be signs of excoriation from scratching.

Dermatitis can appear anywhere. The lesions can be localized or widespread, depending on the area and duration of exposure.

TREATMENT

Treatment involves several different approaches. First, the offending agent should be identified and removed. Second, if pruritis is a problem for the patient, then an antihistamine such as benadryl (12.5 to 25 mg 4 times daily) or hydroxine (25 to 50 mg 3 times daily) should be prescribed. Application of a potent topical corticosteroid (Table 18-5) can alleviate pruritis and frequently promotes resolution of symptoms. For severe cases, systemic corticosteroids can be prescribed. Compresses with Burrow's solution can be used for open and weeping lesions.

Table 18-5

Corticosteroid Preparations Used in the Treatment of Dermatitis

Mild strength
   Hydrocortisone 0.5%, 1% (Hytone)
   Triamcinolone acetonide 0.025% (Aristocort,
      Kenalog)
   Fluocinolone acetonide 0.01% (Synalar)
Moderate strength
   Triamcinolone acetonide 0.1% (Aristocort,
      Kenalog)
   Mometasone furoate 0.1% (Elocon)
   Fluocinolone acetonide 0.025% (Synalar)
   Fluticasonepropionate 0.005%, 0.05%
      (Cutivate)
Potent strength
   Betamethasone dipropionate 0.05%
      (Diprolene)
   Fluocinonide 0.05% (Lidex)
   Clobetasol propionate 0.05% (Temovate)
   Desoximetasone 0.25% (Topicort)

Figure 18-9   (Plate 8)

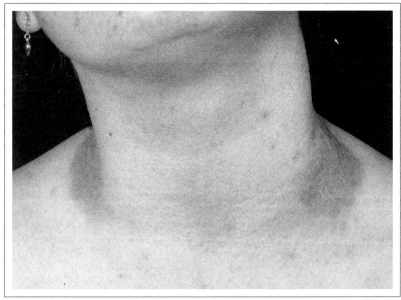

Subacute allergic contact dermatitis: nickel. Red/tan plaques consisting of tiny confluent papules with indistinct borders on the lateral base of the neck recurred whenever a necklace containing nickel was worn. The reaction also commonly occurs when nickel-containing jewelry is worn on the earlobes, wrists, and/or fingers of nickel-sensitized individuals.

Seborrheic Dermatitis

Seborrheic dermatitis is a common skin disorder. It is most frequently seen in areas where sebaceous glands are active including the scalp, face (bridge of the nose, eyebrows, and eyelids), ears, trunk, axilla, groin, and genitals. Seborrheic dermatitis occurs more frequently, and can be more severe, in patients with Parkinson's disease.

PATIENT SYMPTOMS

The most frequent complaint is pruritis. Patients can also complain of dandruff (scaling on the scalp).

PHYSICAL EXAMINATION

Seborrheic dermatitis is characterized by scaling with underlying mild erythema. The scales can be white or yellow and are often described as "greasy" in appearance (Figs. 18-10 and 18-11).

TREATMENT

Low potency corticosteroid preparations or ketoconazole cream are effective in controlling the symptoms and signs of seborrheic dermatitis on the face, trunk, or intertriginous areas.

Over-the-counter (OTC) preparations containing zinc pyrithione, selenium sulfide, or tar are effective in treating seborrheic dermatitis involving the scalp. If not controlled by these OTC preparations, ketoconazole (2%) shampoo and/or corticosteroid-containing shampoos can be substituted.

Xerosis

Xerosis or xerotic dermatitis refers to dryness of the skin. The exact cause is unknown. It is felt to be

Figure 18-10   (Plate 9)

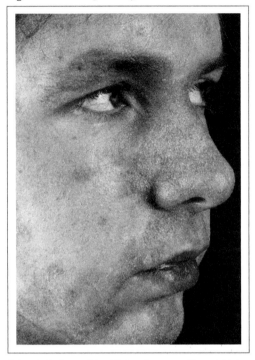

Seborrheic dermatitis with involvement of nasolabial folds, cheeks, eyebrows, and nose.

Figure 18-11   (Plate 10)

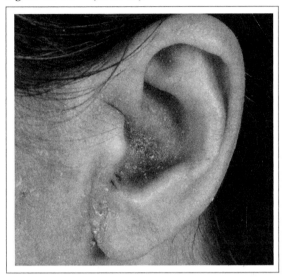

Seborrheic dermatitis of the ear lobe. The ear canal is also involved.

secondary to decreased water content or sebum production of the skin. Xerosis is worse during the winter months when humidity levels are lower.

PATIENT SYMPTOMS

The main complaint is that of pruritis. The skin can become inflamed as the result of chronic itching. This condition is also called erythema craquele and can have the appearance of reticulated erythema and scaling.

TREATMENT

The most effective treatment is topical emollients. Adding oils to a patient's bath water is usu-

ally not recommended in the elderly because the oil can be a safety hazard by creating a slippery surface. Excessive bathing can worsen the condition. A variety of topical emollient preparations are available. They are best applied immediately after bathing to trap the moisture. Environmental humidification can also be helpful. If erythema craquele is present, topical corticosteriods can be applied until the inflammation resolves.

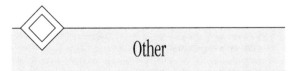

Other

Seborrheic Keratosis

Seborrheic keratosis is a common, benign lesion in the elderly. Usually, the number of keratoses increases gradually with age. A sudden increase in

Figure 18-12 (Plate 11)

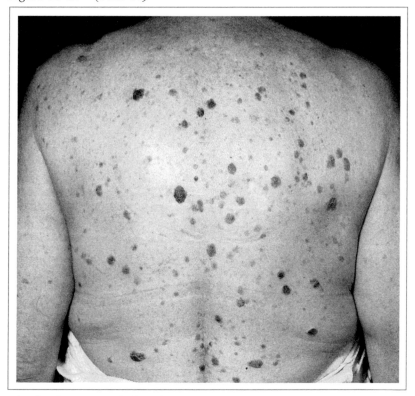

Seborrheic keratoses, multiple. Multiple brown, warty papules and nodules on the back, having a "stuck on" appearance.

the number of lesions (Leser-Trelat sign) can be associated with an internal malignancy (e.g., lung, prostate, colon, or breast).

PATIENT SYMPTOMS

Patients usually complain of local irritation or that the keratosis catch on clothing. They are frequently worried that these lesions are malignant.

PHYSICAL EXAMINATION

Seborrheic keratoses usually appear on the trunk, but can also appear in other areas, such as the extremities. They are usually multiple, raised reddish-brown to black lesions (Fig. 18-12). When a keratosis has multiple colors, it can be confused with melanoma (Fig. 18-13). Keratoses can vary in size from a few millimeters to several centimeters. Although adherent, keratoses can have a "stuck on" appearance. The lesions are round to oval with well-demarcated borders.

TREATMENT

Seborrheic keratoses are usually readily removed by curettage or freezing with liquid nitrogen. They can also be surgically removed. Because some seborrheic keratoses can have the appearance of a melanoma, suspicious lesions should be biopsied

Figure 18-13   (Plate 12)

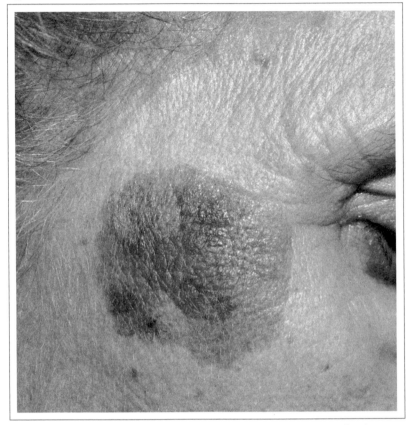

Seborrheic keratosis, solitary. A very large, slightly raised, keratotic, brown, flat plaque on the temple in an older female. The differential diagnosis includes lentigo maligna and lentigo maligna melanoma.

or removed and the specimen sent to pathology to confirm the diagnosis.

Rosacea

Rosacea is a chronic disorder that affects the skin of the face. Heat, spicy foods, alcohol, or sunlight can precipitate flushing. Females are affected more frequently than men. Rhinophyma refers to a hypertrophic disfiguration of the nose and surrounding skin that occurs in some patients with long-standing rosacea. It affects men more frequently.

PATIENT SYMPTOMS

Patients can complain of flushing of the face, intermittent itching, comedones, pustules, or a sensation of warmth.

PHYSICAL EXAMINATION

The primary areas affected are the nose, cheeks, and center of the forehead (Figs. 18-14 and 18-15). In the early stages of rosacea, there are papules and telangiectasia. As the disease progresses, pustules and nodules can form. Blepha-

Figure 18-14   (Plate 13)

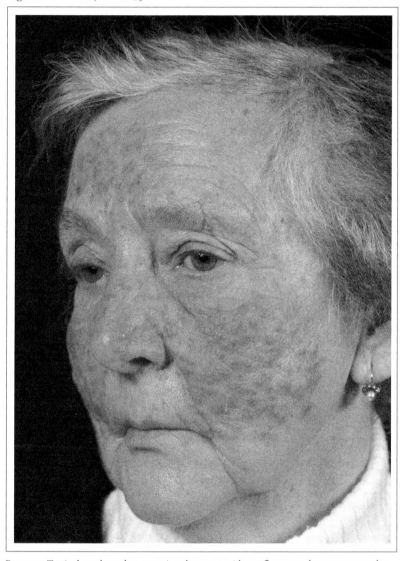

Rosacea. Typical moderately severe involvement with confluent erythematous papules
and pustules on the forehead, cheeks, and nose. Note the absence of comedones
that are typically seen with acne vulgaris.

ritis and conjunctivitis are frequent complications
of rosacea.

Rhinophyma is manifested by enlargement of
the nose (Fig. 18-16). The nose can also have a
copper-red color.

TREATMENT

Patients should avoid agents that precipitate
or aggravate flushing. Topical antibiotics such
as metronidazole gel or cream (0.75%) applied

Figure 18-15

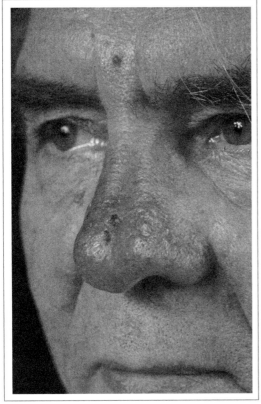

Rosacea. Mild involvement with few erythematous
papules and crusts and striking erythema,
and telangiectasias of the nose (early rhinophyma).

Figure 18-16   *(Plate 14)*

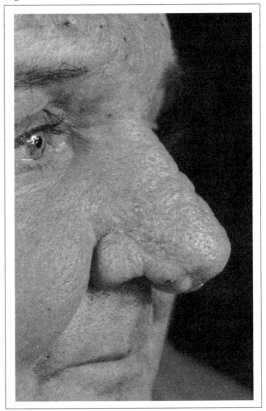

Rosacea. Long-standing disease with edema and
hyperplasia of the tissues of the nose (rhinophyma),
cheeks, and forehead.

twice daily or erythromycin gel are often effective. If topical antibiotics are ineffective, then oral antibiotics such as tetracycline can be added. Once the rash is controlled, the patient can take a once-daily dose of tetracycline for maintenance treatment. Oral isotretinoin has been used for patients with severe cases unresponsive to the previously described treatments.

Senile Purpura

Senile purpura is a black-blue discoloration that appears primarily on the extensor surface of the hands and forearms. Thinning and loss of sub-

cutaneous connective tissue with age results in increased fragility of the skin. This leads to spontaneous rupture of subcutaneous blood vessels. No treatment is required. Patients need to be reassured that senile purpura is a benign process and that the lesion will heal spontaneously.

Drug Eruptions

Drug eruptions are common in the elderly population and can mimic the appearance of many other disorders. They can vary in severity from mild (exanthematous reactions, fixed drug reactions) to life-threatening (acute hypersensitivity reactions with anaphylaxis, Stevens-Johnson syndrome/toxic epidermal necrolysis). The same drug can have the ability of causing different types of reactions.

The pathophysiology of drug eruptions varies. Some are due to immediate-type hypersensitivity reactions (urticarial reactions). The patient can have an immediate reaction if they have been exposed to the offending drug in the past, or they can have a delayed reaction as they become sensitized to a medication during it's administration over a period of time. Drug eruptions can also occur on the basis of cell-mediated responses or deposition of immune complexes (serum sickness or vasculitis). In some drug reactions, the etiology is unknown.

SYNDROMES TO CONSIDER

Table 18-6 lists the common categories of drug eruptions by their appearance. Drugs that are commonly implicated in drug eruptions are listed in Table 18-7.

EXANTHEMATOUS DRUG REACTIONS Exanthematous drug reactions are also called morbilliform drug or maculopapular drug reactions. They are a type of hypersensitivity drug reaction. The patient becomes sensitized to the drug either through previous exposure or during the course of taking the medication. Reactions can either be early, occurring within days of exposure to the offending agent, or late, occurring days to several weeks after exposure to the sensitizing drug.

Exanthematous drug reaction can be the initial presentation of more serious conditions such as Stevens-Johnson syndrome. In this syndrome, patients can initially present with a flu-like illness including fever. Next, the patient develops generalized lesions on the skin and mucous membranes. The patient eventually experiences desquamation with loss of the epidermis. There can be involvement of the kidneys, gastrointestinal tract, and lungs.

Table 18-6

Common Types of Drug Eruptions/Categories of Drug Eruptions

CATEGORY	DISTRIBUTION	APPEARANCE	COMMENTS
Morbilliform, exanthematous	Symmetric, generalized	Red, macular and/or papular	Most common type of drug reaction
Drug-induced acute urticarial/ angioedema	Localized, regional, generalized	Wheals, urticaria, swelling in deep dermal structures (most pronounced on face, tongue)	Urticaria are transient, recurrent; May be accompanied by life-threatening anaphylactic reaction
Drug hypersensitivity syndrome	Symmetric, generalized	Red, macular and/or papular	Differentiated from exanthematous by its late onset (weeks after exposure) and systemic involvement
Fixed drug eruption	Localized (most common), generalized (randomly distributed)	Macules (most common), plaque, bulla, erosion	If rechallenged with offending drug, rash returns in same location as first reaction
Erythema multiforme (EM), Stevens-Johnson syndrome (SJS), Toxic epidermal necrolysis (TEN)	EM: localized, generalized SJS/TEN: generalized	EM: target lesions SJS/TEN: loss of epidermis	SJS/TEN: initially may have appearance of other drug reactions; may be life-threatening

Table 18-7

Drugs Commonly Implicated in Drug Eruptions

Antibiotics	ACE inhibitiors	Other
Sulfonamides	Calcium channel blockers	Radiographic contrast dye
Amoxicillin	Quinine	Allopurinol
Nitrofurantoin	Quinidine	Barbiturates
Analgesics	Antiseizure	Benzodiazepines
NSAIDs	Carbamazepine	Phenothiazines
Cardiovascular	Phenytoin	Gold salts

Figure 18-17   (Plate 15)

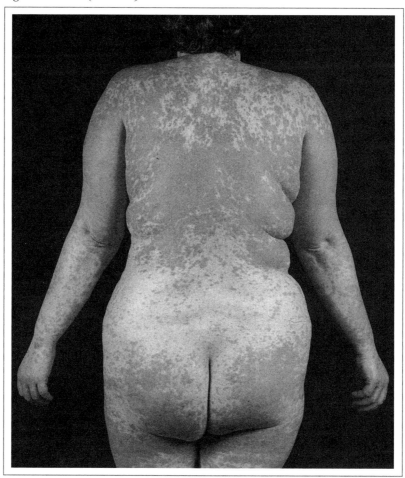

Exanthematous drug eruption: ampicillin. Symmetrically arranged, brightly erythematous macules and papules, discrete in some areas and confluent in others, on the back and extremities.

Starting as macules or papules, exanthematous drug eruptions can become more extensive, with confluence of the rash (Fig. 18-17). The trunk and extremities are almost always involved. The rash can become exfoliative, with desquamation developing during the healing phase.

DRUG-INDUCED ACUTE URTICARIA Urticaria or hives can result from an IgE-mediated immediate hypersensitivity reaction or an immune complex–mediated reaction (Fig. 18-18). It can be associated with a more severe systemic reaction such as anaphylaxis and vascular collapse.

The patient can complain of pruritis. If there is airway involvement, the patient can complain of shortness of breath and wheezing. If angioedema is present, the patient will complain of swelling of the face and/or tongue. If anaphylaxis is present, the patient can complain of wheezing and shortness of breath or can lose consciousness.

DRUG HYPERSENSITIVITY SYNDROME Drug hypersensitivity syndrome (DHS) has several distinguishing characteristics from an erythematous drug eruption. DHS (Fig. 18-19) usually starts weeks after exposure to the offending agent. DHS is a systemic reaction, and in addition to the rash, patients can present with fever, arthralgias, or

Figure 18-18   (Plate 16)

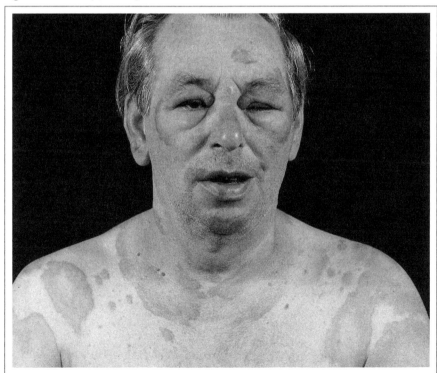

Drug-induced urticaria: penicillin. Large, urticarial wheals on the face, neck, and trunk, with angioedema in the periorbital region.

Figure 18-19   (Plate 17)

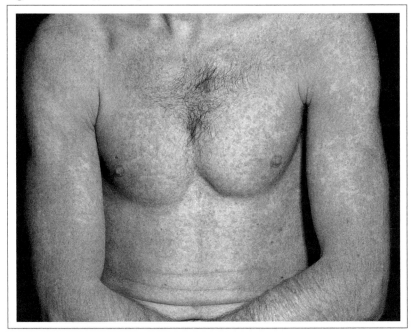

Drug hypersensitivity syndrome: phenytoin. Symmetric, bright-red, exanthematous eruption, confluent in some sites; the patient had associated lymphadenopathy.

lymphadenopathy. This condition can be difficult to diagnose. Eosinophilia or elevation of liver enzymes can help establish the diagnosis.

FIXED DRUG ERUPTION   Fixed drug eruptions can present as a single, localized skin lesion or a generalized rash (Fig. 18-20). If the patient has taken the offending medication in the past, they may relate that the skin lesion(s) is in the same location as during the previous reaction.

ERYTHEMA MULTIFORME/STEVENS-JOHNSON SYNDROME/ TOXIC EPIDERMAL NECROLYSIS   Erythema multiforme (EM) can be present in a variety of forms from mild to severe. The most severe form is the Stevens-

Johnson syndrome. EM can also be caused by infections such as herpes simplex and mycoplasma. The classic appearance of EM is an oval or round erythematous lesion with central clearing (target lesion), although EM can also present as macules, vesicles, or bullae. EM can be localized or generalized and symmetric. (Fig. 18-21).

PATIENT SYMPTOMS

Drug eruptions can be mild, causing no or few symptoms (pruritis, discomfort, and mucous membrane ulcerations), to severe and life-threatening (shortness of breath, wheezing, hypotension, and extensive skin exfoliation).

PHYSICAL EXAMINATION

Table 18-6 lists the classical skin manifestations and distribution of the different types of drug eruptions.

TREATMENT

The treatment for all drug eruptions is to remove the offending agent. Occasionally, the patient may be taking multiple medications that could cause drug eruptions. In this case, all potential offending drugs should be discontinued. This can require substituting medications of equal therapeutic benefit.

Avoiding the offending medication will prevent recurrent, and potentially more severe, reactions.

Symptoms of pruritis can be treated with an antihistamine. Topical corticosteroids are not indicated in the treatment of drug eruptions. Oral corticosteroids should be avoided in patients with mild reactions.

Severe reactions can require immediate treatment (anaphylaxis, bronchospasm) and possibly hospitalization. Systemic corticosteroids, adrenergic agents, inhaled bronchodilators, and parenteral antihistamines are often required to treat severe drug reactions.

Figure 18-20   (Plate 18)

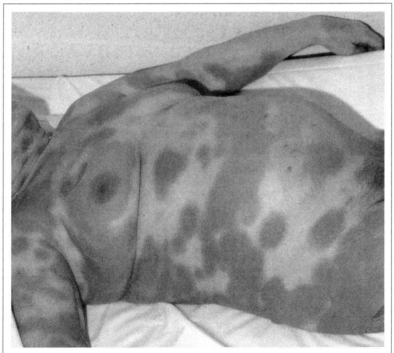

Generalized fixed drug eruption: tetracycline. Multiple, confluent, violaceous-red, oval erythematous areas, some of which later became bullous. The eruption may be difficult to distinguish from toxic epidermal necrolysis.

Figure 18-21   (Plates 19 and 20)

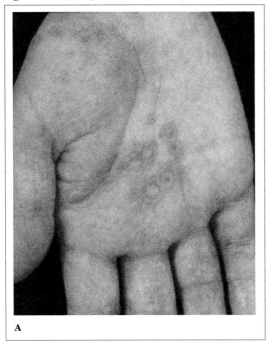

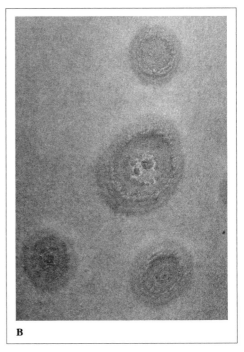

Erythema multiforme minor. **(A)** Papular, urticarial, and vesicular target lesions in acral distribution. **(B)** Herpes iris of Bateman. *(Courtesy of Dr. K. Wolff.)*

Bibliography

Elewski BE: Once-weekly fluconazole in the treatment of onychomycosis: introductions. *J Am Acad Dermatol* 38:S73, 1998.

Feldman SR, Fleischer AB Jr, McConnell RC: Most common dermatologic problems identified by internists, 1990–1994. *Arch Intern Med* 158:726, 1998.

Fitzpatrick TB, Eisen AZ, Wolff K, et al: *Dermatology in General Medicine*, 4th ed. New York: McGraw-Hill; 1993.

Fitzpatrick TB, Johnson RA, Wolff K, et al: Color Atlas and Synopsis of Clinical Dermatology. *Common and Serious Diseases*, 3rd ed. New York: McGraw-Hill; 1997.

Fleischer AB Jr, Feldman SR, McConnell RC: The most common dermatologic problems identified by family physicians, 1990–1994. *Fam Med* 29:648, 1997.

Jackson JL, Gibbons R, Meyer G, et al: The effect of treating herpes zoster with oral acyclovir in preventing postherpetic neuralgia: a meta-analysis. *Arch Int Med* 157:909, 1997.

Kaminer MS, Gilchrest BA: Aging of the skin. In: Hazzard WR, Blass JP, Ettinger WH Jr., et al (eds): *Principles of Geriatric Medicine and Gerontology.* New York: McGraw-Hill, 1999; 573–590.

Levit E, Scher R: Onychomycosis: avoiding indefinite, improper management. *Patient Care* 33:197, 1999.

Lubeck DP: Measuring health-related quality of life in onychomycosis. *J Am Acad Dermatol* 38:S64, 1998.

Maibach HI, Sadick NS, Webster C: A practical approach to managing dermatitis. *Patient Care* 33:65, 1999.

Rowbotham M, Harden N, Stacey B, et al: Gabapentin for the treatment of postherpetic neuralgia: a randomized controlled trial. *JAMA* 280:1837, 1998.

Volmink J, Lancaster T, Gray S, et al: Treatments for postherpetic neuralgia: a systematic review of randomized controlled trials. *Fam Practice* 13:84, 1996.

Aubrey L. Knight

Skin Ulcers

Overview: How Common Are Skin Ulcers?

Identification and management of skin ulcers is a common and challenging problem. Most patients with chronic ulcers are older and have multiple chronic medical problems, making wound prevention and therapy for the skin condition difficult. The three most common chronic ulcers encountered among the geriatric population are pressure ulcers, chronic venous and arterial leg ulcers, and diabetic neuropathic ulcers. All of these wounds are encountered in the office and in long-term care settings. Pressure ulcers of stage II or greater occur among 5 to 29.5 percent of hospitalized patients, 2 to 23 percent of long-term care patients, and 8.7 to 20 percent of patients in home care. Diabetic neuropathic ulcers are encountered among 15 percent of patients with diabetes and account for 6 to 20 percent of all hospitalizations of persons with diabetes.

Principal Diagnoses

Multiple studies of chronic leg ulcers show that 60 to 80 percent have a venous component, 10 to 30 percent an arterial component, and 10 to 20 percent have combined arterial and venous components. Chronic venous and arterial ulcers are difficult to heal, and if they heal, they recur at a rate in excess of 60 percent. Other less common chronic skin wounds include pyoderma gangrenosum, vasculitis, squamous cell carcinoma, basal cell carcinoma, and several cutaneous infectious diseases (Table 19-1). Of these, pyoderma gangrenosum warrents particular attention in the care of older patients.

Table 19-1
Causes of Chronic Skin Ulcers

Vascular
Venous stasis
Arterial
Vasculitis
Thromboangiitis obliterans
Neoplastic
Squamous cell
Basal cell
Mycosis fungoides
Kaposi's sarcoma
Infectious
Deep fungal (histoplasmosis, cryptococcosis)
Bacterial (diphtheria, anthrax, tularemia)
Mycobacterial
Sexually transmitted (syphilis, chancroid)
Viral (herpes)
Protozoal (leishmaniasis, amebiasis)
Miscellaneous
Neuropathic diabetic ulcer
Pressure ulcer
Pyoderma gangrenosum
Trauma
Bites (brown recluse spider)

Pressure Ulcers

Pressure ulcers are the visible evidence of pathologic changes in the blood supply of the dermis. The incidence of pressure ulcers is greatest among patients with spinal cord injuries or cerebrovascular disease and among the bedbound elderly population. Among patients with spinal cord injuries, lack of mobility and loss of vasomotor tone contribute to the high incidence of pressure ulceration. Eight percent of deaths in spinal cord injury hospitals are attributed to pressure ulcers.

Among elderly patients, the skin changes of aging are the primary predisposing factor to the development of pressure ulcers. With aging there are decreases in the blood supply to the skin, a flattening of the epithelial layers, decreases in the subcutaneous fat, and decreases in the cutaneous skin sensitivity. Other factors that contribute to the likelihood of development of pressure sores include debility, volume depletion, increases or decreases in body weight, anemia, renal insufficiency, malignant disease, sedation, major surgery, nutritional and vitamin deficiencies, and various metabolic disorders. Elder abuse and neglect should be considered when pressure ulcers are encountered, particularly if multiple or repeated pressure ulcers develop without other explanation.

LOCATION

Pressure ulcers develop in focal areas over bony prominences. Ninety percent of the wounds occur on the lower half of the body. The sacrum, ischial tuberosities, greater trochanter, and heels are the most likely locations. Pressure ulcers may, however, occur over any bony prominence, including elbows, occiput, scapulae, and spinous processes.

MECHANISMS

Four major etiologic mechanisms are involved in the development of pressure ulcers: pressure, friction, shearing forces, and moisture. Pressure is concentrated wherever weight-bearing areas come in contact with surfaces. There is an inverse relation between amount of pressure and time. Pressure must be applied before skin damage occurs. Relief of pressure before the occurrence of irreversible tissue damage is the goal for patients at risk of pressure ulcers. Studies with animals as subjects have demonstrated that ischemic histologic changes in the muscle occur after 2 h of external pressure. This finding forms the basis for the practice of turning patients who cannot turn themselves every 2 h.

Friction is the force created when two surfaces move across each other, as would occur when maneuvering a patient in the bed. Friction leads to injury to the epidermal layers of the skin, which is particularly vulnerable among the elderly.

Shearing forces are caused by the sliding of adjacent surfaces. Shearing compromises capillary flow. The subcutaneous layer is particularly vulnerable to the effects of shearing forces. Elevation of the head of the bed by more than 30 degrees produces shear in the sacral and coccygeal regions.

Moisture, resulting in skin maceration, increases the risk of skin breakdown. It most often is caused by urinary incontinence or perspiration.

Venous Stasis Ulcers

Venous stasis ulceration occurs in the setting of venous insufficiency followed by edema. Venous insufficiency occurs when venous return in the veins of the lower extremity is impaired by venous valve dysfunction or venous dilatation. Deep venous thrombosis is a common precursor to these venous changes. As a result of valve dysfunction and venous dilatation, blood pools in the deep venous system. The pooling causes venous hypertension and dilatation of the perforating and superficial veins. The largest perforators are at the malleoli, where stasis dermatitis and ulceration are most prevalent.

Before there is frank ulceration, stasis dermatitis occurs. Stasis dermatitis is an eczematous skin eruption. Venous stasis and ulceration do not occur among all patients with venous insufficiency, suggesting that other, unknown factors have a role. Before ulceration develops there can be acute or chronic inflammation of the skin. Acute inflammation can occur during the winter as a result of skin dryness and scratching or as a sudden appearance of an eczematous eruption resembling cellulitis. In either case, weeping and crusting can result, predisposing the patient to ulceration. Recurrent bouts of acute inflammation in poorly vascularized areas cause chronic skin and subcutaneous changes. The skin becomes fibrotic and thickened with postinflammatory hyperpigmentation. Despite the skin thickening and as a result of poor vascularity, skin with chronic venous stasis inflammation has a higher likehood of ulceration.

Arterial Ulcers

Arterial ulceration is caused by atherosclerosis of the limb vessel leading to decreased oxygenation and ischemia of the skin. Ischemia can develop acutely because of embolus or thrombus or chronically because of effects of decreased blood flow from peripheral vascular atherosclerosis.

Neuropathic Diabetic Ulcers

Diabetic ulceration is the result of diabetic neuropathy and vascular insufficiency. These ulcerations tend to occur on the plantar aspect of the foot but can occur elsewhere in the lower extremities. Vascular disease with diminished blood supply and repetitive trauma without appropriate pain sensation cause skin damage and impaired healing. Other factors include ill-fitting shoes and foot deformities caused by simultaneous motor weakness of the flexor and extensor muscles and proprioceptive defects.

Other Ulcers

Of the many skin conditions that can cause ulceration, pyoderma gangrenosum is worthy of consideration in the care of older patients. Pyoderma gangrenosum is deep, undermined ulcers that develop in the lower extremities of patients with inflammatory bowel disease or rheumatoid arthritis. The pathogenesis is unclear, but because the ulcers tend to occur when the inflammatory bowel disease or arthritis is active, immunologic or vasculitic factors are likely. Control of the underlying disease is associated with better healing of the skin wounds than is local treatment of the wound.

Typical Presentation

The patient's history and symptoms can assist in determining the exact cause of chronic skin wounds. For example, a patient with long-standing diabetes who has an ulcer on a lower extremity may have venous ulcers or neuropathic ulcers. Ulcers that occur over bony prominences, especially among patients at risk, are considered pressure ulcers. If these ulcers then do not heal with relief of the pressure and appropriate attention to the sore, a biopsy should be performed to rule out other conditions, including cancer.

Ulcers that begin as minor trauma or as small pustules may represent pyoderma gangrenosum or the bite of a brown recluse spider. An ulcer that has substantial surrounding edema likely represents venous ulceration. A history of trauma, frequently very minor trauma, often accompanies venous ulceration.

An ulcer in the lower extremity accompanied by pain may be an arterial or venous ulcer. Venous ulcers often cause dull, constant pain that is relieved with elevation of the extremity. The more intense pain of arterial ulceration does not improve and is sometimes made worse with elevation. A painful ulcer that develops in a patient with ulcerative colitis, regional enteritis, uveitis, or rheumatoid arthritis may represent pyoderma gangrenosum.

Physical Examination

The physical examination should focus on the wound and the surrounding areas. Patients with skin ulcers frequently have comorbidities; a complete examination is advisable. The clinician should focus on examining the cardiovascular and musculoskeletal systems. When examining the extremities of patients with chronic leg ulcers, assessing of joint mobility is helpful in determining the best mode of treatment. The appearance of the extremity should be described, including the presence of varicosities and abnormal pigmentation. Varicosities and abnormal pigmentation suggest venous insufficiency. The presence of peripheral pulses also should be documented. The absence of posterior tibial and dorsalis pedis pulses suggests but does not confirm peripheral vascular disease. Pulses may be difficult to palpate, especially in the presence of peripheral edema.

The location of the ulcer is the first and often the most important clue in determining the cause of a chronic wound. Ulceration caused by chronic venous insufficiency usually occurs on the medial aspects of the ankles. Pressure ulcers occur over bony prominences. The most common locations of pressure ulcers are the sacrum, heels, ankles, and greater trochanters and ischial tuberosities. Neuropathic diabetic ulcers typically are plantar and occur at the points where weight bearing is greatest. Arterial ulcers are located primarily on the toes and pretibial areas. Pyoderma gangrenosum almost always occurs on the lower extremities. Characteristics of the wounds also assist in determining the cause.

The ulcer should be fully described in the medical record. The exact location and morphologic characteristics of the ulcer should be documented. The ulcer should be measured serially and documented. As described later, the ulcer edge can indicate the type of ulcer and progress with healing. Important characteristics of the wound edge include whether it is a rolling or jagged edge, the depth at the edge, and the presence of epithelialization at the edge. The ulcer base should be assessed as to the presence or absence of granulation or necrotic tissue.

Pressure Ulcers

The clinical appearance of a pressure ulcer varies and depends on the extent of damage to skin and underlying tissue. The most widely used staging scheme divides pressure ulcers into four categories. This is an adaptation of the Shea classification scheme that was modified in 1989 by the National Pressure Ulcer Advisory Panel and adopted by the Agency for Health Care Policy and Research (AHCPR) Pressure Ulcer Guideline Panels and published in the AHCPR Clinical Practice Guidelines for Pressure Ulcers.

A stage I pressure ulcer is an acute inflammatory response in the layers of the skin. A stage I pressure ulcer manifests as a well-defined area of soft-tissue swelling and erythema over a bony prominence. The skin remains intact. The classic description of a stage I pressure ulcer is nonblanchable erythema.

A stage II pressure ulcer (Fig. 19-1) is an extension of the inflammatory response that manifests as an abrasion, shallow crater, or blister in the skin. This can involve the epidermis, dermis, or both but does not extend beyond the dermis. There is often surrounding erythema or induration.

A stage III pressure ulcer is an inflammatory response that progresses into the subcutaneous layers and represents full-thickness skin loss. There is often a rolling edge. One finds an irregular, full-thickness ulcer extending into the subcutaneous tissue surrounded by erythema and induration. There is often a draining, necrotic base. The damage does not extend through the fascia, but undermining of adjacent tissue may be present.

A stage IV pressure ulcer (Fig. 19-2) penetrates the deep fascia, eliminating the last barrier to extensive spread. Stage IV ulcers can involve the muscle, bone, and other supporting structures. Stage IV pressure ulcers may lead to osteomyelitis or septic arthritis.

Venous Stasis Ulcers

Venous ulcers (Fig. 19-3) can be deep or superficial and often have a sharp border. The surrounding tissue is often edematous and erythematous. The chronic changes of venous insufficiency cause the affected skin to have a firm, woody quality. There

Figure 19-1   (Plate 21)

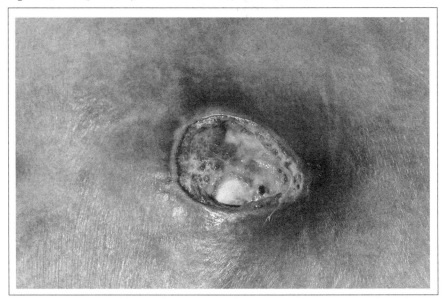

Stage II pressure ulcer.

Figure 19-2   (Plate 22)

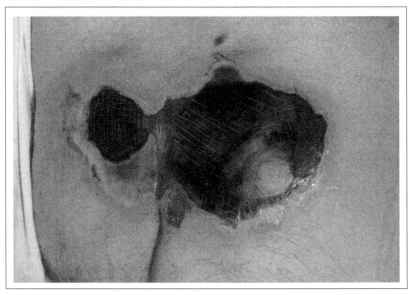

Stage IV pressure ulcer.

Figure 19-3   (Plate 23)

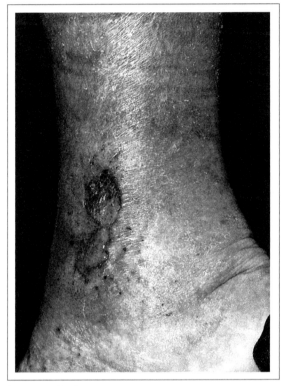

Venous stasis ulcer.

Figure 19-4   (Plate 24)

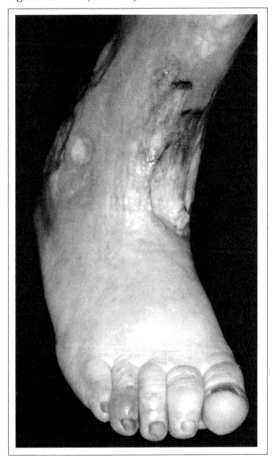

Arterial ulcer.

often is brown staining of the skin that represents hemosiderin. It occurs when red blood cells leak out of the surrounding veins.

Arterial Ulcers

Arterial ulcers (Fig. 19-4) tend to have a punched-out appearance with a gray base. These ulcers are frequently deep, and fascia, tendon, periosteum or bone may be visible in the wound. The surrounding skin is often cold and atrophic.

Neuropathic Diabetic Ulcers

Neuropathic diabetic ulcers often are deep and are surrounded by hyperkeratotic skin. Altered motor nerve function leads to muscle atrophy,

tendon shortening, and foot deformities. These deformities and poorly fitting shoes cause callus formation over pressure points. Trauma to the calluses or fissuring of the callus often begins the process of ulcer formation.

Other Types of Ulcers

An ulcer with bluish overhanging edges and extensive necrosis at the edges suggests pyoderma gangrenosum. Pyoderma gangrenosum also is associated with considerable undermining. Ulcers arising in nodules, particularly in locations other than the lower extremities, are suggestive of primary cancers of the skin or metastasis to the skin. Other causes of nodular ulcers include primary syphilis, primary tuberculosis, sporotrichosis, coccidioidomycosis, and leishmaniasis.

Ancillary Tests

No specific laboratory tests are necessary in the evaluation of skin ulcers. However, several tests can be useful in selected circumstances. These include skin biopsy, cultures, tests for osteoporosis, and tests of arterial circulation.

Biopsy

When there is confusion about the diagnosis or when the location of the wound is not consistent with the major types of wounds, a skin biopsy with pathology review should be performed. If there is deterioration or a lack of progression after 12 weeks, wound biopsy should be performed.

Cultures

Wound cultures are used only to assist in the selection of appropriate antibiotics. Wound cultures should not be obtained routinely because colonization is common and is not associated with delayed healing. Wound cultures should be obtained only when local or systemic infection is suspected. The AHCPR Pressure Ulcer Guideline suggests that quantitative cultures be obtained when pressure ulcers are not responding to appropriate care.

Tests for Osteomyelitis

When osteomyelitis is suspected, especially in neuropathic diabetic ulcers, timely diagnosis is both important and challenging. The standard of care is pathologic examination of the bone. Lewis

et al recommend a combination of radiograph, white blood cell count, and erythrocyte sedimentation rate for the diagnosis of osteomyelitis. If all results are positive, there is a 69 percent positive predictive value. Grayson et al recommend probing for bone during initial examination of a person with diabetes who has a pedal ulcer. In their study, there was a 66 percent sensitivity and an 89 percent positive predictive value for osteomyelitis when bone was palpated and probed. Bone scans and white blood cell–labeled nuclear scans are helpful, but the findings can be confusing in the presence of infection or inflammation of the surrounding skin.

Tests of Arterial Circulation

When patients have chronic leg ulcers that do not fit the criteria for pressure ulcers and pulses cannot be felt, the clinician should assess the arterial system with a handheld Doppler device. The ankle-brachial pressure index (ABPI) of both lower extremities is the most reliable test to detect arterial insufficiency. Patients with an ABPI of 0.8 or less should be assumed to have arterial disease. ABPI is not helpful in the diagnosis of microvascular disease. Ancillary tests such as arteriography and Doppler plethysmography are helpful in certain clinical situations. Arteriography can assist in delineating the extent of arterial disease and determining whether revascularization surgery might be beneficial in the healing of chronic arterial ulceration. Doppler ultrasonography can be used to identify the presence of venous thrombosis or sites of valvar incompetence. Duplex ultrasonography allows direct visualization of the venous system of the lower extremity and can help identify flow through the venous valves.

Other Tests

The presence of a chronic ulcer can be the first indication of a systemic illness. Blood glucose level should be measured for patients who are not known to have diabetes but have a wound that could be a neuropathic diabetic ulcer. Erythrocyte sedimentation rate should be measured for patients with an ulcer that could be pyoderma gangrenosum, especially if accompanied by weight loss and diarrhea or hematochezia.

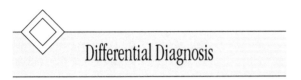

Differential Diagnosis

Although pressure ulcers, venous ulcers, and diabetic ulcers are the most common skin ulcers,

there are other considerations when skin ulcers are encountered. The use of an algorithm can guide the clinician in determining the cause of skin ulcers (Fig. 19-5). Injury from frostbite, burns, or cutaneous trauma can cause skin ulcers. Infections such as cutaneous leishmaniasis, syphilis, cutaneous diphtheria, tuberculosis, and anthrax can cause chronic skin wounds, usually associated with regional lymphadenopathy.

Isolated noduloulcerative lesions may be encountered with such deep fungal diseases as sporotrichosis, coccidioidomycosis, histoplasmosis, and cryptococcosis. The diagnosis is best confirmed with culture or biopsy at the edge of the

Figure 19-5

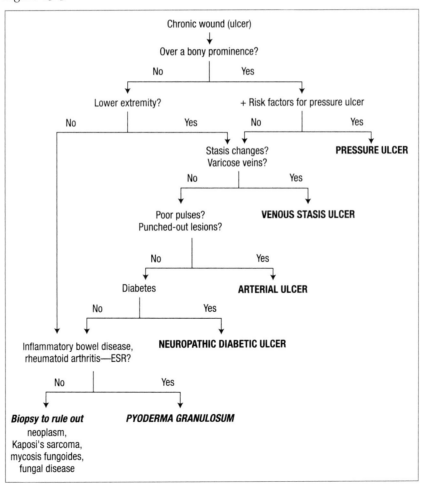

Differential diagnosis algorithm.

lesion. The cutaneous ulcers of deep fungal diseases are more likely encountered among patients who are immunocompromised.

Patients with severe obliterative peripheral arterial disease and types of vasculitis such as systemic lupus erythematosus and Raynaud's phenomenon may have ulceration due to tissue infarction. Ulceration of the lower extremities also can occur with sickle cell anemia, thalassemia, and hereditary spherocytosis. Other conditions that cause neuropathic ulcers similar to those of diabetes are tabes dorsalis, leprosy, and hereditary sensory radicular neuropathy.

Pyoderma granulosum is an indolent ulcer with necrotic edges that frequently occurs among patients with ulcerative colitis or regional enteritis. The development and healing of these lesions often parallels the activity of the associated disease.

Chronic, nonhealing ulcers, especially with unusual shapes, may be a manifestation of abuse, either by caregivers or representing self-abuse. These lesions are most often caused by lighted cigarettes or acid.

Patients with advanced mycosis fungoides can have deep skin ulcers due to destruction by T-cell lymphocytes. Skin ulceration usually occurs in the terminal stage of this condition.

Biopsy to rule out cancer should be performed on any nonhealing ulcer, especially if the location and clinical features are not those of venous ulceration, pressure ulceration, or diabetic ulcer. Skin cancers such as basal cell carcinoma, squamous cell carcinoma, or Kaposi's sarcoma can manifest as a nonhealing skin ulcer.

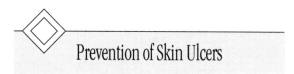

Prevention of Skin Ulcers

Once a skin ulcer develops, regardless of the type, treatment can be difficult. For this reason, prevention of ulceration is important.

Pressure Ulcers

As many as 95 percent of pressure ulcers are preventable. Prevention should be a priority for caregivers and health care providers when caring for persons at risk of pressure ulcers. The strategy for prevention includes recognizing the risk, decreasing the effects of pressure, improving nutritional status, and preserving the integrity of the skin. In long-term care, pressure ulcers are used as an indicator of quality of care. The development of a pressure ulcer is not always, however, the result of poor nursing care.

Several assessment tools are designed to quantify the risk of pressure ulcer (Fig. 19-6). Once patients are deemed at high risk of pressure ulcers, measures should be undertaken to protect the skin. Repositioning bedbound patients at least every 2 h is essential in preventing ulcers. Patients being repositioned should be lifted, not dragged or slid, from a bed or wheelchair to avoid friction and damage to the epidermis. At the time of repositioning, the skin should be evaluated for nonblanchable erythema or skin breakdown.

Routine skin care should include keeping the skin clean and free of stool, urine, and moisture. Special pads and beds are available and are intended to alter the pressure exerted on bony prominences. Table 19-2 lists support surfaces and characteristics. Smaller support surfaces such as gel pads, foam cushions, and sheepskin pads are practical for use in specific areas.

Special beds and mattresses aid in the preventing and management of pressure ulcers. These beds tend to use air or buoyancy to keep the patient's weight evenly distributed. Such devices, although helpful in certain circumstances, should not be relied on as a substitute for basic nursing care.

Venous Stasis Ulcers

Venous stasis is a pathophysiologic process in the development of venous ulceration. Patients such as those with varicose veins or a history of venous thrombosis are at particular risk of the chronic skin changes that predispose one to venous ulceration. These patients and those with known venous disease should be encouraged to exercise and when not active to keep the lower extremities elevated. Exercise and elevation protect the microvascular system of the skin of the lower legs by stimulating emptying of the veins. Wearing support stockings or bandages can facilitate the effect of exercise. Support stockings are worn during the day when the legs are dependent and removed at night when the patient is asleep. Losing weight and stopping smoking can be important in preventing venous ulceration. Persons with venous stasis changes should be especially careful to avoid trauma to the lower extremities, as trauma nearly always precedes skin breakdown among susceptible persons. Diuretics can be prescribed to decrease peripheral edema when conservative measures fail.

Arterial Ulcers

Prevention of arterial ulcers involves recognition of the risk and minimizing risk factors, including smoking. There is no evidence that the use of pentoxifylline or antiplatelet agents can prevent the development of arterial ulcers. Revascularization should be considered when appropriate. Patients with poor arterial circulation should practice aggressive attention to skin care.

Neuropathic Diabetic Ulcers

The most important factor in preventing neuropathic diabetic ulcers is good glycemic control. Proper foot care also is important. Patients with diabetes should be instructed on proper examination and identification of changes in the feet. The clinician should examine the feet completely at least once a year. Feet should be kept clean and dry at all times. Shoes should fit properly, and patients with diabetic neuropathy should not walk barefoot. Patients should inspect their feet frequently for calluses, blisters, and abrasions and consult a physician when there are abnormalities.

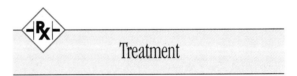

Treatment

The overall goal of treatment is to create an environment that enhances soft-tissue viability and promotes wound healing. In most cases this

Table 19-2
Characteristics for Classes of Support Surfaces

PERFORMANCE CHARACTERISTIC	SUPPORT SURFACE				
	AIR FLUIDIZED	LOW AIR LOSS	STATIC FLOTATION	FOAM	STANDARD MATTRESS
Increased support area	Yes	Yes	Yes	Yes	No
Low moisture retention	Yes	Yes	No	No	No
Reduced heat accumulation	Yes	Yes	No	No	No
Shear reduction	Yes	?	Yes	No	No
Pressure reduction	Yes	Yes	Yes	Yes	No
Dynamic	Yes	Yes	No	No	No
Cost	High	High	Low	Low	Low

SOURCE: Adapted from Bergstrom N, Bennett MA, Carlson CE: *Treatment of Pressure Ulcers*. Clinical Practice Guideline, No. 15. AHCPR publication No. 95-0652, Rockville, MD, US Department of Health and Human Services, Public Health Service, Agency for Healthcare Policy and Research, 1994.

involves removing devitalized tissue and instituting measures aimed at restoring blood supply to the affected area, cleaning and disinfecting the wound, and improving the overall health of the patient. Referral to a dermatologist or surgeon often is necessary. Table 19-3 lists the indications for referral for the different types of skin ulcers.

Pressure Ulcers

Effective therapy for pressure ulcers is best accomplished with a team approach. The first step is assessment of the patient and of the ulcer, because treatment varies with the extent of the ulcer. Assessing the patient involves evaluating overall health and nutrition. In assessing overall health, the clinician looks for risk factors that make healing difficult. The psychosocial state of the patient and family are assessed to assure that the environment is conducive to carrying out the prescribed treatment plan.

NUTRITIONAL ASSESSMENT

Assessment of the nutritional state involves taking a diet history and assessing the ability to achieve an adequate intake (Chap. 16). Anthropometric measurements and laboratory studies such as serum albumin are helpful in assessing the nutritional state. A serum albumin level less than 3.5 g/dL is an indication of malnutrition. The nutritional needs of patients with pressure ulcers are 30 to 35 kcal/kg per day and up to 2 g of protein per kilogram per day. This may have to be modi-

fied for patients with renal insufficiency. When there is evidence of inadequate dietary intake, nutritional support with oral nutritional supplements should be instituted. Every effort should be made to encourage achieving nutritional adequacy orally, but if this means of dietary supplementation is not feasible or successful, nutritional support with tube feedings or total parenteral nutrition (TPN) may be necessary. When possible, the gastrointestinal tract should be used, and TPN should be reserved for patients who are nutritionally depleted and who cannot tolerate gastrointestinal feedings. TPN should be considered carefully because it is not always appropriate for debilitated patients or those with terminal illnesses.

ULCER ASSESSMENT

Assessment of the ulcers should be systematic. The location, size including depth, and presence of undermining, exudate, or necrosis should be recorded. The best way to document assessment and change over time is with the use of an assessment guide. Fig. 19-6 is a sample pressure ulcer assessment guide and is available in the AHCPR Clinical Practice Guideline for pressure ulcer treatment. Whether in the hospital, long-term care, or a home health setting, the patient and the pressure ulcer should receive periodic and regular assessment.

The major etiologic factor in the development and progression of pressure ulcers is prolonged direct pressure. Measures should be undertaken to reduce the pressure and forces on the tissue. The distribution of pressure, friction, and shear on the

Table 19-3

Specialty Referral in Skin Ulcers

WOUND TYPE	INDICATION FOR REFERRAL	TIMING OF REFERRAL	TYPE OF SPECIALIST
Pressure ulcer	Stage III or IV; clean	Late	Plastic surgeon
Venous ulcer	Refractory	Late	Plastic surgeon
	Superficial venous disease	Early	Vascular surgeon
Arterial ulcer	Occlusive arterial disease	Early	Vascular surgeon
Pyoderma gangrenosum	Diagnostic uncertainty	Early	Dermatologist

Figure 19-6   Pressure ulcer assessment guide.

Patient Name: _____ **Date:** _____ **Time:** _____

Ulcer 1:			
Site_____			
Stage[a]			
Size (cm)			
Length_____			
Width_____			
Depth_____			

Ulcer 1:
Site_____
Stage[a]
Size (cm)
  Length_____
  Width_____
  Depth_____

	No	Yes
Sinus tract	___	___
Tunneling	___	___
Undermining	___	___
Necrotic tissue	___	___
Slough	___	___
Eschar	___	___
Exudate	___	___
Serous	___	___
Serosanguineous	___	___
Purulent	___	___
Granulation	___	___
Epithelialization	___	___
Pain	___	___
Surrounding skin:	___	___
Erythema	___	___
Maceration	___	___
Induration	___	___

Ulcer 2:
Site_____
Stage[a]
Size (cm)
  Length_____
  Width_____
  Depth_____

	No	Yes
Sinus tract	___	___
Tunneling	___	___
Undermining	___	___
Necrotic tissue	___	___
Slough	___	___
Eschar	___	___
Exudate	___	___
Serous	___	___
Serosanguineous	___	___
Purulent	___	___
Granulation	___	___
Epithelialization	___	___
Pain	___	___
Surrounding skin:	___	___
Erythema	___	___
Maceration	___	___
Induration	___	___

Description of ulcer(s):

_____

_____

Indicate Ulcer Sites:

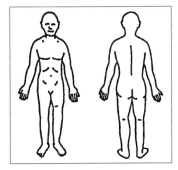

Anterior   Posterior
(Attach a color photo of the
pressure ulcer[s] [Optional]).

[a]Classification of pressure ulcers:
Stage I: Nonblanchable erythema of intact skin, the heralding lesion of
skin ulceration. In individuals with darker skin, discoloration of
the skin, warmth, edema, induration, or hardness may also be
indicators.
State II: Partial-thickness skin loss involving epidermis, dermis, or both.
Stage III: Full-thickness skin loss involving damage to or necrosis of
subcutaneous tissue that may extend down to, but not through,
underlying fascia. The ulcer presents clinically as a deep crater
with or without undermining adjacent tissue.
Stage IV: Full-thickness skin loss with extensive destruction, tissue
necrosis, or damage to muscle, bone, or supporting structures
(e.g., tendon or joint capsule).

affected tissue is called *tissue load*. All direct interventions should be directed at reducing the magnitude of tissue load so that there is support of tissue healing. As is true with prevention of pressure ulcers among patients at risk, the most expedient means of reducing pressure is frequent turning. Especially when patients need total assistance with turning, this becomes a difficult and expensive nursing intervention. Pressure-reducing devices have been developed as a result of the lack of success with adherence to turning schedules. These devices can be categorized as *static* or *dynamic*. Static devices include foam bed overlays, air mattresses, and foam or gel pads. Dynamic devices are devices whereby alternating pressure promotes equalization of pressure over the entire body surface.

Factors besides pressure, friction, and shear should be controlled. Patients should be encouraged to be as mobile as possible. Pain, altered mental state, medications, and significant concomitant illness can affect a patient's mobility. Efforts should be undertaken to minimize the effects of these factors. Moisture contributes to the development of pressure ulcers and hinders the healing of the ulcers. One of the few indications for chronic use of an indwelling urinary catheter is urinary incontinence with a sacral pressure ulcer.

Assessment of Infection

Most open pressure ulcers are colonized with numerous bacteria, many of which are not pathogenic. Routine cultures of an ulcer are not necessary and often lead to the treatment of non-pathogenic bacteria and subsequent drug resistance. However, if infection is present, it inhibits the healing of an ulcer. When clinical signs suggest the presence of infection, such as increased wound pain, foul odor, erythema, exudate, and increasing size of the wound despite appropriate care, wound cultures should be obtained and appropriate antibiotic treatment initiated. The most commonly encountered organisms in pressure ulcers are *Pseudomonas aeruginosa, Providencia* species,

Staphylococcus aureus, and *Bacteroides* species. Empiric antibiotic selection should be effective in treating these organisms. The AHCPR guidelines suggest a 2-week trial of topical antibiotics for clean pressure ulcers that are not healing or continue to produce exudate for 2 to 4 weeks of care. When there is evidence of systemic infection such as bacteremia, cellulitis, or osteomyelitis, systemic antibiotics should be used.

Wound Management

There are several important goals in the care of a wound. The overall goal is to create an environment that promotes healing. To accomplish this, necrotic tissue must be removed, the wound environment must be kept moist, and the wound must be shielded from further damage. As these aspects are attended to and bacterial contamination and infection are controlled, the wound environment should be conducive to healing.

Some topical agents are cytotoxic and have been shown to delay wound healing. These include povidone-iodine, hydrogen peroxide, and acetic acid. These cytotoxic agents should be avoided.

Necrotic debris delays wound healing, and devitalized tissue supports the proliferation of pathologic organisms. There are several acceptable methods of debridement. *Sharp debridement* involves the use of sharp instruments such as a scalpel or scissors to remove devitalized tissue. This is the preferred method when there are large areas of thick, devitalized tissue. *Enzymatic* or *autolytic debridement* with agents such as collagenases, fibrinolysin, and trypsin is slower than sharp debridement but is often helpful when the necrotic tissue is thin. Mechanical debridement techniques include wet-to-dry dressings, whirlpool baths, and wound irrigation. Data suggest that heel ulcers with dry eschar need not be debrided. As long as pressure can be relieved, even with necrotic covering, the heel ulcer will heal. If, however, there is drainage or other evidence of infection, the eschar should be removed and antibiotic therapy begun, if indicated.

WOUND DRESSINGS

The wound must be cleansed and the wound environment kept moist. Dressings or treatments that lead to drying of the ulcer bed are detrimental to wound healing. A wound bed is kept hydrated with the use of moisture-retentive dressings that prevent wound desiccation and promote granulation. It is important to protect the surrounding skin from maceration while keeping the ulcer bed moist. Maceration of the surrounding normal skin renders the skin more likely to break down.

Many materials are available as dressings on pressure ulcers. The purposes of dressings on skin ulcers are protection from trauma or contamination, creation of the ideal environment for healing, absorption of drainage, and application of medications. The material selected as a dressing should accomplish the appropriate goals for the individual wound. Table 19-4 lists the types of dressings available and the specific indications for use. Dry gauze should be used for protection and wet-to-dry gauze dressings for mechanical debridement. Continuously moist gauze dressings keep the ulcer bed moist and are ideal when the wound should and can be inspected frequently. The dressing must be changed often enough to ensure that the gauze does not become dry. If it does become dry, granulation tissue may be removed with dressing changes. Care must be taken that the moist dressing be placed on the ulcer bed and not on the surrounding skin.

Selecting the best dressing is an individual decision based on the characteristics of the wound and the availability of services. In the home health setting, using dressings that must be changed two to three times a day is not practical. The presence or absence of exudate is another important factor in choosing the proper dressing material. If there are large amounts of exudative drainage, an absorbent dressing should be used.

OCCLUSIVE DRESSINGS There has been rapid development and marketing of other forms of dressings broadly categorized as occlusive dressings. When continuously moist gauze is compared with occlusive dressings, healing of pressure ulcers has been similar. The main advantage of occlusive dressings is the decreased frequency needed for dressing changes. This makes them particularly useful in home care. Occlusive dressings can be divided into categories of polyurethane films, polymer foams, hydrocolloids, hydrogels, and alginates. Table 19-4 lists the proprietary names and indications for use for the different types of dressings.

FILMS Polyurethane films (OpSite, Tegaderm, Bioclusive) are synthetic, semipermeable, and transparent. They offer protection from friction and moisture damage. Studies have shown excellent wound healing and decreased nursing time. Because of the adhesive properties, however, there can be damage to the wound and surrounding skin.

FOAMS Polymer foams (Allevyn, Lyofoam) are absorbent and provide padding. Because they are not adherent, the dressing often has to be taped. Foam dressings have to be changed more frequently, especially if there is copious drainage.

OTHER DRESSINGS Hydrocolloid dressings (Duo-Derm, Tegasorb, Restore) are adhesive and similar to ostomy barrier products. They are not adherent to the wound bed and cause no damage to wound epithelialization. A wound managed with a hydrocolloid dressing is kept in a serous exudate, often leading caregivers to assume that the wound is draining more. The exudate produced by the hydrocolloid enhances healing.

Hydrogels (Vigilon, Elasto Gel) are hydrophilic polymers that are nonadherent. They are cooling to the skin and may improve pain control. They are, however, a poor barrier and may promote the growth of *Pseudomonas* organisms and yeast.

Alginate dressings (Sorbsan, Kaltostat, Fibracol, Tegagen) are naturally occurring polysaccharides found in seaweed. They are highly absorbent in exudative wounds and are particularly suited to this type of wound. Care must be taken so that

Table 19-4

Dressing Materials

Dressing Category	Proprietary Name	Use
Gauze dressings	—	
Dry	—	Absorption of heavy exudate
Wet-to-dry	—	Mechanical debridement in wounds with thin necrosis
Continuously moist	—	Protection; useful when frequent examination of the wound is desirable
Polyurethane film	OpSite, Tegaderm, Bioclusive	Good protection of the wound and surrounding skin from trauma, friction, and moisture
Foams	Allevyn, Lyofoam	Protection and padding; absorbent and nonadherent
Hydrocolloid	DuoDerm, Tegasorb, Restore	Absorbent and nonadherent; protection from trauma, friction, and moisture; saves nursing time because it can stay on for 3–5 days
Hydrogel	Vigilon, ElastoGel	Used as a delivery system for topical medications; conforms well to wound
Alginate	Sorbsan, Kaltostat, Fibracol, Tegagen	Highly absorbent and nonadherent

alginate dressings are applied before the wound dries to avoid damage to epithelialization.

OTHER TREATMENTS

Other interventions have been proposed for the management of pressure ulcers, including electrical stimulation, hyperbaric oxygen, ultrasound, and laser irradiation. Electrical stimulation is the only adjuvant therapy with sufficient supporting evidence to warrant consideration for use. Electrical stimulation involves direct placement of 5 milliamperes of current on a pad on the wound for up to 60 mins twice a day. Electrical stimulation should be reserved for stage II, III, and IV wounds that have proved unresponsive to conventional therapy. Other adjunctive therapies,

including zinc, vitamin C, vasodilators, hormones, serotonin inhibitors, and growth factors, have been investigated. There is little evidence of the effectiveness of these therapies.

SURGICAL TREATMENT

Surgical management of pressure ulcers includes primary closure, skin grafting, and skin musculocutaneous flaps. More research is needed to determine clear criteria for selecting patients for operative repair. There are, however, some general guidelines that can help in selecting patients who will likely benefit from surgical repair. Patients should receive preoperative counseling about the procedure, the expected outcome, and the required postoperative follow-up care. Patients in medically stable condition and adequately nourished who have stage III or IV wounds that are clean and refractory to standard therapy should be considered for surgical repair. Patients who are considered for surgical repair must be willing to adhere to intensive postoperative care.

Venous Stasis Ulcers

MANAGEMENT OF EDEMA

The most important intervention for preventing and managing venous stasis ulcers is controlling edema. This protects the microvascularity of the skin by allowing better drainage of the venous system. This can be accomplished by means of graduated compression, elevation, and exercise. Other measures used to manage the wound will be ineffective if edema is not controlled. It is important to emphasize the importance of exercise and elevation. The patient must understand that exercise is important and instructed that, when sitting or lying, the legs should be elevated above the level of the heart. Unna's boots, graded elastic stockings, or pneumatic compression devices are effective adjuncts to exercise and elevation.

Unna's boots are bandages impregnated with zinc oxide. They should be applied when there is little inflammation of the surrounding skin, ideally early in the morning when edema is minimal. They are applied from the foot to just below the knee in a pressure-gradient manner. The boot can be left on for 7 to 10 days and replaced until there is healing. If there is marked inflammation or infection, such a boot should not be applied, because the wound and surrounding skin must be evaluated more than once a week. Diuretics sometimes are necessary to control edema among patients with venous stasis ulcers.

MANAGEMENT OF INFLAMMATION

A second important consideration in the management of venous stasis ulcers is attending to inflammation in the skin surrounding the ulcer. A group V topical steroid (triamcinolone acetonide 0.1% cream or betamethasone valerate 0.1% cream), wet compresses (Burow's solution), or both are useful in controlling inflammation. Ulcers may be contaminated with various bacteria, but routine administration of either topical or systemic antibiotics does not improve wound healing. As with pressure ulcers, routine culture often leads to treatment of nonpathologic bacteria and subsequent drug resistance. When there is cellulitis of the surrounding skin or infection within the wound, topical or systemic antibiotics are useful in wound healing. The most common organisms in venous ulcers are β-hemolytic *Streptococcus pyogenes* and *Pseudomonas pyocyanea*.

DEBRIDEMENT AND DRESSINGS

Healing requires a bed of healthy granulation tissue that is present only when necrotic tissue is removed. Devitalized tissue can be removed in several ways. Necrotic eschar and crust should be surgically removed with care not to disturb the healthy underlying granulation tissue. Thin necrotic tissue, exudate, and slough often are difficult to remove surgically. This tissue can be softened and removed with wet-to-dry saline dressings.

Care must be taken to keep the surrounding tissue from becoming macerated and not to remove granulation tissue from the ulcer bed when the dressing is removed. Other products such as absorbing granules or paste (Debrisan wound cleaning paste or DuoDerm hydroactive granules), proteolytic enzyme ointments (Elase, Collagenase), and occlusive film dressings (DuoDerm, CGF, Coverderm) are effective in removing exudate and slough but should be discontinued once healthy granulation tissue predominates. Table 19-4 lists several products and classes of products that can be used in certain situations to manage venous ulcers or pressure ulcers.

SYSTEMIC THERAPY

Systemic therapy aimed at improving blood flow to the affected area has been studied with some success noted. Pentoxifylline (Trental) has a specific blood flow–promoting effect and has been shown, in limited trials, to improve healing of venous stasis ulcers. This therapy, however, is not universally accepted as standard treatment.

SURGICAL TREATMENT

Skin grafting may be needed to complete healing but should generally be reserved for ulcers that have failed to heal after 6 to 12 months of standard care. Skin grafting does not address the underlying pathologic process, however, so recurrence rates are high. Injecting sclerosing solution into varicose veins or vein stripping may be helpful to some patients with chronic venous ulcers. Surgical intervention in the superficial venous system is most helpful when the deep venous system is normal. Surgery must be followed by aggressive graduated compression on the legs to minimize or eliminate peripheral edema.

OTHER TREATMENTS

Measures should be undertaken to improve the overall health of a patient with venous stasis ulcers. Nutrition is important in wound healing. If venous stasis ulcers do not respond to these conservative measures, skin grafting becomes an option.

Arterial Ulcers

Arterial ulcers are difficult to heal unless the blood flow to the area of the ulcer can be improved. Unlike those with venous ulceration, patients with arterial ulcers need early surgical referral for local care and evaluation for revascularization. In the meantime, patients should be instructed to stop smoking. Aspirin, 325 to 650 mg/d, dipyridamole, 50 to 100 mg four times a day, or pentoxifylline, 400 mg three times a day may be indicated in certain situations. Care should be taken in local therapy for arterial ulcers. Dry eschar should be removed carefully from the wound edges every 2 to 3 days and wet dressings applied. Meticulous foot

protection, lower extremity elevation, and avoidance of weight bearing should be recommended.

Neuropathic Diabetic Ulcers

The same principles of management of venous ulcers apply to management of neuropathic diabetic ulcers. Infection is a common and potentially disastrous complication among patients with diabetes and neuropathic ulcers. For this reason, antibiotics should be used earlier in treatment than when a patient has another form of chronic ulcer. Mild infections can be managed with outpatient administration of broad-spectrum antibiotics. More severe infections that might be life threatening or limb threatening often require hospitalization and parenteral administration of broad-spectrum antibiotics. In one study, the cure rates were 85 percent with intravenous ofloxacin followed by oral ofloxacin for a total of 3 weeks and 83 percent with intravenous ampicillin/sulbactam followed by oral amoxicillin/clavulanate for a total of 3 weeks. When osteomyelitis is suspected, bone culture or removal is recommended, followed by antibiotic therapy for at least 6 weeks. Diabetic ulcers should be debrided and cleaned frequently. As with venous stasis ulcers, edema should be managed. Activity should be limited during the acute treatment phase of neuropathic diabetic ulcers.

Pyoderma Gangrenosum

Underlying systemic diseases such as inflammatory bowel disease or rheumatoid arthritis should be sought and appropriately managed when the typical lesion of pyoderma gangrenosum is encountered. The most commonly studied therapy for pyoderma gangrenosum is oral prednisone, 40 to 60 mg a day tapered after several weeks. Other possible treatments are occlusive dressings, hyperbaric oxygen, dapsone, and cyclophosphamide. Cyclosporine has been used successfully in refractory cases.

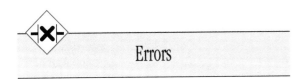

Errors

Factitious Ulcers

The cause of chronic ulcers usually is multifactorial. With a careful history and physical examination, the clinician should be able to determine the primary cause of the ulcer. However, some patients have factitious ulcers. Factitious ulcers are self-inflicted. They are uncommon, but the clinician needs to have a high index of suspicion when a patient has a nonhealing ulcer and no obvious local or systemic cause or when the patient derives some benefit from having an ulcer. The ulcers tend to occur among patients with psychiatric disorders, substance abuse, or disorders associated with chronic pruritus.

Cultures

The use of cultures in the management of skin ulcers is controversial. Skin ulcers are invariably colonized with bacteria. Swab cultures give information only about bacteria colonizing the surface and will lead to confusion about appropriate treatment. The most effective method of managing wound colonization and preventing infection is wound cleansing and debridement with careful attention to infection control procedures. Systemic antibiotics should only be used when there is evidence of soft-tissue infection, systemic infection, or osteomyelitis.

Topical Agents

There are claims that a multitude of topical agents and dressings have healing properties in the management of skin ulcers. Despite little or no evidence to support such claims, clinicians still prescribe these agents. Studies should be reviewed closely to determine the actual effect of the agent used, as opposed to the increased attention that often accompanies such trials. Some topical agents may actually cause harm to the wound. Many skin cleansers or antiseptic agents, including povidone-iodine, iodophor, hydrogen peroxide, and sodium hypochlorite, are toxic to skin.

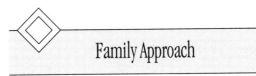

Family Approach

The care of skin ulcers often requires caregiver assistance. Caregivers may be the staff at long-term care facilities or the families of patients living at home (see Chap. 4). Knowledge of methods of prevention and treatment is important for caregivers. Although home health practitioners offer assistance to patients and families, many needs can only be met by the full-time caregivers. Family members should be included in any education aimed at the patient. Identifying educational needs often is a difficult process. The level of understanding of the family caregivers should be assessed and the educational programs tailored appropriately. The physical ability of the family caregiver also has to be assessed; caregivers of these patients are frequently frail themselves. The financial status of the family should be assessed. Family must be involved in decisions concerning interventions and the cost. Many of the interventions are expensive and are not covered by Medicare or conventional insurance.

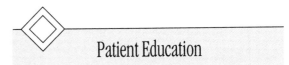

Patient Education

Education is one of the most important aspects in the care of patients with skin ulcers. Education empowers patients to understand the disease and positively affect their health. Educational efforts should be aimed at preventing and controlling the wound and the disease that contributed to the wound. The amount of time required for education depends on the learner and the amount of educational content. Large amounts of information cannot be presented at one time, so efforts at education for hospitalized patients and their caregivers should be begun before the return to independent living.

Pressure Ulcers

All patients with pressure ulcers or who are at risk of pressure ulcers should know how to identify risk factors and how to recognize early pressure changes in the skin. The AHCPR publication, *Preventing Pressure Ulcers: A Patient's Guide,* is a helpful adjunct to individual patient education. Patients at risk of pressure ulcers need to know how to perform a basic skin examination. They should understand the importance of pressure relief and the intended purpose of the special beds and pads that are being used. Patients with pressure ulcers or who are at risk of pressure ulcers should inform the health care provider when there is new skin breakage, redness or warmth in the surrounding skin, new or foul-smelling drainage, or fever.

Venous Stasis Ulcers

Patients with venous stasis ulcers or who are at risk of venous stasis ulcers should be reminded of the importance of controlling edema in preventing and managing venous ulcers. Patients should be encouraged to exercise to stimulate muscle activity and venous return. Smoking cessation should be encouraged.

Neuropathic Ulcers

Patients with diabetes or who are at risk of neuropathic ulcers frequently need specially molded shoes because they have severely deformed feet. They should be instructed about the potential

harm in using heating pads and hot water bottles. Other activities that can cause trauma, such as walking barefoot and stepping into tubs of hot water, should be avoided. The use of topical lubricants should be emphasized to treat dry skin. Maceration between the toes should be avoided. Patients with diabetes should inspect their feet frequently and seek medical attention if there is any change. They should also be instructed not to use chemicals or sharp objects or remove corns or calluses. Smoking also is a risk factor in the development of neuropathic diabetic ulcers, so smoking cessation should be encouraged.

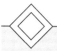

Emerging Concepts

Two new medications have been studied and approved to manage certain skin ulcers. Human platelet-derived growth factor has been approved as a gel for managing lower extremity neuropathic diabetic ulcers that extend into the subcutaneous tissue or beyond. It has not yet been approved for use in other types of skin ulcers. Granulocyte colony stimulating factor (G-CSF) by perilesional injection has been reported to be effective therapy for refractory pyoderma granulosum. G-CSF also has been used in the management of neuropathic diabetic ulcers. Results of clinical trials with growth factors such as human growth factor and G-CSF have been disappointing, and these products are not yet approved for use in the care of wounds.

Cost Analysis

Most patients with chronic ulcers have multiple medical problems, so determining the cost of care for the ulcer while controlling other factors is difficult. In one study, it was estimated that the cost per ulcer episode for patients with diabetes and leg ulcers was $4595. The authors concluded that the high cost of managing diabetic foot ulcers is an argument for strategies to improve care. The most efficacious and cost-effective strategy would be to improve methods of assessing risk and then preventing the development and progression of the wounds.

Bibliography

Alinovi A, Bassissi P, Pini M: Systemic administration of antibiotics in the management of venous ulcers. *J Am Acad Dermatol* 15:186, 1986.

Allman RM, LaPrade CA, Noel LB, et al: Pressure sores among hospitalized patients. *Ann Intern Med* 105:337, 1986.

Bergstrom N, Bennett MA, Carlson CE: *Treatment of Pressure Ulcers.* Clinical Practice Guideline No. 15. AHCPR publication No. 95-0652. Rockville, MD, US Department of Health and Human Services, Public Health Service, Agency for Health Care Policy and Research, 1994.

Clarke M, Kadhom HM: The nursing prevention of pressure sores in hospital and community patients. *J Adv Nurs* 13:365, 1989.

Colwell JC, Foreman MD, Trotter JP: A comparison of the efficacy and cost-effectiveness of two methods of managing pressure ulcers. *Decubitus* 6:28, 1992.

Douglas WS, Simpson NB: Guidelines for the management of chronic venous leg ulceration: report of a multidisciplinary workshop. *Br J Dermatol* 132:446, 1995.

Foresman PA, Payne DS, Becker D, et al: A relative toxicity index for wound cleansers. *Wounds* 5:226, 1993.

Grayson ML, Gibbons GW, Balogh K: Probing to bone in infected pedal ulcers: a clinical sign of underlying osteomyelitis in diabetic patients. *JAMA* 273:721, 2995.

Habif TP: *Clinical Dermatology,* 3rd ed. St. Louis, Mosby; 1996; 74.

Holzer SE, Camerota A, Martens L, et al: Costs and duration of care for lower extremity ulcers in patients with diabetes. *Clin Ther* 20:169, 1998.

Husain T: An experimental study of some pressure effects on tissues with reference to the bedsore problem. *J Pathol Bacteriol* 66:347, 1953.

Kolari PJ, Pekanmaki P: Intermittent pneumatic compression in the healing of venous ulcers. *Lancet* 2:1108, 1986.

Langemo DK, Olson B, Hunter S, et al: Incidence of pressure sores in acute care, rehabilitation, extended care, home health, and hospice in one locale. *Decubitus* 2:42, 1989.

Lewis VL Jr, Baily MH, Pulawski G, et al: The diagnosis of osteomyelitis in patients with pressure sores. *Plast Reconstr Surg* 81:229, 1988.

Lipsky BA, Baker PD, Landon GC, et al: Antibiotic therapy for diabetic foot infections: comparison of two parenteral-to-oral regimens. *Clin Infect Dis* 24:643, 1997.

Mancini, L, Ruotolo V: The diabetic foot: epidemiology. *Rays* 22:511, 1997.

Meehan M: Multisite pressure ulcer prevalence survey. *Decubitus* 3:14, 1990.

National Pressure Ulcer Advisory Panel: Pressure ulcers: incidence, economics, risk assessment—Consensus development conference statement. *Decubitus* 2:24, 1989.

Panel for the Prediction and Prevention of Pressure Ulcers in Adults: Clinical Practice Guideline, No. 3. AHCPR publication no. 92-0047. Rockville, MD, US Department of Health and Human Services, Public Health Service, Agency for Health Care Policy and Research, 1992.

Panel for the Prediction and Prevention of Pressure Ulcers in Adults: *Consumer Version, Clinical Practice Guideline, No. 3.* AHCPR publication No. 92-0048. Rockville, MD, US Department of Health and Human S ervices, Public Health Service, Agency for Health Care Policy and Research, 1992.

Rousseau P: Pressure ulcers in the aged: a preventable problem. *Contin Care* 17:35, 1988.

Scottish Intercollegiate Guidelines Network. The Care of Patients with Chronic Leg Ulcer. Publication No. 26. 1998. http://www.sign.ac.uk. Accessed January 27, 2000.

Shea JD: Pressure sores: classification and management. *Clin Orthop* 112:89, 1975.

Shpiro D, Gilat D, Fisher-Feld L, et al: Pyoderma granulosum treated with perilesional granulocyte-macrophage colony stimulating factor. *Br J Dermatol* 138:368, 1998.

Waterlow J: The Waterlow card for the prevention and management of pressure sores: toward a pocket policy. *Care, Science and Practice* 6:8, 1988.

Weitgasser H; The use of pentoxifylline (Trental) in the treatment of leg ulcers: a double blind trial. *Pharmacotherapeutica* 3:143, 1983.

Young L: Pressure ulcer prevalence and associated patient characteristics in one long-term care facility. *Decubitus* 2:52, 1989.

Chapter

20

Dizziness

Alan M. Adelman

Dizziness is a common complaint of patients seen in the ambulatory care setting. Thirty percent of individuals over the age of 65 years report dizziness. In younger individuals, dizziness is frequently a benign, self-limited illness, but this is not necessarily true for the elderly person. A history of syncope and/or falls is common in elderly individuals who report dizziness. Falls (see Chap. 14) and syncope can not only be associated with severe illnesses but can lead to serious injury.

Overview: How Common Is Dizziness in the Office Practice?

Dizziness is a common presenting complaint in primary care. It is the 13th leading reason for visits to general internists. There are approximately 6 million visits per year for dizziness. It accounts for over 1 percent of office visits to physicians.

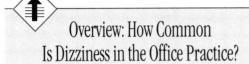

Principal Diagnoses

There are several potential etiologic categories to consider when a patient presents with dizziness. These include vestibular, cardiovascular, psychogenic, multifactorial, and other causes. (Table 20–1).

Vestibular

Vestibular causes can be subdivided into central and peripheral etiologies. Peripheral vestibular problems are the most common cause of dizziness in the primary care setting, resulting in 30 to 50 percent of the cases of dizziness.

Table 20-1

Causes of Dizziness

Peripheral
    Benign paroxysmal positional vertigo
    Labyrinthitis
    Meniere's disease
Central
    Cerebrovascular ischemia
    Tumors
    Multiple sclerosis
    Parkinson's disease
    Cerebellar disease
Cardiovascular
    Orthostatic hypotension
    Carotid sinus hypersensitivity
    Aortic stenosis
    Idiopathic hypertrophic subaortic stenosis
    Arrhythmia
Psychogenic
    Anxiety
    Depression
    Somatoform disorders
Multifactorial
Other
    Acute blood loss
    Cervical spondylosis
    Peripheral neuropathies
    Medications (e.g., antihypertensives, lithium, Dilantin, benzodiazepines, neuroleptics, aminoglycosides, and antidepressants)
    Idiopathic

PERIPHERAL

BENIGN POSITIONAL VERTIGO Benign positional vertigo (BPV) is the single most common cause of dizziness in the elderly. It is an episodic, self-limited condition that is produced by sudden head movements or changes in body position such as rolling over in bed. BPV is thought to be due to an accumulation of debris in the semicircular canals. The movement of this debris is believed to stimulate the vestibular mechanism, resulting in the patient's symptoms. BPV is sometimes temporally related to a viral illness and resulting inflammation.

LABYRINTHITIS Labyrinthitis is another self-limited, peripheral vestibular cause of dizziness. It generally lasts for days to several weeks. It is caused by or related to a viral infection. Labyrinthitis is believed to be due to an inflammation of the vestibular nerve.

MENIERE'S DISEASE The classic triad of tinnitus, hearing loss, and vertigo defines Meniere's disease. This syndrome usually develops at a younger age and is an uncommon cause of dizziness in the elderly. The cause is believed to be recurrent episodes of endolymphatic hypertension resulting in cochlear hair cell atrophy. Episodes of Meniere's disease are usually self-limited, but frequently repetitive. Eventually, an individual can reach a chronic "burned out" phase in which the hearing loss can be profound, but episodes of dizziness cease.

CENTRAL

Central vestibular causes of dizziness are uncommon, with a prevalence of less than 10 percent in the elderly with dizziness. Cerebrovascular ischemia (strokes, transient ischemic attacks), tumors (acoustic neuroma, cerebellar), multiple sclerosis, migraine, and Parkinson's disease are examples of central vestibular causes of dizziness. As age increases, cerebrovascular ischemia becomes a more prevalent cause of dizziness.

Patients with a central cause for their dizziness rarely have dizziness as their only symptom. New-onset dizziness that is associated with other symptoms (headache, visual disturbances, or neurologic symptoms), however, should suggest a potentially serious central nervous system pathologic process; further evaluation, including CNS imaging, is usually appropriate.

Cardiovascular

Cardiovascular disease is an important cause of dizziness. This disorder is also important because of potentially life-threatening consequences if the underlying disease is not treated. Examples of cardiovascular causes of dizziness are orthostatic hypotension, cardiac arrhythmia, cardiomyopathy, aortic stenosis, carotid sinus hypersensitivity, and hypertrophic subaortic stenosis. The common pathophysiology of this group of disorders is decreased blood flow to the brain, and resultant dizziness. If blood and oxygen flow to the brain drops too low, syncope can result. Dizziness can be a warning symptom of, or precede, syncope.

In a recent study, Lawson and associates reported that cardiovascular causes were more frequent than vestibular causes of dizziness among primary care ambulatory elderly patients. Nearly half of the patients had a cardiovascular cause for their dizziness, with carotid sinus hypersensitivity alone or in combination with other disorders being the most frequent cause. They also reported that patients with a chief complaint of dizziness (described as lightheadedness, pallor, and the need to sit or lie when symptoms occurred) and a history of cardiovascular disease had symptoms that were more likely to be secondary to a cardiovascular cause than any other causes.

Multifactorial

It can be difficult to determine a specific cause for an elderly individual's symptom of dizziness, because dizziness in an elderly person can have multiple contributing causes. Among elderly men, up to 50 percent of patients have multiple causes for their dizziness. This should not be surprising since elderly individuals usually have multiple chronic medical conditions and are taking multiple medications. An example is the older person with multiple sensory deficits who complains of lightheadedness or unsteadiness on his or her feet. It can be difficult to identify a specific cause for their complaint in the presence of multiple medical conditions (e.g., Parkinson's disease, congestive heart failure, and hypertension) and the concomitant use of multiple pharmacologic agents. Each of these medical conditions can be associated with symptoms of dizziness (orthostatic hypotension, cerebral hypoperfusion, and hypoxia), and pharmacologic agents can further compound these physiologic effects. Orthostatic hypotension (a decline of systolic blood pressure of $\geq$ 20 mmHg on standing) can occur in older persons on an idiopathic basis and can occur among older patients with autonomic neuropathy secondary to Parkinson's disease, diabetes mellitus, or progressive supranuclear palsy.

Psychogenic

Psychogenic causes, such as anxiety, depression, and somatoform disorders, are common and can account for up to one-quarter to one-third of the cases of dizziness in the primary care setting. Hyperventilation, which is a manifestation of panic disorder or other anxiety disorders, can also cause dizziness. Several studies have suggested that psychogenic causes of dizziness are less prevalent than in a younger population.

Other

MEDICATIONS

Other causes of dizziness include medications (e.g., antihistamines, lithium, anticholinergic agents, benzodiazepines, neuroleptic agents, aminoglycosides, and antidepressants), infections, and metabolic disorders (see Table 20-1). Antihypertensive agents (β-blockers, α-blockers, ACE inhibitors, and diuretics) can frequently cause orthostatic hypotension.

CERVICAL DIZZINESS

Cervical dizziness is caused by compression of the vertebral artery by an osteophytic spur, which results in decreased blood supply to the brainstem. As with BPV, this type of dizziness can be provoked by looking up or turning of the head.

IDIOPATHIC

In a number of cases, no cause for the patient's dizziness is found. Lawson and colleagues reported that they were unable to identify a specific cause for the patient's dizziness in nearly 25 percent of the cases.

Key History

There are numerous terms patients use to describe dizziness including dizziness, lightheadedness, woozy, spinning, unsteadiness, whirling, and faintness. Drachman and Hart classified dizziness into four symptom categories: vertigo, presyncope, dysequilibrium, and lightheadedness. Although these categories correspond to the major causes of dizziness (vestibular, cardiovascular, multifactorial, and psychogenic, respectively), the fit is not exact. For example, a patient who complains of lightheadedness can have a multifactorial cause and not a cardiovascular cause.

Vertigo

Patients with vertigo describe a sensation that the surrounding environment is spinning or revolving. The underlying cause of this type of dizziness is usually vestibular, such as labyrinthitis or benign postural vertigo. Patients state that their vertigo is elicited by rolling over in bed. Vertigo produced by rolling over in bed has a sensitivity of 40 percent for BPV. Rapid head movements or gazing upward, such as reaching for objects on upper shelves of cabinets, can produce vertigo. Patients can also complain of vertigo when bend-ing over to tie their shoes. Rapid turn of the neck inducing dizziness can also suggest cervical spondylosis. Associated symptoms can include nausea and vomiting. It is unusual for the patient to lose consciousness with this type of dizziness. Patients with Meniere's disease will also often complain of tinnitus.

If patients who present with vertigo are less than 69 years of age and have no neurologic deficits, the likelihood of a serious cause of their dizziness is low (negative predictive value [NPV] 88 percent, likelihood ratio negative [LR−] 0.3). The opposite, however, is not a good predictor of a serious cause of dizziness. With the absence of vertigo, age greater than 69 years, and a neurologic deficit present, the positive predictive value (PPV) of this triad is only 40 percent (likelihood ratio positive [LR+] 1.5).

Presyncope

Presyncope is defined as faintness or a woozy sensation. Patients state that they felt as if they were about to pass out. The pathogenesis of presyncope is believed to be decreased cerebral blood flow. The underlying cause of this type of dizziness is usually cardiovascular such as orthostatic hypotension. If orthostatic hypotension is the culprit, patients will complain of dizziness within seconds to minutes upon arising or standing. Patients also complain that their legs were rubbery or almost "gave way." Associated symptoms can include nausea and diaphoresis.

Dysequilibrium

Dysequilibrium refers to a sense of unsteadiness or imbalance. The cause is usually due to a single or multiple sensory deficits. Other conditions (mostly central nervous system disorders) that affect mobility, such as Parkinson's disease, stroke, and multiple sclerosis, can also contribute to the sensation of dysequilibrium. Patients will usually complain of this type of dizziness with ambulation.

Lightheadedness

Lightheadedness is described as a vague or indefinable sensation. This type of dizziness is without the characteristics of the previous three categories. The underlying cause can be difficult to determine. Psychogenic causes of dizziness are often found in these patients. Patients may complain of feeling like they are in a constant "fog." If there truly is a psychogenic cause, the patient may also complain of symptoms of depression (e.g., feeling down, difficulty sleeping), anxiety (e.g., nervousness), or panic attacks (e.g., hyperventilation, palpitations). Patients with somatoform disorders can complain of chest pain, headache, or abdominal pain.

Other Symptoms

After having the patient describe his or her symptom of dizziness, it is important to ask about other symptoms and obtain a complete list of prescription and over-the-counter medications. Important questions for the history are shown in Table 20-2. Many medications, such as alcohol, tricyclic antidepressants, anticonvulsants, antiparkinsonian agents, or anticholinergic agents, can cause dizziness. Other medications can lead to hypotension and dizziness such as diuretics and antihypertensive agents.

The timing of symptoms can be helpful. Patients who complain of vertigo upon first arising in the morning (matutinal vertigo) usually have a periph-

Table 20-2

Important Questions to Determine the Cause of Dizziness

What is the timing of the dizziness? When does it occur?
Are there any other otologic symptoms such as tinnitus or hearing loss?
Are there any neurologic symptoms such as weakness, difficulty with speech, or diplopia?
Is there any symptom pattern?
What medications are taken?

eral vestibular cause for their dizziness. This symptom has a sensitivity of 51 percent and a specificity of 69 percent.

The presence of other otologic symptoms can help differentiate between the many causes of dizziness. Patients with Meniere's disease have the classic triad of dizziness, tinnitus, and hearing loss. In addition, these individuals will usually have a history of recurrent episodes.

Patients should be asked about the presence of neurologic symptoms such as weakness, visual disturbance (e.g., diplopia), focal sensory loss, dysarthria, or gait disturbance. Whereas patients with a stroke or transient ischemic attack may complain of dizziness, dizziness is rarely the only symptom. Vertebrobasilar transient ischemic attacks (TIAs) can present with episodic dizziness, but usually patients will also complain of other neurologic symptoms.

Asking the patient about the pattern of symptoms or what elicits the symptom of dizziness can also help to differentiate between the causes of dizziness. Patients with benign positional vertigo complain of vertiginous type of dizziness, especially with rapid movements of the head or looking up. Labyrinthitis can be found in patients with a cold or flu-like illness. In general, dizziness due to a peripheral vestibular problem is of short duration (days to several weeks), whereas dizziness caused by a central problem is longer in duration. Palpitations or chest pain can be described in patients with presyncopal dizziness.

Physical Examination

Since the cause of dizziness in primary care is usually either self-limited or peripheral vestibular, or both, the examination can be relatively brief. The purpose of the examination is twofold. The primary purpose is to rule out more serious causes of dizziness such as a cardiac arrhythmia or orthostatic hypotension. Another purpose is to search for physical findings that can confirm a vestibular cause for the dizziness. The five components of

this brief examination are: brief examinations of the ears, heart, and nervous system; examination of the vestibular system; and measurement of blood pressure (Table 20-3).

Blood Pressure

Blood pressure should be checked in the supine, sitting, and standing positions. Pressures are obtained 1 to 2 min after each position change. A fall in systolic blood pressure of more than 20 mmHg, or a fall in diastolic blood pressure of more than 10 mmHg, is diagnostic of orthostatic changes. With a change in position, the clinician should inquire about a sensation of lightheadedness or dizziness. If a neurocardiogenic cause for dizziness is suspected, tilt-table testing can be performed.

Ear Examination

Hearing loss occurs in Meniere's disease, and hearing can be briefly examined with the whisper test. Patients are asked to identify words whispered by the examiner. The auditory canal and tympanic membrane should be visualized. Chronic otitis media and cholesteatoma are causes of dizziness. A rare cause of vertigo is the Ramsay Hunt syndrome, which presents with vesicles in the auditory canal, facial weakness, deafness, and sometimes, pain in the ear.

Cardiac Examination

The heart should be auscultated and the rhythm evaluated. Arrhythmias can be a cause of dizzi-

Table 20-3
The Five Components of the Brief Dizziness Examination

Blood pressure
Examination of the ears
Cardiac examination
Vestibular examination
Neurologic examination

ness. Aortic stenosis that reduces cardiac output and blood flow to the brain, especially with activity, can cause dizziness.

Vestibular Examination

The detection of nystagmus is the focus of the vestibular examination. The examiner should look for spontaneous nystagmus. If not present, the examiner should attempt to elicit nystagmus. Horizontal or rotatory nystagmus usually points to a vestibular cause for the dizziness. Vertical nystagmus points to a central nervous system cause for the dizziness.

SPONTANEOUS NYSTAGMUS

First, the eyes should be examined with the patient looking straight ahead. Next, the eyes should be moved through their full range of motion. Gaze-evoked nystagmus refers to the elicitation of nystagmus when the eyes are deviated from looking straight ahead. Pathologic nystagmus can usually be elicited at deviations from central gaze between 30 and 45 degrees. Physiologic nystagmus can be produced at the extremes of deviation.

HALLPIKE MANEUVER

The Hallpike maneuver is used to elicit nystagmus. The appearance of nystagmus with this maneuver points to a peripheral vestibular cause for the dizziness such as BPV or labyrinthitis.

The Hallpike maneuver is performed by having the patient lie supine with the head hyperextended over the edge of the examination table. With the head turned 30 degrees to either the right or left, the patient is asked to sit up quickly. The maneuver is then repeated with the head deviated in the opposite direction. The examiner observes the eyes for nystagmus and should inquire about the symptom of dizziness.

The examiner may also perform the head-shaking maneuver to elicit nystagmus. This maneuver is performed by having the patient close

the eyes and shake the head back and forth approximately 10 to 20 times. Upon opening the eyes, the examiner observes for the presence of nystagmus.

The elicitation of nystagmus usually indicates a peripheral cause of vertigo, particularly BPV. Sensitivity of this test is between 50 to 78 percent. The absence of this sign does not rule out BPV. Patients with both a positive Hallpike maneuver and vertigo or vomiting have a high likelihood of having a peripheral cause for their dizziness (LR − 7.8, PPV 85 percent). Lack of either one of these findings has a negative predictive value of 68 percent (LR − 0.6).

Neurologic Examination

A brief neurologic examination should be performed, with particular emphasis on cerebellar function and gait.

Ancillary Tests

There is no routine battery of tests for the evaluation of dizziness. Multiple studies have reported the low yield from diagnostic testing. Testing should be guided by the patient's symptoms and the response to therapy. In most cases, a peripheral vestibular cause for the dizziness will be present and the patient's symptoms will resolve spontaneously. This being the case, no further testing is warranted.

Cardiovascular testing including electrocardiogram, 24-h Holter monitoring, tilt-table, echocardiogram, and stress testing are of low yield in patients with a normal cardiac examination and in the absence of syncope. If orthostatic hypotension due to anemia is suspected, a hematocrit should be ordered. Neuroimaging can be of value if a tumor or cerebrovascular disease is suspected. Audiometry should be performed if hearing loss is present.

When dizziness is persistent and a vestibular cause is suspected, specialized vestibular function tests such as electronystagmography, brainstem auditory evoked responses, or rotatory chair testing may be warranted. Referral to an otolaryngologist may also be warranted if the dizziness becomes persistent. Several studies have reported the low yield from routine referral.

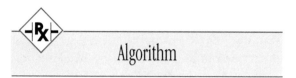

Algorithm

Figure 20-1 shows an algorithm for the evaluation of dizziness. The algorithm addresses the most frequent causes of dizziness in the elderly population. A thorough history and physical examination forms the basis of the algorithm. Cardiovascular causes should be considered if the patient has orthostatic changes or if there is a history of syncope or falls. BPV and other vestibular problems are a frequent cause of dizziness. The symptom of vertigo, vomiting associated with vertigo/dizziness, or a positive Hallpike maneuver are clues to a vestibular cause of the dizziness. The presence of neurologic signs and/or symptoms suggests a central cause. Psychogenic causes of dizziness in the elderly are not as frequent as in a younger population. The presence of psychiatric symptoms or a history of a psychiatric disorder, however, can suggest a psychogenic cause. Finally, dizziness can be caused by multiple factors. It can be difficult to separate the contribution of each. If there are several potential causes for an elderly individual's dizziness, each should be addressed separately.

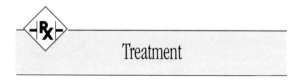

Treatment

The treatment for the patient's dizziness should be directed at the specific cause. Since the most

Figure 20-1

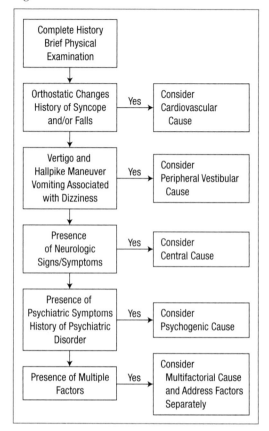

Algorithm for the evaluation of dizziness.

common cause for dizziness is vestibular, this section focuses on the treatment of this group of diagnoses. Because orthostatic hypotension is relatively frequent, its treatment is also addressed.

Vestibular Dizziness

WATCHFUL WAITING

Frequently dizziness due to a vestibular cause will spontaneously resolve without therapy. Dizziness secondary to labyrinthitis will resolve in 1 to 2 weeks.

PHARMACOLOGIC THERAPY

Several medications are available for the treatment of dizziness. Although they are commonly prescribed, their effectiveness has not been rigorously tested. They can also worsen or prolong the patient's dizziness because dizziness is one of their side effects. Although of undocumented benefit, meclizine (Antivert) 12.5 to 25 mg three times daily is frequently prescribed. Prochlorperazine (Compazine) 5 mg three to four times daily or other phenothiazines can be tried. Benzodiazepines can also relieve dizziness and are considered drugs of first choice for severe vertigo.

HABITUATION EXERCISES

Habituation exercises can be effective for persistent dizziness from a vestibular cause. By deliberately repeating the head movements that elicit the symptom of vertigo, the patient can lessen or eliminate the symptom. These exercises are meant to stimulate the vestibular system and then promote compensation. It is usually recommended that the patient repeat the exercises several times per day to achieve the full benefit of the exercise.

CANALITH REPOSITIONING PROCEDURE

This procedure, also known as the Epley maneuver, can be used for persistent BPV. The purpose of the maneuver is to reposition debris in the semicircular canal that can be causing the patient's dizziness.

Orthostatic Hypotension

The initial treatment of orthostatic hypotension is to eliminate the cause or exacerbating factors such as drugs or volume depletion. Diuretics and antihypertensives are the most common drugs implicated in orthostatic hypotension. Patients should be advised to make positional shifts slowly, such as standing or rising from bed in the morning, and wait several moments before starting to ambulate. Support stockings can help to prevent pooling of blood in lower extremities and alleviate the dizziness associated with sudden positional changes. Fludrocortisone acetate (Florinef) or ephedrine can also be used if the previously described measures fail.

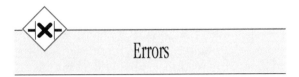

Errors

Overuse of Meclizine in the Treatment of Dizziness

Meclizine is overprescribed in the treatment of dizziness. It is frequently overprescribed for vestibular causes of dizziness (that can be self-limited), and often when the exact cause of the dizziness is unknown. Not only has the effectiveness of meclizine for vestibular causes of dizziness not been proven, but its value in other causes of dizziness is also not proven. Meclizine has anticholinergic effects and can cause drowsiness, dry mouth, and urinary retention.

Overuse of Laboratory Testing

Several studies of dizziness have demonstrated the low yield of laboratory and cardiovascular testing unless specifically suggested by the history and physical examination. Despite these reports, clinicians continue to order a battery of tests to "rule out" disease. Clinicians should refrain from this "shotgun" approach and be guided by the history and physical examination. This latter approach will identify the majority of causes for a patient's complaint of dizziness.

Overuse of the Diagnosis of Labyrinthitis

In many studies, the most frequent cause of dizziness is peripheral vestibular or labyrinthitis. Attributing a patient's complaint of dizziness to this cause can lead to delay or failure to search for other diagnoses.

Missing the Diagnosis of Orthostatic Hypotension

The diagnosis of orthostatic hypotension can be missed if the blood pressure is not taken appropriately. Many clinicians take a standing blood pressure immediately upon the patient coming to a standing position. The onset of orthostatic hypotension can be delayed, with the blood pressure falling only after prolonged standing. The diagnosis of orthostatic hypotension can be missed if the examiner does not wait at least 2 min before checking the blood pressure after a position change. If orthostatic hypotension is strongly suspected, it is not unreasonable to have the patient stand for up to 10 min before taking the standing blood pressure.

Emerging Concepts

Lawson and associates recently reported that almost 50 percent of elderly patients in a primary care setting with dizziness had a cardiovascular cause for their symptom. Given the high prevalence of cardiovascular disease in the elderly population, the results are not surprising. Many patients who reported dizziness had mild orthostasis. Whether or not future studies confirm the findings of Lawson and colleagues, clinicians need to be vigilant about cardiovascular causes of dizziness. Falls or syncope in association with dizziness should increase the clinician's suspicion of a cardiovascular cause of the patient's dizziness.

Bibliography

Colledge NR, Barr-Hamilton RM, Lewis SJ, et al: Evaluation of investigations to diagnose the cause of dizziness in elderly people: a community-based controlled study. *BMJ* 313:788, 1996.

Davis LE: Dizziness in elderly men. *J Am Geriatr Soc* 42:1184, 1994.

Derebery MJ: The diagnosis and treatment of dizziness in Otolaryngology for the Internist. *Med Clin North Am* 83:163, 1999.

Drachman DA, Hart CW: An approach to the dizzy patient. *Neurology* 22:323, 1972.

Epley JM: The canalith repositioning procedure: for treatment of benign paroxysmal positional vertigo. *Otolaryngol Head Neck Surg* 107:399, 1992.

Froehling DA, Silverstein MD, Mohr DN, et al: Does this dizzy patient have a serious form of vertigo? *JAMA* 271:385, 1994.

Khan A, Kroenke K: Diagnosis and treatment of the dizzy patient. *Primary Care Case Rev* 2:3, 1999.

Kroenke K, Hoffman RM, Einstadter D: A rational approach to the dizzy patient. *J Clin Outcome Management* 4:33, 1997.

Kroenke K, Lucas CA, Rosenberg ML, et al: Causes of persistent dizziness: a prospective study of 100 patients in ambulatory care. *Ann Intern Med* 117: 898, 1992.

Lawson J, Fitzgerald J, Birchall J, et al: Diagnosis of geriatric patients with severe dizziness. *J Am Geriatr Soc* 47:12, 1999.

Sloane PD, Dallara J: Clinical research and geriatric dizziness: the blind men and the elephant (editorial). *J Am Geriatr Soc* 47:113, 1999.

Sullivan M, Clark MR, Katon WJ, et al: Psychiatric and otologic diagnoses in patients complaining of dizziness. *Arch Intern Med* 153:1479, 1993.

Troost BT, Patton JW: Exercise therapy for positional vertigo. *Neurology* 42:1441, 1992.

Index

Page numbers followed by *t* indicate tables; page numbers followed by *f* indicate figures.

ISBN 0-07-000518-4
90000

9 780070 005181